Systemic Factors Affecting Prognosis and Outcomes of Dental Treatment

Editor

DAVIS C. THOMAS

DENTAL CLINICS OF NORTH AMERICA

www.dental.theclinics.com

October 2024 • Volume 68 • Number 4

ELSEVIER

1600 John F. Kennedy Boulevard • Suite 1800 • Philadelphia, Pennsylvania, 19103-2899

http://www.dental.theclinics.com

DENTAL CLINICS OF NORTH AMERICA Volume 68, Number 4
October 2024 ISSN 0011-8532, ISBN: 978-0-443-24692-0

Editor: John Vassallo; j.vassallo@elsevier.com
Developmental Editor: Akshay Samson

Dental Clinics of North America (ISSN 0011-8532) is published quarterly by Elsevier Inc., 360 Park Avenue South, New York, NY 10010-1710. Months of issue are January, April, July, and October. Business and Editorial Offices: 1600 John F. Kennedy Boulevard, Suite 1800, Philadelphia, PA 19103-2899. Periodicals postage paid at New York, NY and additional mailing offices. Subscription prices are $333.00 per year (domestic individuals), $100.00 per year (domestic students/residents), $396.00 per year (Canadian individuals), $100.00 per year (Canadian students/residents) $463.00 per year (international individuals), and $200.00 per year (international students/residents). For institutional access pricing please contact Customer Service via the contact information below. International air speed delivery is included in all *Clinics* subscription prices. All prices are subject to change without notice. Orders, claims, and journal inquiries: Please visit our Support Hub page https://service.elsevier.com for assistance.

Reprints. For copies of 100 or more, of articles in this publication, please contact the Commercial Reprints Department, Elsevier Inc., 360 Park Avenue South, New York, NY 10010-1710. Tel.: 212-633-3874; Fax: 212-633-3820; E-mail: reprints@elsevier.com.

The Dental Clinics of North America is covered in *MEDLINE/PubMed (Index Medicus), Current Contents/Clinical Medicine, ISI/BIOMED* and *Cinahl.*

Contributors

EDITOR

DAVIS C. THOMAS, BDS, DDS, MSD, MSc Med, MSc
Associate Clinical Professor; Program Director, Clinical Preceptorship in General
Dentistry, Rutgers School of Dental Medicine, Newark, New Jersey, USA; Clinical
Associate Professor of Dentistry, Rochester Medical School, Rochester, New York, USA;
Adjunct Associate Professor, The University of Western Australia, Perth, Australia

AUTHORS

VARSHA AGNIHOTRI, DMD, MBS
Associate Dentist, Tend Rockefeller Center, New York, New York, USA

SOWMYA ANANTHAN, BDS, DMD, MSD
Associate Professor, Center for Temporomandibular Disorders and Orofacial Pain,
Rutgers School of Dental Medicine, Newark, New Jersey, USA

KAINAT ANJUM, BDS, MSc
Clinical Preceptor, Rutgers School of Dental Medicine, Newark, New Jersey, USA

LOVELY MUTHIAH ANNAMMA, BDS, MDS, PhD
Assistant Professor, College of Dentistry, Ajman University, Ajman, United Arab Emirates

ANIL ARDESHNA, DMD, MDS
Diplomate, American Board of Orthodontics, Associate Professor, Director of Research,
Department of Orthodontics, Rutgers School of Dental Medicine, Newark, New Jersey,
USA

**RAMESH BALASUBRAMANIAM OAM, BSc, BDSc (UWA), MS, Cert Orofacial Pain
(UK), Cert Oral Medicine (Penn), MRACDS (OralMed), ABOP, FOMAA**
Associate Professor, Discipline Lead in Oral Medicine, The University of Western Australia
Dental School, The University of Western Australia, Nedlands, Western Australia, Australia

FATMA BANDAY, BDS, MS
General Dentist, Rutgers School of Dental Medicine, Newark, New Jersey, USA

DEPTI BELLANI, BDS, MDS
Private Practice, Navi Mumbai, India

DIPTI BHATNAGAR, BDS, MDS
Professor and Head, Department of Oral Medicine and Radiology, Rayat Bahra Dental
College and Hospitals, Punjab, India

JITENDRA CHAWLA, BDS, MDS
Assistant Professor, Department of Dentistry, All India Institute of Medical Sciences,
Mangalagiri. Dist. Guntur, Andhra Pradesh, India

ANNA COLONNA, DDS, MSC
Lecturer, Department of Medical Biotechnologies, School of Dentistry, University of Siena, Siena, Italy

JANANI DAKSHINAMOORTHY, MTech, PhD
Scientific Head, GeneAura Pvt. Ltd, Chennai, India

THAO THI DO, DDS, MSc, PhD
Associate Dean, Faculty of Odonto-Stomatology, Can Tho University of Medicine and Pharmacy, Can Tho, Vietnam

ELI ELIAV, DMD, PhD
Dean, Eastman Institute for Oral Health, University of Rochester Medical Center, Rochester, New York, USA

CARLA Y. FALCON, DMD, MDS
Diplomate, American Board of Endodontics, Associate Professor, Department of Endodontics, Rutgers School of Dental Medicine, Newark, New Jersey, USA

MAHNAZ FATAHZADEH, DMD, MSD
Professor and Director, Division of Oral Medicine, Department of Diagnostic Sciences, Rutgers School of Dental Medicine, Newark, New Jersey, USA

AMRITA GOGIA, BDS, MDS
Senior Consultant and Head, Department of Dental Sciences, Medanta - The Medicity, Gurugram, Haryana, India

SUMIT GUPTA, BDS, MDS
Diplomate, American Board of Orofacial Pain, Private Practice, Rak Dental Care & Implant Centre, Ras Al Khaimah, United Arab Emirates

SUNIL SURESH HARIKRISHNAN, MDS
Private Practice, Prosthodontics and Orofacial Pain Specialist, Doha, Qatar

VERONICA ITURRIAGA, DDS, MSC, PhD
Assistant Professor, Department of Integral Adult Care Dentistry, Temporomandibular Disorder and Orofacial Pain Program, Sleep and Pain Research Group, Faculty of Dentistry, Universidad de La Frontera, Temuco, Chile

MYTHILI KALLADKA, BDS, MSD
Assistant Professor, Orofacial Pain and Temporomandibular Disorders, Eastman Institute for Oral Health, Rochester, New York, USA

JUNAD KHAN, DDS, MSD, MPH, PhD
Associate Professor, Program Director, Orofacial Pain and Temporomandibular Disorders, Eastman Institute for Oral Health, Rochester, New York, USA

OLGA A. KORCZENIEWSKA, PhD
Assistant Professor, Department of Diagnostic Sciences, Center for Orofacial Pain and Temporomandibular Disorders, Rutgers School of Dental Medicine, The State University of New Jersey, Newark, New Jersey, USA

DAMIAN J. LEE, DDS, MS
Chair, Department of Prosthodontics, Tufts University School of Dental Medicine, Boston, Massachusetts, USA

UPASANA LINGAIAH, BDS, MDS
Associate Professor, Department of Oral Medicine and Radiology, VS Dental College and Hospital, Bengaluru, India

DANIELE MANFREDINI, DDS, MSc, PhD
Professor, Department of Medical Biotechnologies, School of Dentistry, University of Siena, Siena, Italy

ASHER MANSDORF, DDS, MA
Clinical Assistant Professor of Dental Medicine, Board Certified Orofacial Pain, Board Certified Dental Anesthesia, Touro College of Dental Medicine, Woodmere, New York, USA

STANLEY MARKMAN, DDS, DABOP, FOFP
Assistant Clinical Professor, Orofacial Pain, Rutgers School of Dental Medicine, Newark, New Jersey, USA

ANU PRIYA GURUSWAMY PANDIAN, BDS, MDS
Associate Dentist and Consultant Endodontist, Durga Dental, Chennai, Tamil Nadu, India

SRISHTI PAREKH, BDS, MDS
Private Practice, Mumbai, India

JAIMIN PATEL, BDS, MDS
Chief Implantologist and Orofacial Pain Specialist, 32 PEARLS: Multispeciality Dental Clinics & Implant Center, Ahmedabad, Gujarat, India

JACK PIERMATTI, DMD, FACP
Associate Professor, Post Graduate Prosthodontics, Nova Southeastern University College of Dental Medicine, Davie, Florida, USA

PRIYANKA KODAGANALLUR PITCHUMANI, BDS, MS
Clinical Assistant Professor, Department of Periodontics, University of Iowa College of Dentistry and Dental Clinics, Iowa City, Iowa, USA

VAISHNAVI PRABHAKAR, BDS, MDS
PhD Candidate, Department of Dental Sciences, Dr.M.G.R Educational and Research Institute, Chennai, India

SAMUEL Y.P. QUEK, DMD, MPH
Professor, Department of Diagnostic Sciences, Rutgers School of Dental Medicine, Newark, New Jersey, USA

RACHANA HEGDE, BDS, MS
Adjunct Associate Professor, University of Utah, Salt Lake City, Utah, USA

KARTIK R. RAMAN, BDS, MDS, FOFP
Former Associate Professor and PG Guide, CSMSS Dental College Aurangabad, Aurangaba, Maharashtra, India

ANJALI RAVI, BDS
DMD Candidate, Class of 2026, University of Pittsburgh School of Dental Medicine, Pittsburgh, Pennsylvania, USA

PAUL EMILE ROSSOUW, BSc, BCHD(Dent), BCHD-Hons (Child Dent), MCHD (Ortho), Cert (Ortho), PhD (Dental Science), FRCD(C)
Professor and Chairman, Division of Orthodontics and Dentofacial Orthopedics, University of Rochester, Eastman Institute for Oral Health, Rochester, New York, CSA

LINDA SANGALLI, DDS, MS, PhD
Assistant Professor, College of Dental Medicine - Illinois, Midwestern University, Downers Grove, Illinois, USA

SAURABH K. SHAH, BDS, PGDMLS
Private Practice, Mumbai, India

KARPAGAVALLI SHANMUGASUNDARAM, BDS, MDS
Professor and Head, Department of Oral Medicine and Radiology, Seema Dental College and Hospital, Rishikesh, Uttarakhand, India

STEVEN R. SINGER, DDS
Professor and Chair, Department of Diagnostic Sciences, Rutgers School of Dental Medicine, Newark, New Jersey, USA

GAYATHRI SUBRAMANIAN, PhD, DMD
Associate Professor, Department of Diagnostic Sciences, Rutgers School of Dental Medicine, Newark, New Jersey, USA

ANDREW SULLIVAN, DDS
Chair, Rutgers School of Dental Medicine, Newark, New Jersey, USA

DAVIS C. THOMAS, BDS, DDS, MSD, MSc Med, MSc
Associate Clinical Professor; Program Director, Clinical Preceptorship in General Dentistry, Rutgers School of Dental Medicine, Newark, New Jersey, USA; Clinical Associate Professor of Dentistry, Rochester Medical School, Rochester, New York, USA; Adjunct Associate Professor, The University of Western Australia, Perth, Australia

PRISLY THOMAS, BDS, MDS
Diplomate, American Board of Orofacial Pain, Assistant Professor, Believers Church Medical College Hospital, Kerala, India

MANISH VALIATHAN, BDS, MDS, DDS, MSD
Professor, Department of Orthodontics, Case Western Reserve University, Cleveland, Ohio, USA

NICOL VELASQUEZ, DDS
Permanent Teaching Staff, Department of Integral Adult Care Dentistry, Temporomandibular Disorder and Orofacial Pain Program, Sleep and Pain Research Group, Faculty of Dentistry, Universidad de La Frontera, Temuco, Chile

FENGYUAN ZHENG, BDS, PhD
Director, Advanced Education Program in Prosthodontics, Department of Restorative Sciences, Division of Prosthodontics, University of Minnesota School of Dentistry, Minneapolis, Minnesota, USA

VINCENT B. ZICCARDI, DDS, MD, FACS
Professor and Chair, Department of Oral and Maxillofacial Surgery, Rutgers School of Dental Medicine, Associate Dean of Hospital Affairs, Newark, New Jersey, USA

Contents

> Clinicians who place and restore implants are always concerned about the
> success and longevity of the same. There are several local and systemic
> factors that affect osseointegration and the health of the peri-implant tis-
> sues. In this study, we review the systemic factors that can affect implant
> survival, osseointegration, and long-term success. The study highlights
> the importance of delineating, and taking into consideration these sys-
> temic factors from the planning phase to the restorative phase of dental
> implants. A thorough medical history, including prescription and over-
> the-counter medications, is vital, as there may be numerous factors that
> could directly or indirectly influence the prognosis of dental implants.

> This review delves into the effects of autoimmune conditions like rheuma-
> toid arthritis, inflammatory disorders such as irritable bowel syndrome,
> cardiovascular disease, diabetes, infectious ailments like human immuno-
> deficiency virus, and their medications on periodontal therapy outcomes. It
> also explores the influence of hormones. Understanding these systemic
> factors is crucial for optimizing periodontal health and treatment efficacy.
> The review underscores the necessity of considering these variables in pe-
> riodontal care. Other vital systemic factors are addressed elsewhere in this
> special edition.

> This study gives an insight into certain systemic conditions and factors
> such as nutrition, age, hematological disorders, hypertension, smoking,
> obesity, and metabolic syndrome that have a notable effect on the perio-
> dontium. The review highlights the importance of taking these factors into
> consideration in periodontal therapy and their impact on the prognosis of
> periodontal therapies. The other systemic factors are discussed in detail
> elsewhere in the special issue.

> Stress is a process that activates neuronal, metabolic, and neuroendocrine mechanisms. The individual's response may be determined by variables such as genetic factors, environmental conditions, sex, and age, among others. These responses are critical for survival, and the involvement of the hypothalamic–pituitary–adrenal axis is necessary for adaptation, which through counter-regulatory mechanisms seeks to restore homeostasis. Dentists are aware that there are variations in people's response to treatment, and there are many patients in whom dental treatment generates an important source of stress, which in many cases leads to treatment avoidance behavior.

> The appearance of coronavirus disease 2019 (COVID-19) and other emerging infections has significantly impacted the field of dentistry, leading to widespread changes in practices and protocols. This has included the implementation of strict infection control measures, such as meticulous use of personal protective equipment, minimizing aerosol-generating procedures, and the adoption of teledentistry to reduce in-person contact. To date, the complete impact of delays in dental care caused by lockdowns has yet to be determined. The challenges faced during the COVID-19 pandemic have propelled innovation, shaping a new era of dentistry focused on safety against novel and re-emerging infections.

> This study provided an overview of the knowledge on the main sleep-related disorders and conditions affecting the prognosis of dental treatment: sleep bruxism (SB), obstructive sleep apnea (OSA), and gastroesophageal reflux disease (GERD). Current scientific evidence seems to suggest that these phenomena (ie, SB, OSA, GERD) belong to a circle of mutually relating sleep disorders and conditions where dental practitioners can play a key role in diagnosis and treatment.

> Genetics plays a significant role in determining an individual's susceptibility to dental diseases, the response to dental treatments, and the overall prognosis of dental interventions. Here, the authors explore the various genetic factors affecting the prognosis of dental treatments focusing on dental caries, orthodontic treatment, oral cancer, prosthodontic treatment, periodontal disease, developmental disorders, pharmacogenetics, and genetic predisposition to faster wound healing. Understanding the genetic

underpinnings of dental health can help personalize treatment plans, predict outcomes, and improve the overall quality of dental care.

Sumit Gupta, Anil Ardeshna, Paul Emile Rossouw, and Manish Valiathan

This article explores the intersection of various systemic conditions with orthodontic treatment. Renal diseases, including chronic kidney disease and renal transplant, present challenges such as delayed tooth eruption and gingival overgrowth, necessitating careful orthodontic planning and collaboration with physicians. Liver diseases, particularly hepatitis, heighten the risk of periodontal disease and mandate strict infection control measures during orthodontic procedures. Ehlers-Danlos syndrome poses challenges related to collagen fragility, rapid tooth movement, and orthodontic relapse. Autoimmune diseases like diabetes mellitus and juvenile idiopathic arthritis require tailored orthodontic approaches considering oral complications and joint involvement.

Anil Ardeshna, Sumit Gupta, Paul Emile Rossouw, and Manish Valiathan

This article explores the various challenges systemic conditions can pose before and during orthodontic treatment. Cardiovascular conditions like infective endocarditis require antibiotic prophylaxis before certain orthodontic procedures are started. Patients with bleeding disorders require special considerations in regards to viral infection risk and maintenance of excellent atraumatic oral hygiene. Orthodontists play an important role in early identification of signs and symptoms of eating disorders and should deal with these patients sensitively. Congenital disorders, craniofacial anomalies, and nutritional deficiencies require special considerations and should be addressed appropriately before orthodontic treatment is started.

Davis C. Thomas, Junad Khan, Sowmya Ananthan, and Mythili Kalladka

There are several factors that affect a patient's experience of pain. These include both local and systemic factors. The systemic factors that affect patients' dental and orofacial pain experience include, but not limited to, hormonal, nutritional, systemic infections, neurodegenerative, and autoimmune, among others. Comprehensive medical history is essential to delineate any possible systemic factors affecting pain experience. A thorough review of systems should form the foundation, since multiple factors can affect the prognosis of pain management. This would facilitate early recognition and trigger prompt referrals to the appropriate medical professionals. This helps to reduce the health care burden.

Mythili Kalladka, Stanley Markman, Kartik R. Raman, and Asher Mansdorf

Many psychological factors may have a significant bearing on an individual's oral health and success of dental treatments. Overall, these factors may result in the avoidance of dental visits, emergency-based dental appointments, noncompliant dental behavior, the utilization of multiple oral health care providers, and poor oral health. These factors may affect the quality of life of individuals and may lead to patient dissatisfaction, poor prognosis, and failure of dental treatment. Multiple psychological factors may affect the dentist and the patient. Those factors may alter the prognosis for successful dental treatment. Physician empathy is fundamental in developing long-term physician–patient trust.

The field of restorative and prosthetic dentistry focuses on restoring lost tooth structures and replacing missing teeth and lost tissue to restore or improve esthetics and oral health. Many systemic factors such as metabolic, bone, autoimmune, cardiovascular, and endocrine disorders can affect healing procedures, and bone density and impact oral health. Hence patients suffering from systemic disease when treated for prosthodontic rehabilitation can have negative prognostic outcomes. The commonest prosthodontic treatments that can be affected include dental implants, fixed prostheses, and removable prostheses. Understanding and managing these systemic factors play a key role in the success of prosthodontic treatment.

This article gives valuable insight into the effect of selected groups of medications on dental treatment outcome and prognosis. The review emphasizes the importance of thorough medical history, which may have an impact on the prognosis of dental treatment. We discuss drugs acting on the central nervous system, gastrointestinal tract, respiratory tract, endocrine system, and bone metabolism among others. Other pertinent drugs are discussed elsewhere in this special issue.

Today, it is common for medically complex patients who are receiving multiple medications, to seek routine and emergent dental care. It is essential for the practitioner to recognize and comprehend the impact of such medications on the patient's ability to tolerate the planned dental treatment and on dental treatment outcomes. An active appraisal of current literature is essential to stay abreast of emerging findings and understand their treatment implications. This article outlines the process of such active critical appraisal, illustrating key paradigms of the models that describe the impact of medications on treatment outcomes.

Healing process in the oral cavity is influenced by a range of systemic factors. More specifically, patient health status, medications, habits, and nutritional state play crucial roles in dental healing. Additionally, the body's immune response, inflammation, and overall well-being are key determinants in wound repair. Understanding these systemic factors is essential for dental professionals to optimize patient care, minimize complications, and achieve successful healing.

The successful outcome of endodontic treatment is dependent on the immune response and the reparative potential of the individual. Alteration in the host immune response is a common characteristic shared by both apical periodontitis and systemic diseases. Although infection-induced periapical lesions occur in a localized environment, numerous epidemiologic studies in the last few decades have investigated the potential association between endodontic disease pathogenesis and systemic diseases. The goal of this review is to identify common systematic factors and discuss the effect they may or may not have on the prognosis and outcome of endodontic therapy.

DENTAL CLINICS OF NORTH AMERICA

FORTHCOMING ISSUES

RECENT ISSUES

SERIES OF RELATED INTEREST

Atlas of the Oral and Maxillofacial Surgery Clinics
https://www.oralmaxsurgeryatlas.theclinics.com/

Oral and Maxillofacial Surgery Clinics
https://www.oralmaxsurgery.theclinics.com/

THE CLINICS ARE AVAILABLE ONLINE!
Access your subscription at:
www.theclinics.com

Dedication

When I was invited by *Dental Clinics of North America* to be the guest editor for this special edition, my heart was filled with gratitude to all my teachers/gurus who were instrumental in guiding me to be the teacher and mentor I have become. Therefore, I strongly felt that this entire issue should be dedicated to all those teachers. I may not have some of their full names, however, I have attempted to do my justice in remembering them with reverence and indebtedness.

As I entered Bachelor of Dental Surgery (BDS), my undergraduate course in dentistry, at Manipal College of Dental Surgery (MCODS) in India, I was slightly apprehensive of how much rigor I would have to go through to graduate from the best dental school in India. However, all my teachers at MCODS facilitated the best learning environment and experience for me. Dr. C N Chandrashekhar of the physiology department was my first inspiration. He was instrumental in sparking and rekindling my innate interest in physiology and medicine. Dr. Shakuntala R Pai, as she explained cadaver dissections, really inspired me to learn clinical anatomy. Dr. Rajendra Holla, professor of pharmacology, inspired me to love this tough, volatile subject and take up the challenge of trying to excel in it. I still vividly remember him walking into the class with impeccable, crisp clothing, looking like he walked out of a men's body building magazine! He inspired the entire class to learn the subject of Pharmacology.

Dr. Balasubramaniam, Unit 5 medicine chief, was exceptional. Dr. Mohan Alexander (OFMS), Dr. B H Sripathi Rao (OFMS), Dr. S R Prabhu (Oral Medicine Oral Pathology), Dr. Vijay Raghavan (Oral Radiology), Dr. Keerthilata Pai (OMR), Dr. Mahalinga Bhat (Periodontology), and Dr. Macchado (General Surgery) were some of our outstanding teachers who have inspired me. This list is by no means complete and all inclusive, but only reflects some of my gurus who influenced me to the greatest extent. I bow before all my teachers who made me the clinician, author and mentor who I humbly think I have become today. To them I dedicate this special Dental Clinics of North America issue.

Dent Clin N Am 68 (2024) xiii
https://doi.org/10.1016/j.cden.2024.07.009
dental.theclinics.com
0011-8532/24/© 2024 Elsevier Inc. All rights are reserved, including those for text and data mining, AI training, and similar technologies.

Preface

Systemic Factors Affecting Prognosis in Dentistry

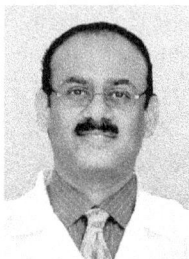

Davis C. Thomas, BDS, DDS, MSD, MSc Med, MSc
Editor

Dentistry has gone through explosive changes in terms of technology over the past few decades. Advances in science and technology have helped dental clinicians in achieving outstanding levels of diagnosis, treatment planning, and prognosis. However, the influence of the systemic factors in a patient that can robustly affect, and possibly alter, the course and outcomes of treatment, and treatment prognosis, is sometimes overlooked. Recent literature is rich with succinct publications that point to the significant effects of systemic conditions, illnesses, and medications affecting the prognosis and outcomes of dental treatment.

The supporting hard and soft tissues of teeth and restorations, including implants, are greatly influenced by the effects of systemic factors. This knowledge has prompted leading professional dental organizations to incorporate systemic diseases, such as diabetes, and habits, such as smoking, as part of treatment planning and in determining the prognosis, and thereby treatment outcomes. Predicting prognosis based on the existing systemic factors is becoming the new norm based on which the clinician could choose to alter the choice of treatment, and have an informed decision from the patients, enabling them to set realistic treatment goals. For example, the latest literature on some of the commonly used medications, such as proton pump inhibitors, antidepressants, and certain antibiotics, such as clindamycin, posing an increased risk of implant failure must be considered in gauging the prognosis of these cases. Similar literature has also evolved regarding systemic factors affecting the healing of periapical tissues of endodontically treated teeth. Similar effects of systemic factors on such treatment modalities as orthodontics, periodontal treatment, pain management, and restorative dentistry are also emerging in the recent literature.

This special issue of *Dental Clinics of North America* brings together the world's leading experts in this field. I am honored and privileged to be the editor of this issue.

Dent Clin N Am 68 (2024) xv–xvi
https://doi.org/10.1016/j.cden.2024.07.008
0011-8532/24/© 2024 Published by Elsevier Inc.

My interactions with these amazing clinicians and experts in their fields that have transpired over the past several months, culminating in this valuable special issue, have been phenomenal and enriching. It has been my distinct honor and pleasure to have associated with this exquisitely high-level scholastic group of contributors. The result of these collaborations, and the quality of articles produced in this special issue, is truly gratifying.

I wish to thank all our mentors, colleagues, residents, students, and all the contributors, without whose constant support and encouragement this quality special issue would not have been possible. I also thank my friends and family for their support during the time I was away from them. My immense gratitude to Mr John Vassallo, Mr Akshay Samson, and the entire *Dental Clinics of North America* team for their continued and constant support.

Davis C. Thomas, BDS, DDS, MSD, MSc Med, MSc
Rutgers School of Dental Medicine
Newark, NJ, USA

Rochester Medical School
Rochester, NY, USA

The University of Western Australia
Perth, Australia

E-mail address:
davisct1@gmail.com

Systemic Factors Affecting Prognosis of Dental Implants

Davis C. Thomas, BDS, DDS, MSD, MSc Med, MSc[a],*,
Depti Bellani, BDS, MDS[b], Jack Piermatti, DMD[c],
Priyanka Kodaganallur Pitchumani, BDS, MS[d]

KEYWORDS

- Implant prognosis • Implant failure • Dental implants • Osseointegration
- Implant survival • Implant success • Implant stability

KEY POINTS

- Endocrine factors seem to be the most vibrant affecting implant prognosis, out of the systemic factors published in this regard to date.
- Smoking seems to be a crucial factor with both systemic and local effects contributing to implant failure.
- Medication classes negatively affecting dental implant prognosis include selective serotonin reuptake inhibitors and proton pump inhibitors.
- In general, systemic factors that may hamper and interfere with proper oral hygiene maintenance seem to be contributing to implant failure.
- Prophylactic antibiotics given prior to implant surgery seem to strongly favor implant survival rates.

INTRODUCTION

In medicine, all patients for planned surgical procedures are evaluated carefully for the preoperative assessment of possible systemic factors that can affect the prognosis, both during and after surgery. Following the same principle, in the recent past dental literature, several authors have looked at these systemic factors that may predict and affect implant success, survival, and prognosis. Although the literature seems not so robust in all the various possible factors, emerging evidence points out to a number of succinct systemic factors that can significantly affect both the short-term and long-term prognosis of dental implants.

[a] Department of Diagnostic Sciences, Center for Temporomandibular Disorders and Orofacial Pain, Rutgers School of Dental Medicine, Newark, NJ, USA; [b] Private Practice, Navi Mumbai, India; [c] Nova Southeastern University College of Dental Medicine, FL, USA; [d] Department of Periodontics, University of Iowa College of Dentistry and Dental Clinics, Iowa City, IA 52242, USA
* Corresponding author. Department of Diagnostic Sciences, Rutgers School of Dental Medicine, 110 Bergen Street, Newark, NJ 07103.
E-mail address: davisct1@gmail.com

Dent Clin N Am 68 (2024) 555–570
https://doi.org/10.1016/j.cden.2024.07.001
0011-8532/24/© 2024 Elsevier Inc. All rights are reserved, including those for text and data mining, AI training, and similar technologies.
dental.theclinics.com

The available medical/dental/implant literature seems to indicate a crucial role played by several factors including, but not limited to, medications (selective seroto-nin reuptake inhibitor [SSRI] and proton pump inhibitor [PPI]), endocrine disorders, and systemic factors affecting the patient's ability to maintain optimal oral hygiene, as the key players in determining implant prognosis. The effect of smoking seems to be both local and systemic, and a cumulative effect results in poor implant prog-nosis. Researchers and clinicians seem to prefer deferring implant placement until such a point that the patient has either successfully quit smoking or reduced the habit significantly to help the clinician's comfort placing the implant. Some clinicians, within their individual rights, totally reject the proposal for surgical implants if the patient re-fuses to quit smoking. Systemic factors that affect a patient's manual dexterity and/or mental capability to maintain optimal oral hygiene can adversely affect the prognosis of dental implants. These include conditions such as Down's syndrome, movement disorders, rheumatoid arthritis, and other conditions that pose a physical and/or cognitive challenge. Even in this new medical era of trying to limit antibiotic usage, the latest literature seem to indicate that prophylactic antibiotic usage is improving implant success rates and prognosis. The authors have enumerated the most salient systemic factors that have been proposed and shown to be affecting the prognosis of dental implants.

HEMATOLOGICAL DISORDERS

Since local tissue bleeding could potentially impact the implant surgical procedures, implementing a systematic protocol in these cases is paramount for the proper healing and patient comfort.[1–3] It must be noted that most of the related literature in this regard has been extrapolated from the data dealing with surgical tooth extraction and post-extraction healing.[4] Individuals who suffer from infections, idiopathic purpura, radia-tion therapy, bone marrow suppression, or cancers (such as leukemia) may be at risk for platelet deficiency. Platelet deficiency is associated with the high risk of bleeding.[5] A potentially serious complication of dental implant placement in these pa-tients, which happens infrequently, is upper airway obstruction brought on by severe hemorrhage from the tissues in the floor of the mouth.[6] Due to the potential for lingual artery involvement as a result of inferior alveolar canal perforation or lingual cortical plate involvement, the first mandibular premolar position is the most dangerous place to place dental implants.[7–9]

In the field of oral implantology, blood disorders are among the most serious con-ditions. Prolonged healing, reduced bone density, and prolonged healing times are all consequences of anemia. This patient population has a high rate of intraoperative bleeding, which could lead to increased discomfort and postoperative edema. The risk of secondary infections is elevated in association with it. Chronic infections are common, which reduces the long-term implant survival rate. A number of com-plications caused by leukocyte disorders may jeopardize the implant's success. Among these, infection is the most frequent (it can happen at any point in the course of treatment). The uncertainty of postsurgical edema and secondary infection is elevated, and intraoperative bleeding is common, similar to what happens to patients who have anemia.[10] von-Willebrand disease appears to have some association with implant failure, although the effect seems to be once the implant has been "loaded."[11] Well-controlled leukemia is no longer considered an absolute contraindi-cation for dental implants.[12] Both bone reparative situations showed that osteogen-esis is "sensitive" to anemia and/or the associated conditions, causing a delay in bone healing.[13]

OSTEOPOROSIS

Multiple studies including systematic review with meta-analysis showed no difference in the survival rate of implants in groups of patients with and without osteoporosis. This was true at the implant level as well as the patient level.[14,15] However, many of the studies show that the patients with osteoporosis have increased peri-implant bone loss compared to non-osteoporotic group.[14] Research suggests that parenteral bisphosphonates cause implant failure by hampering osseointegration.[16] Recent literature shows that osteoporosis by itself is not a contraindication for implant placement. However, it has been suggested that patients with osteoporosis may need a higher level of maintenance of the bone surrounding the implants, due to possible increased susceptibility to bone loss.[14,15,17–19]

ENDOCRINE FACTORS AND THEIR RELATIONSHIP TO DENTAL IMPLANT PROGNOSIS

The endocrine system regulates all biological functions of the body, utilizing hormones as chemical messengers released into the bloodstream, targeting specific receptors in order to elicit a physiologic response. The major endocrine glands include the hypothalamus, pituitary, pineal, pancreas, ovaries, testes, thyroid, parathyroids, and the adrenals. Abnormalities of any of these glands or the receptors of their respective hormones may manifest as metabolic disruption. Endocrine disorders can cause a myriad of metabolic disease states; however, this section focuses on those disorders that impact the prognosis and treatment outcomes of dental implants.

Melatonin

There is increasing evidence in the literature for the efficacy of topical melatonin in increasing the bone-implant contact, and thereby promoting osseointegration and reducing late implant failure.[20–23] The mechanism by which melatonin brings about these apparent positive effects is thought to be by reducing bone resorption.[20] Local application of melatonin at the osteotomy site was shown to improve the implant stability and minimize the crestal bone resorption.[24] The addition of melatonin into autogenous bone graft material was shown to increase bone density and thereby improve the hard and soft tissue characteristics around immediate implants placed in the esthetic zone.[25,26] It must be noted that the role of melatonin in dental implant success remains equivocal. Further focused studies are necessary in this regard.

Insulin

With respect to this section, our discussion will be limited to diabetes mellitus (DM). This condition has a definite negative impact on all oral surgical procedures and the resultant healing process. The main tenant of implant success is dependent on strict glycemic control.[27–29] There is current evidence suggesting that increased glycosylated hemoglobin (HbA1C) levels are associated with increased bleeding on probing around dental implants.[30] Patients with DM were shown to have more implant-related complications as compared to patients without DM.[30] It must be noted that DM is associated with an increased incidence of peri-implantitis, while there was a lack of association with peri-implant mucositis.[31] However, a relatively recent systematic review looking at the relationship between DM and peri-implantitis also reported inconclusive correlation between the two.[32] With regard to osseointegration, HbA1c levels were not correlated with implant stability at 1 year after implant placement.[32] With reference to DM and implant survival, the same study found that most of the implant failures occurred within the first 12 months upon prosthetic loading of the implant.[32] A recent systematic review with meta-analysis of observational studies concluded that patients with DM were more likely to have higher risk of peri-implantitis.[26] Further, some studies show increased failure rates of dental implants in patients with DM,[33,34] while others show no significant difference in failure rates among patients with DM.[35] Since there is no clear-cut distinction between failure rates of patients with and without DM , the prudent clinician must ensure strict control of the disease prior to dental implant surgery. The single most effective evaluation of a patient's diabetes control is the HbA1c and should be checked in all patients with DM prior to dental implant surgery.

Estrogen

Earlier studies regarding the role of estrogen on implant healing had shown that lower hormonal levels were associated with compromised implant healing, specific to the maxilla, not observed in the mandible.[36] The same study also showed that postmenopausal women who were not on hormonal supplements had higher failure rates.[36] Estrogen deficiency was shown to induce osteoporosis, which negatively affected machined implant osseointegration.[37] However, contradicting literature based on animal studies does not indicate an increased failure rate in osteoporotic animals, nor does it show increased failure rates in female individuals with estrogen deficiency.[38]

Thyroid Hormones

Patients being treated for thyroid cancer, utilizing radioiodine therapy are advised to wait for 2 weeks after cessation of the treatment, for surgical implant placement.[39] There was no significant difference between the survival rates of implants in patients with thyroid diseases as compared to healthy controls.[40] A recent study suggested that hypothyroidism does not pose a risk for implant failure. On the contrary, the authors have proposed that reduction in the bone metabolic rate in hypothyroidism may be protective of the dental implant.[41]

Parathyroid Hormone

Parathyroid hormone (PTH) plays a crucial role in maintaining calcium homeostasis and bone remodeling. It has been hypothesized that various concentrations and varying duration of exposure to PTH may induce diverse effects on bone remodeling. PTH is believed to induce bone apposition by downregulating sclerostin expression in osteocytes.[42] Some studies suggest that serum PTH levels may be an indicator predicting the condition of the bone around the implant, in conjunction with other factors.[43] However, a relatively recent systematic review concluded that PTH supplementation shows promising levels of efficacy on implant osseointegration.[42] The same study also warrants further investigation in application in humans.

VITAMIN D

Although termed as a vitamin, structurally vitamin D is a sterol, with effects similar to those of corticosteroids, robustly affecting immunomodulation.[44] It is considered an important cofactor in bone metabolism. Although earlier suggestions were made as to the important role vitamin D plays in the success of dental implants, the more recent focused systematic reviews seem to indicate otherwise. Short-term follow-up studies have shown that vitamin D deficiency results in mild marginal bone loss; however, it lacks solid evidence.[45–47] Long-term follow-up has been suggested to investigate the effects of vitamin D levels on implant stability.

MEDICATIONS AFFECTING DENTAL IMPLANT PROGNOSIS
Cardiovascular Medications

The utilization of antihypertensive medications correlates with an increased survival rate of osseointegrated implants. The elevated survival rate of osseointegrated dental implants has been linked to the utilization of antihypertensive drugs, which can be attributed to their influence on bone metabolism.[48] Beta-blockers, thiazide diuretics, angiotensin-converting enzyme (ACE) inhibitors, and angiotension receptor blockers (ARBs), among other antihypertensive medications, exert beneficial effects on bone health.[49,50] Bone cells express beta-adrenergic receptors, notably beta-2 receptors, which when activated, promote bone resorption and inhibit bone formation.[51] Indeed, in addition to their cardiovascular impact, beta-blockers hinder the activity of beta-2 receptors involved in bone resorption, leading to enhanced bone accumulation.[52] Hence, beta-blockers have demonstrated favorable impacts on bone structure, metabolism, and the healing process.[48] This may be beneficial for implant survival, although not shown in studies. Thiazide diuretics act by inhibiting the thiazide-sensitive sodium chloride cotransporter located in the distal tubules of the kidney, which reduces the excretion of calcium and consequently promotes calcium absorption.[53] Reduced urinary calcium excretion may result in elevated serum calcium levels, potentially leading to decreased PTH levels and subsequently reducing bone turnover, resulting in beneficial effects on bone mineral density (BMD).[54] Additionally, thiazide diuretics may exert a direct beneficial impact on BMD by influencing the proliferation and differentiation of osteoblasts.[55] ACE inhibitors and ARBs suppress ACE activity, subsequently influencing bone metabolism[56]; ARBs can also significantly increase BMD by inhibiting bone resorption.[57] Gingival enlargement may manifest around dental implants, particularly in rehabilitative scenarios for individuals who have undergone head and neck cancer treatment. Clinicians should consider the possibility of gingival enlargement in hypertensive patients prescribed calcium channel blockers before proceeding with implant placement. Whether this drug-influenced gingival enlargement affects prognosis of implants has not been shown.[58] The utilization of renin–angiotensin system (RAS) inhibitors is linked to increased implant stability upon implant exposure subsequent to implant therapy compared to individuals who do not use these inhibitors.[59] RAS inhibitors were shown in animal studies to decrease periodontal inflammation and cause an increase in the volume of the alveolar bone.[60] Given that the success of osseointegrated implants relies heavily on bone formation and remodeling, individuals using antihypertensive drugs who have undergone dental implant treatment may experience advantages. Angiotensin II type 1 receptor blockers (ARBs) and ACE inhibitors have demonstrated the ability to inhibit the release of osteoclast-activating mediators via angiotensin II type 1 receptors on osteoblasts.[61,62] They also enhance blood flow in bone marrow capillaries, elevate free Ca^{2+} ion levels in plasma while reducing parathormone levels,[63] and overall mitigate the detrimental effects of angiotensin II on bones, particularly the activation of osteoclasts by angiotensin II.[56,64,65] Propranolol likely improves bone healing and osseointegration by reducing the number of osteoclasts, increasing collagen production, and promoting mineralization.[66] Antihypertensive medications like beta-blockers or ACE inhibitors might also have a beneficial impact on reducing the rate of implant failure.[67–69] Statins exhibit a notable positive influence on the process of implant osseointegration.[70] Recent human studies have shown that the systemic oral intake of lipophilic statins, such as simvastatin, led to an increase in BMD.[71] Simvastatin, a semisynthetic derivative of lovastatin, was observed to exert a beneficial influence on bone metabolism.[72] Levels of bone alkaline phosphatase, C-terminal telopeptide of type I collagen, and osteocalcin rose concurrently with the elevation in BMD.[73–77] The intriguing potential impact of antihypertensive medications on dental implant osseointegration arises when contemplating their beneficial effects on bone formation, remodeling, and reduced risk of bone fractures.[67] Implant survival rates in individuals with cardiovascular disease may be equivalent to or greater than those observed in healthy patients.[78] There is no conclusive evidence that cardiovascular diseases by themselves are contraindications for implant placement.[17]

Immunosuppressants

Cyclosporin A (CsA), an immunosuppressant, may impact the process of bone remodeling and inhibit osteoblast cell activity, which may reduce the likelihood of proper bone healing.[79,80] According to recent research, taking CsA prior to implant surgery can disrupt the osseointegration around implants and lower bone quality, which may lower the prognosis of implants.[81] The use of CsA hinders bone healing process around implant placement and increases bone loss.[82] The potential for developing osteoporosis secondary to CsA therapy has been mentioned in the literature.[83] Immunosuppressive medications may have an adverse effect on the long-term prognosis of dental implants.[17,79]

Bisphosphonates

Systemic bisphosphonates have been linked to osteonecrosis of the jaw (ONJ).[84] Due to the possibility of bisphosphonate-induced ONJ, it is advised that these patients are carefully evaluated, and risk assessment performed prior to surgical intervention including implants.[84,85] A position paper supporting the term medication-related ONJ rather than bisphosphonate-induced ONJ was released in 2017 by the American Association of Oral and Maxillofacial Surgeons.[86] In patients receiving oral antiresorptive medicines for longer than 3 years, the rate of medication-related ONJ can reach as high as 0.5% after dental extractions. Currently, there is a lack of robust literature to contraindicate implant placement in patients taking bisphosphonates. However, dentists who place implants must understand the risk associated with treating patients receiving intravenous or oral bisphosphonate therapy.[79]

Nonsteroidal Anti-inflammatory Drugs

These medications inhibit the cyclooxygenase enzymes, thereby reducing prostaglandin synthesis, a crucial process for healthy bone formation and repair.[87,88] A retrospective study showed a significant reduction in success rates of implants with concomitant nonsteroidal anti-inflammatory drug (NSAID) treatment. The same study also showed less than ideal results for patients who were on NSAIDs prior to implant placement.[17,89,90] Given the evidence available so far, further careful evaluation may warranted for patients being treated for dental implants.

Antidepressants

SSRIs have been associated with a higher rate of implant failure.[91–93] It is thought to be a result of these medications decreasing the bone turnover and inducing greater destruction of bone.[92] SSRIs have been linked to decreased BMD and an increase in bone fractures.[69] Serotonin receptors are ubiquitous, presenting in multiple tissues including, but not limited to, brain, neurons, the gastrointestinal tract, blood platelets, and bone. Reduced bone density results from blocking serotonin reuptake, which also causes an increase in osteoclast differentiation and a decrease in osteoblast prolifer-ation.[17] Because of their anti-anabolic skeletal effects, SSRIs have been shown to negatively impact trabecular microarchitecture and BMD.[68] It is prudent to further evaluate patients on SSRIs for the appropriateness and risks of dental implants.

Proton Pump Inhibitors

A class of medications known as PPIs works by reducing the amount of gastric acid produced. However, some authors have proposed an association between PPIs and a higher risk of bone fractures, possibly due to changes in absorption of cal-cium.[67] Long-term PPI use can lower acidity, which can negatively impact the absorp-tion of calcium, magnesium, iron, and vitamin B12.[67,68] Emerging literature seems to indicate an association between PPI treatment and implant failure.[67–69,94,95]

Glucocorticoids

Glucocorticoids act on osteoblasts causing apoptosis and promoting the differentia-tion of adipocytes from bone marrow cells, which may suggest that these medications have a deleterious effect on bone remodeling. Long-term use of systemic corticoste-roids may also have a deleterious effect on osseointegration of dental implants.[96–98] Long-term corticosteroid therapy seems to be reported in the literature as a strong relative contraindication to dental implant placement.[69,99]

Prophylactic Antibiotics

The latest literature seems to indicate that prophylactic antibiotic usage is improving implant success rates and prognosis. In a relatively recent narrative review on the sub-ject, the authors recommend a prophylactic regimen somewhat similar to the prophy-lactic infective endocarditis regimen to prevent early implant failure. However, they add that the use of antibiotics has no statistically significant effect on postoperative infections after implant placement.[100] Similar results were reported in meta-analysis performed recently on the topic.[101,102] A network meta-analysis of randomized control trials also have come to the same conclusions.[103] Although the exact mechanism of the protective nature of prophylactic antibiotics on surgical implants is not known, the plausible explanation seems to be the antibiotic's effect in eradicating initial bac-terial colonization and subsequent development of infection.[100] The recent consensus report from the Spanish group of implantologists also seems to ratify this same philos-ophy.[104] Interestingly, allergy to penicillin/amoxicillin is being shown as more condu-cive to implant failure.[105–107] The mechanism of this phenomena is unknown but proposed to have to do with the use of alternate antibiotics for prophylaxis in patients with penicillin allergy.

PSYCHIATRIC DISORDERS

There are some significant inconsistencies in the evaluation of implants in patients with neuropsychiatric disorders. In general, psychiatric disorders and mental disabil-ities are not shown to be a strong contraindication for dental implant placement.[108,109] Many of these patients may have related habits or physical/mental limitations that may impact the factors such as oral hygiene, thereby affecting implant prognosis.[109,110] However, treatment with implants can be a beneficial option for patients with such dis-abilities, provided that oral hygiene is maintained.[111–113] Patients with conditions, such as schizophrenia and obsessive-compulsive disorder, showed a similar trend toward higher implant failure.[114]

MOVEMENT DISORDERS

Patients with movement disorders may have a lower implant survival rate, more early, rather than late failures seem to occur. Rather than the direct effect of movement disorders, the associated relative inability to maintain oral hygiene may be a more significant factor leading to possible implant failure.[115] In patients with acquired and congenital neurologic disabilities, there were no higher implant failures observed.[116] In a recent meta-analysis, patients with neuropsychiatric disorders were found to have a higher propensity for implant failure, primarily due to inability to maintain proper oral hygiene.[117]

GENETIC DISORDERS

Some genetic disorders such as Down's syndrome may negatively impact dental implant prognosis, due to impairments in immunity, combined with cognitive impairment.[115,116,118–121] Other characteristics of these patients include macroglossia, parafunctional habits, and a history of periodontal disease, thereby conceivably affecting implant survival. The majority of failures, however, seem to occur prior to implant loading, that is, during the osseointegration phase.[115,119–122]

SMOKING

From the available current literature, it appears that smoking affects implant prognosis negatively, due to its local and systemic effects. The risk of implant failure has been found to be higher in smokers as compared to nonsmokers.[123,124] The amount of marginal bone loss was found to be significantly higher in smokers as compared to the controlled group of nonsmokers.[125,126] In addition to these, the postoperative infection risk was also found to be higher in smokers, compared to controls.[127,128] It is interesting to note that most of the literature points out to an increased marginal bone loss secondary to smoking at the implant site.[129] Traditionally (maybe anecdotally) implantologists are increasingly likely to defer or choose to refuse implant placement in smokers.

SUMMARY

The analysis of the most recent literature regarding implant prognosis and failures seems to reveal the importance of, and the role played by, systemic factors. The astute clinician has to carefully consider the systemic factors and elucidate a complete medical history from the patient to aid in succinct treatment planning and take appropriate precautions preoperatively, intraoperatively, and postoperatively to ensure optimal implant prognosis.

CLINICS CARE POINTS

- The planning phase of dental implants must include a careful evaluation and consideration of systemic factors that can potentially affect implant prognosis.
- A sound knowledge of the latest literature showing the effect of these systemic factors on implant prognosis is paramount to plan and manage any possible potential complications with dental implants.
- Patient cooperation and compliance with instructions regarding variables potentially under the control of the patient are also a significant factor in deciding implant prognosis.
- The clinician should carefully consider the risk–benefit ratio of prophylactic or interventional antibiotic therapy.

ACKNOWLEDGMENTS

None.

DISCLOSURE

D. C. Thomas, D. Bellani, J. Piermatti, and P. Kodaganallur Pitchumani declare no conflict of interest. There was no funding for this study. Statement of institutional review board approval or waiver: Institutional review and approval were not necessary for this study.

REFERENCES

1. Gornitsky M, Hammouda W, Rosen H. Rehabilitation of a hemophiliac with implants: a medical perspective and case report. J Oral Maxillofac Surg 2005; 63(5):592–7.
2. Castellanos-Cosano L, Núñez-Vázquez RJ, Segura-Egea JJ, et al. Protocol for oral implant rehabilitation in a hemophilic HIV-positive patient with type C hepatitis. Implant Dent 2014;23(5):622–5.
3. Gatti PC, Parreira M, Gutierrez Fillol A, et al. Prospective observational study on the clinical behaviour of dental implants in patients with haemophilia. Preliminary results. Br J Oral Maxillofac Surg 2022;60(2):157–61.
4. Bacci C, Schiazzano C, Zanon E, et al. Bleeding disorders and dental implants: review and clinical indications. J Clin Med 2023;12(14).
5. Drews RE. Critical issues in hematology: anemia, thrombocytopenia, coagulopathy, and blood product transfusions in critically ill patients. Clin Chest Med 2003;24(4):607–22.
6. Givol N, Chaushu G, Halamish-Shani T, et al. Emergency tracheostomy following life-threatening hemorrhage in the floor of the mouth during immediate implant placement in the mandibular canine region. J Periodontol 2000;71(12):1893–5.
7. Kalpidis CD, Setayesh RM. Hemorrhaging associated with endosseous implant placement in the anterior mandible: a review of the literature. J Periodontol 2004; 75(5):631–45.
8. Kalpidis CD, Konstantinidis AB. Critical hemorrhage in the floor of the mouth during implant placement in the first mandibular premolar position: a case report. Implant Dent 2005;14(2):117–24.
9. Kiani S, Razav SM, Movahedian B, et al. The effect of common local and systemic conditions on dental implant osseointegration: a review of literature. Avicenna Journal of Dental Research 2015;7(2):4.
10. Gheorghiu IM, Stoian IM. Implant surgery in healthy compromised patients-review of literature. J Med Life 2014;7(Spec Iss 2):7–10. Spec No. 2.
11. Pérez-Fierro M, Castellanos-Cosano L, Hueto-Madrid JA, et al. 2-years retrospective observational case-control study on survival and marginal bone loss of implants in patients with hereditary coagulopathies. Med Oral Patol Oral Cir Bucal 2023;28(6):e572–80.
12. Yu H, Zhou A, Liu J, et al. Management of systemic risk factors ahead of dental implant therapy: A beard well lathered is half shaved. J Leukoc Biol 2021; 110(3):591–604.
13. Giglio MJ, Gorustovich A, Guglielmotti MB. Bone healing under experimental anemia in rats. Acta Odontol Latinoam 2000;13(2):63–72.
14. Lemos CAA, de Oliveira AS, Faé DS, et al. Do dental implants placed in patients with osteoporosis have higher risks of failure and marginal bone loss compared

to those in healthy patients? A systematic review with meta-analysis. Clin Oral Invest 2023;27(6):2483–93.

15. de Medeiros F, Kudo GAH, Leme BG, et al. Dental implants in patients with osteoporosis: a systematic review with meta-analysis. Int J Oral Maxillofac Surg 2018;47(4):480–91.
16. Bazli L, Chahardehi AM, Arsad H, et al. Factors influencing the failure of dental implants: A Systematic Review. Journal of Composites and Compounds 2020; 2(2):18–25.
17. Samara W, Moztarzadeh O, Hauer L, et al. Dental implant placement in medically compromised patients: a literature review. Cureus 2024;16(2):e54199.
18. Perez E, Salinas L, Mendoza R, et al. Osseointegration of dental implants in patients with congenital and degenerative bone disorders: a literature review. J Int Soc Prev Community Dent 2023;13(3):167–72.
19. Shibli JA, Aguiar KC, Melo L, et al. Histological comparison between implants retrieved from patients with and without osteoporosis. Int J Oral Maxillofac Surg 2008;37(4):321–7.
20. Gómez-Moreno G, Aguilar-Salvatierra A, Boquete-Castro A, et al. Outcomes of topical applications of melatonin in implant dentistry: a systematic review. Implant Dent 2015;24(1):25–30.
21. Permuy M, López-Peña M, González-Cantalapiedra A, et al. Melatonin: a review of its potential functions and effects on dental diseases. Int J Mol Sci 2017;18(4).
22. Cutando A, Gómez-Moreno G, Arana C, et al. Melatonin stimulates osseointegration of dental implants. J Pineal Res 2008;45(2):174–9.
23. López-Valverde N, Pardal-Peláez B, López-Valverde A, et al. Role of melatonin in bone remodeling around titanium dental implants: Meta-analysis. Coatings 2021;11(3):271.
24. El-Gammal MY, Salem AS, Anees MM, et al. Clinical and radiographic evaluation of immediate loaded dental implants with local application of melatonin: a preliminary randomized controlled clinical trial. J Oral Implantol 2016;42(2):119–25.
25. Hazzaa HHA, El-Kilani NS, Elsayed SA, et al. Evaluation of immediate implants augmented with autogenous bone/melatonin composite graft in the esthetic zone: a randomized controlled trial. J Prosthodont 2019;28(2):e637–42.
26. Li Y, Lu Z, Sun H. Impact of diabetes mellitus on the poor prognosis in patients with osseointegrated dental implants: a meta-analysis of observational studies. Biotechnol Genet Eng Rev 2023;1–19.
27. Javed F, Romanos GE. Impact of diabetes mellitus and glycemic control on the osseointegration of dental implants: a systematic literature review. J Periodontol 2009;80(11):1719–30.
28. Abdulwassie H, Dhanrajani PJ. Diabetes mellitus and dental implants: a clinical study. Implant Dent 2002;11(1):83–6.
29. Olson JW, Shernoff AF, Tarlow JL, et al. Dental endosseous implant assessments in a type 2 diabetic population: a prospective study. Int J Oral Maxillofac Implants 2000;15(6):811–8.
30. Jiang X, Zhu Y, Liu Z, et al. Association between diabetes and dental implant complications: a systematic review and meta-analysis. Acta Odontol Scand 2021;79(1):9–18.
31. Monje A, Catena A, Borgnakke WS. Association between diabetes mellitus/hyperglycaemia and peri-implant diseases: Systematic review and meta-analysis. J Clin Periodontol 2017;44(6):636–48.
32. Naujokat H, Kunzendorf B, Wiltfang J. Dental implants and diabetes mellitus-a systematic review. Int. J. Implant Dent. 2016;2(1):5.

33. Daubert DM, Weinstein BF, Bordin S, et al. Prevalence and predictive factors for peri-implant disease and implant failure: a cross-sectional analysis. J Periodontol 2015;86(3):337–47.

34. Moy PK, Medina D, Shetty V, et al. Dental implant failure rates and associated risk factors. Int J Oral Maxillofac Implants 2005;20(4):569–77.

35. Al Zahrani S, Al Mutairi AA. Stability and bone loss around submerged and non-submerged implants in diabetic and non-diabetic patients: a 7-year follow-up. Braz Oral Res 2018;32:e57.

36. August M, Chung K, Chang Y, et al. Influence of estrogen status on endosseous implant osseointegration. J Oral Maxillofac Surg 2001;59(11):1285–9 [discussion 1290-1].

37. Du Z, Xiao Y, Hashimi S, et al. The effects of implant topography on osseointegration under estrogen deficiency induced osteoporotic conditions: Histomorphometric, transcriptional and ultrastructural analysis. Acta Biomater 2016;42:351–63.

38. Giro G, Coelho PG, Sales-Pessoa R, et al. Influence of estrogen deficiency on bone around osseointegrated dental implants: an experimental study in the rat jaw model. J Oral Maxillofac Surg 2011;69(7):1911–8.

39. Piciu D, Bran S, Moldovan M, et al. Radioiodine-131 therapy used for differentiated thyroid cancer can impair titanium dental implants: an in vitro analysis. Cancers 2023;15(9).

40. Torrejon-Moya A, Izquierdo-Gómez K, Pérez-Sayáns M, et al. Patients with thyroid disorder, a contraindication for dental implants? a systematic review. J Clin Med 2022;11(9).

41. Ursomanno BL, Cohen RE, Levine MJ, et al. The effect of hypothyroidism on bone loss at dental implants. J Oral Implantol 2021;47(2):131–4.

42. Javed F, Al Amri MD, Kellesarian SV, et al. Efficacy of parathyroid hormone supplementation on the osseointegration of implants: a systematic review. Clin Oral Invest 2016;20(4):649–58.

43. Hadrowicz P, Hadrowicz J, Kozakiewicz M, et al. Assessment of parathyroid hormone serum level as a predictor for bone condition around dental implants. Int J Oral Maxillofac Implants Jul/2017;32(4):e207–12.

44. Cutolo M, Paolino S, Sulli A, et al. Vitamin D, steroid hormones, and autoimmunity. Ann N Y Acad Sci 2014;1317:39–46.

45. Bazal-Bonelli S, Sánchez-Labrador L, Cortés-Bretón Brinkmann J, et al. Influence of serum vitamin D levels on survival rate and marginal bone loss in dental implants: a systematic review. Int J Environ Res Public Health 2022;19(16).

46. Alsulaimani L, Alqarni A, Almarghlani A, et al. The relationship between low serum vitamin D level and early dental implant failure: a systematic review. Cureus 2022;14(1):e21264.

47. Mangano F, Mortellaro C, Mangano N, et al. Is low serum vitamin D associated with early dental implant failure? a retrospective evaluation on 1625 implants placed in 822 patients. Mediators Inflamm 2016;2016:5319718.

48. Pierroz DD, Bonnet N, Bianchi EN, et al. Deletion of β-adrenergic receptor 1, 2, or both leads to different bone phenotypes and response to mechanical stimulation. J Bone Miner Res 2012;27(6):1252–62.

49. Ghosh M, Majumdar SR. Antihypertensive medications, bone mineral density, and fractures: a review of old cardiac drugs that provides new insights into osteoporosis. Endocrine 2014;46(3):397–405.

50. Wu X, Al-Abedalla K, Eimar H, et al. Antihypertensive medications and the survival rate of osseointegrated dental implants: a cohort study. Clin Implant Dent Relat Res 2016;18(6):1171–82.

51. Moore RE, Smith CK 2nd, Bailey CS, et al. Characterization of beta-adrenergic receptors on rat and human osteoblast-like cells and demonstration that beta-receptor agonists can stimulate bone resorption in organ culture. Bone Miner 1993;23(3):301–15.

52. Togari A, Arai M. Pharmacological topics of bone metabolism: the physiological function of the sympathetic nervous system in modulating bone resorption. J Pharmacol Sci 2008;106(4):542–6.

53. Bazzini C, Vezzoli V, Sironi C, et al. Thiazide-sensitive NaCl-cotransporter in the intestine: possible role of hydrochlorothiazide in the intestinal Ca2+ uptake. J Biol Chem 2005;280(20):19902–10.

54. Bolland MJ, Ames RW, Horne AM, et al. The effect of treatment with a thiazide diuretic for 4 years on bone density in normal postmenopausal women. Osteoporos Int 2007;18(4):479–86.

55. Aubin R, Ménard P, Lajeunesse D. Selective effect of thiazides on the human osteoblast-like cell line MG-63. Kidney Int 1996;50(5):1476–82.

56. Rejnmark L, Vestergaard P, Mosekilde L. Treatment with beta-blockers, ACE inhibitors, and calcium-channel blockers is associated with a reduced fracture risk: a nationwide case-control study. J Hypertens 2006;24(3):581–9.

57. Shimizu H, Nakagami H, Osako MK, et al. Angiotensin II accelerates osteoporosis by activating osteoclasts. Faseb J 2008;22(7):2465–75.

58. Quach H, Ray-Chaudhuri A. Calcium channel blocker induced gingival enlargement following implant placement in a fibula free flap reconstruction of the mandible: a case report. Int. J. Implant Dent. 2020;6(1):47.

59. Saravi B, Vollmer A, Lang G, et al. Impact of renin-angiotensin system inhibitors and beta-blockers on dental implant stability. Int. J. Implant Dent. 2021;7(1):31.

60. Santos CF, Morandini AC, Dionísio TJ, et al. Functional local renin-angiotensin system in human and rat periodontal tissue. PLoS One 2015;10(8):e0134601.

61. Mills KT, Stefanescu A, He J. The global epidemiology of hypertension. Nat Rev Nephrol 2020;16(4):223–37.

62. Bromfield S, Muntner P. High blood pressure: the leading global burden of disease risk factor and the need for worldwide prevention programs. Curr Hypertens Rep 2013;15(3):134–6.

63. Lim SS, Vos T, Flaxman AD, et al. A comparative risk assessment of burden of disease and injury attributable to 67 risk factors and risk factor clusters in 21 regions, 1990-2010: a systematic analysis for the Global Burden of Disease Study 2010. Lancet 2012;380(9859):2224–60.

64. Ilić K, Obradović N, Vujasinović-Stupar N. The relationship among hypertension, antihypertensive medications, and osteoporosis: a narrative review. Calcif Tissue Int 2013;92(3):217–27.

65. Lynn H, Kwok T, Wong SY, et al. Angiotensin converting enzyme inhibitor use is associated with higher bone mineral density in elderly Chinese. Bone 2006;38(4):584–8.

66. Al-Subaie AE, Laurenti M, Abdallah MN, et al. Propranolol enhances bone healing and implant osseointegration in rats tibiae. J Clin Periodontol 2016;43(12):1160–70.

67. Aghaloo T, Pi-Anfruns J, Moshaverinia A, et al. The effects of systemic diseases and medications on implant osseointegration: a systematic review. Int J Oral Maxillofac Implants 2019;34:s35–49.

68. Chappuis V, Avila-Ortiz G, Araújo MG, et al. Medication-related dental implant failure: Systematic review and meta-analysis. Clin Oral Implants Res 2018; 29(Suppl 16):55–68.
69. D'Ambrosio F, Amato A, Chiacchio A, et al. Do systemic diseases and medications influence dental implant osseointegration and dental implant health? an umbrella review. Dent J 2023;11(6).
70. Tahamtan S, Shirban F, Bagherniya M, et al. The effects of statins on dental and oral health: a review of preclinical and clinical studies. J Transl Med 2020; 18(1):155.
71. Chuengsamarn S, Rattanamongkoulgul S, Suwanwalaikorn S, et al. Effects of statins vs. non-statin lipid-lowering therapy on bone formation and bone mineral density biomarkers in patients with hyperlipidemia. Bone 2010;46(4):1011–5.
72. Pagkalos J, Cha JM, Kang Y, et al. Simvastatin induces osteogenic differentiation of murine embryonic stem cells. J Bone Miner Res 2010;25(11):2470–8.
73. Montagnani A, Gonnelli S, Cepollaro C, et al. Effect of simvastatin treatment on bone mineral density and bone turnover in hypercholesterolemic postmenopausal women: a 1-year longitudinal study. Bone 2003;32(4):427–33.
74. Rejnmark L, Buus NH, Vestergaard P, et al. Statins decrease bone turnover in postmenopausal women: a cross-sectional study. Eur J Clin Invest 2002;32(8): 581–9.
75. Chan MH, Mak TW, Chiu RW, et al. Simvastatin increases serum osteocalcin concentration in patients treated for hypercholesterolaemia. J Clin Endocrinol Metab 2001;86(9):4556–9.
76. Stein EA, Farnier M, Waldstreicher J, et al. Effects of statins on biomarkers of bone metabolism: a randomised trial. Nutr Metabol Cardiovasc Dis 2001; 11(2):84–7.
77. Fu JH, Bashutski JD, Al-Hezaimi K, et al. Statins, glucocorticoids, and nonsteroidal anti-inflammatory drugs: their influence on implant healing. Implant Dent 2012;21(5):362–7.
78. Schimmel M, Srinivasan M, McKenna G, et al. Effect of advanced age and/or systemic medical conditions on dental implant survival: A systematic review and meta-analysis. Clin Oral Implants Res 2018;29(Suppl 16):311–30.
79. Ouanounou A, Hassanpour S, Glogauer M. The influence of systemic medications on osseointegration of dental implants. J Can Dent Assoc 2016;82:g7.
80. Hwang D, Wang HL. Medical contraindications to implant therapy: part I: absolute contraindications. Implant Dent 2006;15(4):353–60.
81. de Molon RS, Sakakura CE, Faeda RS, et al. Effect of the long-term administration of Cyclosporine A on bone healing around osseointegrated titanium implants: A histomorphometric study in the rabbit tibia. Microsc Res Tech 2017; 80(9):1000–8.
82. Duarte PM, Nogueira Filho GR, Sallum EA, et al. The effect of an immunosuppressive therapy and its withdrawal on bone healing around titanium implants. A histometric study in rabbits. J Periodontol 2001;72(10):1391–7.
83. Cayco AV, Wysolmerski J, Simpson C, et al. Posttransplant bone disease: evidence for a high bone resorption state. Transplantation 2000;70(12):1722–8.
84. Scully C, Madrid C, Bagan J. Dental endosseous implants in patients on bisphosphonate therapy. Implant Dent 2006;15(3):212–8.
85. Marx RE, Sawatari Y, Fortin M, et al. Bisphosphonate-induced exposed bone (osteonecrosis/osteopetrosis) of the jaws: risk factors, recognition, prevention, and treatment. J Oral Maxillofac Surg 2005;63(11):1567–75.

86. Ruggiero SL, Dodson TB, Fantasia J, et al. American Association of Oral and Maxillofacial Surgeons position paper on medication-related osteonecrosis of the jaw–2014 update. J Oral Maxillofac Surg 2014;72(10):1938–56.

87. Pountos I, Georgouli T, Calori GM, et al. Do nonsteroidal anti-inflammatory drugs affect bone healing? A critical analysis. Sci World J 2012;2012:606404.

88. Jones MK, Wang H, Peskar BM, et al. Inhibition of angiogenesis by nonsteroidal anti-inflammatory drugs: insight into mechanisms and implications for cancer growth and ulcer healing. Nat Med 1999;5(12):1418–23.

89. Winnett B, Tenenbaum HC, Ganss B, et al. Perioperative use of non-steroidal anti-inflammatory drugs might impair dental implant osseointegration. Clin Oral Implants Res 2016;27(2):e1–7.

90. Grant BT, Amenedo C, Freeman K, et al. Outcomes of placing dental implants in patients taking oral bisphosphonates: a review of 115 cases. J Oral Maxillofac Surg 2008;66(2):223–30.

91. Shariff JA, Gurpegui Abud D, Bhave MB, et al. Selective serotonin reuptake inhibitors and dental implant failure: a systematic review and meta-analysis. J Oral Implantol 2023;49(4):436–43.

92. Ball J, Darby I. Mental health and periodontal and peri-implant diseases. Periodontol 2000 2022;90(1):106–24.

93. Wu X, Al-Abedalla K, Rastikerdar E, et al. Selective serotonin reuptake inhibitors and the risk of osseointegrated implant failure: a cohort study. J Dent Res 2014; 93(11):1054–61.

94. Chawla BK, Cohen RE, Stellrecht EM, et al. The influence of proton pump inhibitors on tissue attachment around teeth and dental implants: A scoping review. Clin Exp Dent Res 2022;8(5):1045–58.

95. Vinnakota DN, Kamatham R. Effect of proton pump inhibitors on dental implants: A systematic review and meta-analysis. J Indian Prosthodont Soc 2020;20(3): 228–36.

96. Smith RA, Berger R, Dodson TB. Risk factors associated with dental implants in healthy and medically compromised patients. Int J Oral Maxillofac Implants 1992;7(3):367–72. Fall.

97. Cranin AN. Endosteal implants in a patient with corticosteroid dependence. J Oral Implantol 1991;17(4):414–7.

98. Mohammadi A, Dehkordi NR, Mahmoudi S, et al. Effects of drugs and chemo-therapeutic agents on dental implant osseointegration: narrative review. Curr Rev Clin Exp Pharmacol 2022. https://doi.org/10.2174/2772432817666220607 114559.

99. Fujimoto T, Niimi A, Sawai T, et al. Effects of steroid-induced osteoporosis on os-seointegration of titanium implants. Int J Oral Maxillofac Implants 1998;13(2): 183–9.

100. Sharaf B, Dodson TB. Does the use of prophylactic antibiotics decrease implant failure? Oral Maxillofac Surg Clin North Am 2011;23(4):547–50.

101. Chrcanovic BR, Albrektsson T, Wennerberg A. Prophylactic antibiotic regimen and dental implant failure: a meta-analysis. J Oral Rehabil 2014;41(12):941–56.

102. Chen Z, Chen D, Zhang S, et al. Antibiotic prophylaxis for preventing dental implant failure and postoperative infection: A systematic review of randomized controlled trials. Am J Dent 2017;30(2):89–95.

103. Li ZB, Li K. Prophylactic antibiotics can prevent early implant failure, but post-operative antibiotics may not be beneficial for dental implant placement. J Evid Base Dent Pract 2019;19(4):101339.

104. Salgado-Peralvo AO, Garcia-Sanchez A, Kewalramani N, et al. Consensus report on preventive antibiotic therapy in dental implant procedures: summary of recommendations from the Spanish Society of Implants. Antibiotics 2022;11(5).

105. Edibam NR, Lorenzo-Pouso AI, Caponio VCA. Self-reported allergy to penicillin and clindamycin administration may be risk factors for dental implant failure: A systematic review, meta-analysis and delabeling protocol. Clin Oral Implants Res 2023;34(7):651–61.

106. Salgado-Peralvo AO, Peña-Cardelles JF, Kewalramani N, et al. Is penicillin allergy a risk factor for early dental implant failure? a systematic review. Antibiotics 2021;10(10).

107. Salomó-Coll O, Lozano-Carrascal N, Lázaro-Abdulkarim A, et al. Do penicillin-allergic patients present a higher rate of implant failure? Int J Oral Maxillofac Implants 2018;33(6):1390–5.

108. Rogers JO. Implant-stabilized complete mandibular denture for a patient with cerebral palsy. Dent Update Jan-Feb 1995;22(1):23–6.

109. Corcuera-Flores JR, López-Giménez J, López-Jiménez J, et al. Four years survival and marginal bone loss of implants in patients with Down syndrome and cerebral palsy. Clin Oral Invest 2017;21(5):1667–74.

110. Feijoo JF, Limeres J, Diniz M, et al. Osseointegrated dental implants in patients with intellectual disability: a pilot study. Disabil Rehabil 2012;34(23):2025–30.

111. López-Jiménez J, Romero-Domínguez A, Giménez-Prats MJ. Implants in handicapped patients. Med Oral 2003;8(4):288–93.

112. Oczakir C, Balmer S, Mericske-Stern R. Implant-prosthodontic treatment for special care patients: a case series study. Int J Prosthodont (IJP) 2005;18(5): 383–9.

113. Nam H, Sung KW, Kim MG, et al. Immediate implant placement for schizophrenic patient with outpatient general anesthesia. J Dent Anesth Pain Med 2015;15(3):147–51.

114. Castellanos-Cosano L, Corcuera-Flores JR, Mesa-Cabrera M, et al. Dental implants placement in paranoid squizofrenic patient with obsessive-compulsive disorder: A case report. J Clin Exp Dent 2017;9(11):e1371–4.

115. Packer ME. A review of the outcome of dental implant provision in individuals with movement disorders. Eur J Oral Implant 2018;11(Suppl 1):S47–63.

116. Ekfeldt A, Zellmer M, Carlsson GE. Treatment with implant-supported fixed dental prostheses in patients with congenital and acquired neurologic disabilities: a prospective study. Int J Prosthodont (IJP) 2013;26(6):517–24.

117. Bera RN, Tripathi R, Bhattacharjee B, et al. Implant survival in patients with neuropsychiatric, neurocognitive, and neurodegenerative disorders: A meta-analysis. Natl J Maxillofac Surg 2021;12(2):162–70.

118. Cristea I, Agop-Forna D, Martu MA, et al. Oral and periodontal risk factors of prosthetic success for 3-unit natural tooth-supported bridges versus implant-supported fixed dental prostheses. Diagnostics 2023;13(5).

119. De Bruyn H, Glibert M, Matthijs L, et al. Clinical guidelines for implant treatment in patients with down syndrome. Int J Periodontics Restor Dent 2019;39(3):361–8.

120. Najeeb S, Khurshid Z, Siddiqui F, et al. Outcomes of dental implant therapy in patients with down syndrome: a systematic review. J Evid Base Dent Pract 2017;17(4):317–23.

121. Limeres Posse J, López Jiménez J, Ruiz Villandiego JC, et al. Survival of dental implants in patients with Down syndrome: A case series. J Prosthet Dent 2016; 116(6):880–4.

122. Baus-Domínguez M, Gómez-Díaz R, Torres-Lagares D, et al. Retrospective case-control study genes related to bone metabolism that justify the condition of periodontal disease and failure of dental implants in patients with down syndrome. Int J Mol Sci 2023;24(9).
123. Mustapha AD, Salame Z, Chrcanovic BR. Smoking and dental implants: a systematic review and meta-analysis. Medicina 2021;58(1).
124. Naseri R, Yaghini J, Feizi A. Levels of smoking and dental implants failure: A systematic review and meta-analysis. J Clin Periodontol 2020;47(4):518–28.
125. Moraschini V, Barboza E. Success of dental implants in smokers and non-smokers: a systematic review and meta-analysis. Int J Oral Maxillofac Surg 2016;45(2):205–15.
126. Veitz-Keenan A. Marginal bone loss and dental implant failure may be increased in smokers. Evid Base Dent 2016;17(1):6–7.
127. Chrcanovic BR, Albrektsson T, Wennerberg A. Smoking and dental implants: A systematic review and meta-analysis. J Dent 2015;43(5):487–98.
128. Heitz-Mayfield LJ, Huynh-Ba G. History of treated periodontitis and smoking as risks for implant therapy. Int J Oral Maxillofac Implants 2009;24(Suppl):39–68.
129. Radi IA, Elsayyad AA. Smoking might increase the failure rate and marginal bone loss around dental implants. J Evid Base Dent Pract 2022;22(4):101804.

Systemic Factors Affecting Prognosis and Outcomes in Periodontal Disease

Linda Sangalli, DDS, MS, PhD[a], Fatma Banday, BDS, MS[b], Andrew Sullivan, DDS[b], Kainat Anjum, BDS, MSc[b],*

KEYWORDS

- Systemic factors • Periodontal prognosis • Periodontal outcomes
- Systemic medications

KEY POINTS

- Prognosis refers to the predictive assessment of the expected course, duration, and final outcome of a dental disease or condition. It is based on a comprehensive diagnosis and is conducted prior to the development of a treatment plan.
- The prognosis of a dental disease or condition is influenced by various factors include biological aspects such as age, disease severity, and the effectiveness of biofilm control.
- Systemic factors like systemic conditions and genetic predisposition, as well as environmental factors like smoking habits and stress, can also impact the prognosis.
- Local factors such as the presence of biofilm, calculus, and subgingival restorations, as well as anatomic factors like root shape, cervical enamel projections, enamel pearls, root concavities, developmental grooves, root proximity, furcation invasion, tooth mobility, caries, tooth vitality, and root resorption also play a role in determining prognosis.

INTRODUCTION

Within dentistry, *prognosis* can be defined as the predictive estimation of the trajectory, duration, and ultimate outcome of a dental disease or condition, which results from a thorough diagnosis and precedes the formulation of treatment plan.[1] Prognosis is influenced by patients' domains, such as biological (age, disease severity, and effectiveness of biofilm control), systemic (systemic conditions and genetic predisposition), environmental (smoking habits and stress), local (biofilm, calculus, and subgingival restorations), anatomic factors (root shape, cervical enamel projections, enamel pearls, root concavities, developmental grooves, root proximity, furcation invasion,

Funding: None.
[a] College of Dental Medicine, Midwestern University, 555 31st, Downers Grove, IL, USA;
[b] Rutgers School of Dental Medicine, 110 Bergen Street, Newark, NJ, USA
* Corresponding author. 110 Bergen Street, Newark, NJ.
E-mail address: kainat.anjum@rutgers.edu

Dent Clin N Am 68 (2024) 571–602
https://doi.org/10.1016/j.cden.2024.05.001
0011-8532/24/© 2024 Elsevier Inc. All rights reserved, including those for text and data mining, AI training, and similar technologies.

dental.theclinics.com

tooth mobility, caries, tooth vitality, and root resorption), and compliance with recommendations. All of these elements collectively contribute to the comprehensive evaluation of a patient's prognosis in dental care.[2,3]

In dentistry, *outcomes* are defined as results or consequences, and every dental intervention is strategically designed to enhance prognosis and improve the anticipated outcome of a patient's dental health.[4] Treatment planning in dentistry should not only consider professional knowledge but also integrate patient's goals and expectations to establish comprehensive plans aligned with improving oral health.

SYSTEMIC FACTORS AFFECTING PROGNOSIS AND OUTCOME OF PERIODONTAL THERAPY

This review will examine the impact of autoimmune conditions (eg, rheumatoid arthritis [RA]), inflammatory conditions (eg, irritable bowel syndrome), cardiovascular disease, diabetes, infectious diseases (eg, human immunodeficiency virus [HIV]), along with their respective medications, and influence of hormones on prognosis and outcomes of periodontal therapy. Other cardinal systemic factors are discussed elsewhere in this special edition.

Rheumatoid Arthritis

RA is an autoimmune disease characterized by chronic inflammation of hard and soft tissues (tendons, ligaments, cartilage, muscles, and internal organs) and proliferation of synovial membranes in arthrodial joints (typically the small joints of hands, wrists, and feet).[5] RA represents a prototype of autoimmune conditions that affect periodontal prognosis, and it has been selected to exemplify the effect of immunity in periodontics.

Association between rheumatoid arthritis and periodontal disease
Evidence suggests a link between periodontal disease and RA.[6–9] Both conditions are chronic inflammatory diseases characterized by bone and soft tissue destruction,[8,10,11] by sharing similar proinflammatory pathways, including cytokines such as interleukin (IL)-1, IL-6, IL-4, IL-10, tumor necrosis factor (TNF), and prostaglandin E2.[8,10,12–15] As such, individuals with RA exhibit higher inflammatory state than controls, as measured by salivary and serum C-reactive protein (CRP),[16] metalloproteinase (MMP-8), and IL-6.[17,18] Notably, greater MMP-8 levels are associated with greater periodontal disease severity.[18,19] Both conditions share certain risk factors (ie, smoking) and a genetic predisposition such as major histocompatibility complex class II molecules and human leukocyte antigen (HLA)-DR4, associated to RA development and a more rapid periodontal disease progression.[12]

Novel concept of periodontal dysbiosis may indicate a bidirectional link between RA and periodontal disease,[20] so much so that patients with RA have an elevated risk of developing periodontal conditions,[21] especially when seropositive for RA.[22] Prevalence of RA is 6 times higher among patients with periodontal disease (specifically moderate to severe)[23,24] compared to those without any periodontal involvement.[25] Individuals with RA show the presence of bacteria in the synovial fluid of affected joints, potentially correlated with disease severity.[26,27] Some of these have been identified as oral bacteria (such as *Porphyromonas gingivalis*, *Prevotella intermedia*, *Prevotella melaninogenica*, *Tannerella forsythia*, *Aggregatibacter actinomycetemcomitans*, and *Bacteroides forsythus*), suggesting that oral bacteria might be implicated in the etiopathogenesis of RA[20,27–31] for a process involving citrullination.[32,33] *P gingivalis* facilitates certain enzymes known as *P gingivalis* peptidyl arginine deiminase, which can produce citrullinated proteins. This leads to the production of specific anticitrullinated protein antibodies (ACPA), which are directly responsible for the development of

RA.[22,32,34,35] Subsequently, ACPA-positive patients exhibit poor clinical prognosis with greater levels of erosive damage.[33,36] These periodontal pathogens tend to be higher in the oral cavity of individuals with RA.[20,28,29] Increased presence of gram-negative anaerobic species in dental plaque strongly associated with periodontal inflammation and destruction.[33] Moreover, all periodontal parameters indicating periodontal disease severity (such as plaque index [PI], probing depth [PD], bleeding on probing [BOP], and clinical attachment loss [CAL]) were significantly worse in individuals with RA than controls.[7,37] RA disease activity was positively associated with higher periodontal disease severity.[7,37,38] Additionally, nationally representative studies suggested that RA is associated with tooth loss in adults aged less than 60 years compared to healthy controls,[22] after controlling for smoking, sex, dental caries, educational level, and frequency of toothbrushing.[22] However, the same study failed to demonstrate an association between RA and periodontitis after controlling for contributing factors (ie, smoking, educational level, age, dental caries, body mass index, alcohol consumption, physical activity, diabetes mellitus, and frequency of toothbrushing).[22] Another observational study conducted on individuals with early RA observed that tooth loss was associated with seropositive RA, disease severity, and inflammatory erythrocyte sedimentation rate (ESR) marker,[39] which was also confirmed elsewhere.[40] A population-based study supported an increase by 2 fold in tooth loss rate in patients with RA compared with non-RA controls after adjusting for confounders.[9] Tooth loss was also significantly associated with high rheumatoid factor.[41]

Outcomes and prognosis of periodontal therapy in individuals with rheumatoid arthritis

Severe RA can lead to joint pain and limited mobility, thus making it potentially challenging to maintain proper oral hygiene practices, especially in men.[42] Difficulty in brushing, flossing, and regular dental visits can contribute to the worsening of periodontal disease and to ideal outcomes following periodontal therapies.[42] As such, when periodontal treatments are performed in individuals with RA, their abnormal innate and adaptive immune system and oral dysbiosis can also affect the immune response to bacterial infection in the oral cavity resulting in increased periodontal destruction, periodontal inflammation, and disease progression.[33,43–46]

Finally, although some studies claimed that RA should be considered a contraindication for implant surgery[46] possibly due to shared common risk factors and genes such as CD14 and FCGR2B,[47] most of the literature failed to reveal any association between peri-implantitis and RA.[48–50] As a matter of fact, some studies noticed that patients with RA exhibited higher implant survival rate.[51–53] Interestingly, other autoimmune conditions such as connective tissue diseases (ie, scleroderma) and Sjogren syndrome exhibited worse outcomes in terms of bleeding index around implants and increased bone resorption.[53] Similarly, clinical implant parameters such as BOP and alveolar bone loss were greater in individuals with both RA and connective tissue diseases compared to healthy controls.[54]

Periodontal conditions secondary to rheumatoid arthritis medication

Medications used to treat RA and other autoimmune conditions with similar therapeutic management may also impact prognosis and outcomes of periodontal therapy.[55]

Some RA medications may exert direct effects on anti-inflammatory cytokines associated with periodontal disease development.[56] Nevertheless, opposing results are evidenced on the effect of RA medications on periodontal outcomes, as displayed in **Table 1**.

Table 1
Effects of rheumatoid arthritis systemic medications on periodontal outcome and prognosis

Type of RA Medication	Effects on Hampering Periodontal Outcome	Effects on Improved Periodontal Outcome
Chronic use of corticosteroids	Oral side effects (ie, infections, delayed wound healing,[57] immunosuppression, decreased mineral bone density, osteoporosis, alveolar bone loss, inhibition of fibroblast proliferation, and reduced collagen production); inability to control periodontal disease, higher incidence of periodontal disease[58]; and higher incidence of tooth loss.[37,39] Presence of fewer teeth was associated with prednisone intake[40]	Protective effect on the number of teeth[59]
Antirheumatic agents (csDMARDs, anti-B lymphocyte, anti-IL-6R, anti-TNF-α agents, and JAK inhibitors)	—	Improvement of PD, CAL, and GI in patients with RA and periodontitis[60,61]
DMARDs	RA patients with greater tooth loss had 21 time higher odds of taking biological DMARDs compared to RA individuals with greater number of teeth, after adjusting for disease severity[62]	Inhibition of periodontal disease progression[24,63-67] by reducing periodontal inflammatory burden of TNF-α, IL-6, IL-1, IL-17,[10,68] but not salivary MMP-8 concentration[69]
MTX and corticosteroids	RA patients with greater tooth loss exhibited >8 times higher odds of taking MTX compared to RA individuals with greater number of teeth, after adjusting for disease severity.[62] Increased periodontal inflammation was observed in patients with RA treated with MTX[70]	Inhibitory effects on proinflammatory cytokines implicated in periodontal disease development, such as IL-6,[71,72] reactive oxygen species,[72] IL-12A, and reduced gene expression of IL-18[71]
TNF-inhibitors	Individuals with RA on infliximab therapy showed increased gingival inflammation (expect for PD) compared to individuals with RA not on infliximab.[73] Patients with RA on anti-TNF treatment presenting periodontal disease did not show any significant improvement in clinical periodontal parameters.[55,74] Increased periodontal inflammation was observed in patients with RA treated with TNF-inhibitors[70]	Inhibition of periodontal disease in patients with RA[75] with high levels of inflammatory cytokines[76] by reducing periodontal indices of GI, BOP, and PD,[77] especially when coupled with periodontal treatment

Abbreviations: csDMARDs, conventional disease-modifying antirheumatic drugs; MTX, methotrexate; TNF, tumor necrosis factor.

Prognosis and outcome of periodontal therapy secondary to rheumatoid arthritis medications

Periodontal treatment prognosis and outcome have high variability in individuals with RA, according to periodontal disease and RA severity. A meta-analysis concluded that nonsurgical periodontal therapy (NSPT) was equally effective in RA and non-RA individuals with periodontitis.[78] Individuals with RA and periodontitis on conventional disease-modifying antirheumatic drugs (csDMARDs) showed significantly greater reduction in PD and CAL after scaling and root planning (SRP) compared to systematically healthy patients with periodontitis,[79] potentially attributed to decreased systemic inflammation derived from better oral health. Changes in systemic inflammatory markers (ie, plasminogen activator [t-PA] and plasminogen activator inhibitor-2 [PAI-2]) resulted from NSPT, regardless of the systemic status of RA.[80]

Likewise, periodontal treatment in individuals with RA and periodontitis may improve RA severity by decreasing markers of disease activity (ESR, TNF-α, and serologic ACPA),[81–83] levels of antibodies against *P gingivalis* and citrulline.[84] Controlling oral bacterial load and gingival inflammation, the systemic inflammatory burden may decrease, leading to improved RA outcomes.[81]

Hormones

Sex hormones

Female's lifetime is characterized by fluctuation in sex hormonal level. Given the presence of estrogen receptors in gingiva and periodontal ligament,[85] examining how sex hormone fluctuation may impact periodontal therapy is crucial. **Table 2** summarizes how conditions characterized by sex hormone fluctuation influence periodontal status.

Prognosis and outcome of periodontal therapy secondary to sex hormones

Puberty Puberty, characterized by increased levels of progesterone and estrogen, results in growth of the periodontium and presence of bacteria (such as spirochetes) in the periodontal pocket.[102,103] As a result, certain periodontal conditions (dental plaque-induced gingival disease, early onset periodontitis, prepubertal, and juvenile periodontitis) are more prevalent in puberty compared to prepuberty.[104–107] Such periodontal conditions are characterized by specific bacterial species that differ from periodontal conditions in adults, such as *Actinomyces*, *Capnocytophaga*, *Leptotrichia*, and *Selenomonas*.[106] Hormone level fluctuation at this age influences the gingival inflammatory response to dental plaque.[106,108] Nevertheless, either surgical therapy or NSPT is effective in reducing clinical periodontal index values in this age group.[109]

Menstrual cycle and reproductive age Estradiol is the most abundant estrogen in female individuals during their reproductive age. A fluctuation of estrogen/progesterone levels characterizes menstrual cycle,[93,97] in that estrogen levels increase from follicular phase until ovulation; soon after (ie, luteal phase), progesterone increases. Such fluctuation results in changes of bacterial flora in gingival and periodontal tissues. Notably, estrogens have been suggested to be protective and influence the virulence of various gram-negative bacteria.[110]

Increased gingival inflammation has been associated with the menstrual cycle, especially during the menses period.[93,94,98] A significantly higher gingival inflammation has been consistently observed during ovulation and premenstruation compared to menstruation period,[93,97,99] more so among women with baseline gingivitis. However, periodontal treatment addressing chronic gingivitis reverses the inflammation and periodontal changes occurring during menstrual cycle.[97,99]

Table 2
Effects of conditions causing sex hormone fluctuation on periodontal status

Clinical Studies (Year)	Participants	Periodontal Outcome Measures	Main Findings
Oral contraceptive			
Mullally et al,[86] 2007	50 young female individuals (20–35 y) divided in taking oral contraceptive vs controls	PI, GI, PD, CAL, and BOP	Women taking oral contraceptive had significantly deeper PD, greater CAL, and more BOP sites
Brusca et al,[87] 2010	92 female individuals (19–40 y) divided in taking oral contraceptive vs controls	PD, GI, CAL, *Candida* species, *P gingivalis, A actinomycetemcomitans,* and *P intermedia*	Women taking oral contraceptive had significantly higher prevalence of periodontitis, PD, GI, CAL, the presence of *Candida, P gingivalis, P intermedia, A actinomycetemcomitans*
Haerian-Aedakani et al,[88] 2010	70 young female individuals (17–35 y) divided in birth control pill vs controls	PI, GI, PD, CAL, and BOP	Higher level of gingival inflammation and BOP in female individuals taking oral contraceptive; no significant difference in PI, PD, and CAL
Pregnancy			
Offenbacher et al,[89] 2006	67 pregnant women divided in periodontal treatment vs nonperiodontal treatment group	GCF levels of IL-1β, PGE(2), 8-iso, IL-6, serum level of IL-6, sICAM1, sGP130, IL-6sr, CRP, PI, GI, BOP, CAL, and PD	NSPT significantly improved clinical periodontal parameters (CAL, PD, PI, GI, and BOP) and significant decreased *Prevotella nigrescens* and *P intermedia,* serum IL-6sr, GCF IL-1β; NSPT was associated with significant increase in PD, PI, GCF IL-1β, and IL-6 levels
Khairnar et al,[90] 2015	100 pregnant women with periodontitis divided in periodontal treatment vs nonperiodontal treatment group	CRP level	Those who were treated with SRP therapy showed statistically significant reduction in CRP level after delivery, while controls did not exhibit any change

Study	Sample	Parameters	Findings
Penova-Veselinovic et al,[91] 2015	80 pregnant women divided in periodontal treatment vs nonperiodontal treatment group	GCF levels of IL-1β, IL-6, IL-8, IL-10, IL-12p70, IL-17, TNF-α, MCP-1, BOP, CAL, and PD	Significantly reduced GCF levels of IL-1β, IL-10, IL-12p70, IL-6, PD, CAL, and BOP compared to controls following periodontal therapy; MCP-1, IL-8, and TNF-α exhibited gestational age-dependent increase with no treatment response
Yarkaç,[92] 2018	30 pregnant with gingivitis vs 30 nonpregnant women with gingivitis	GCF IL-1β, IL-10 levels, and salivary CgA hormone	Decreased gingival inflammatory indexes following periodontal therapy in both groups, but no change in IL-1β levels in pregnant women
Menstrual cycle			
Machtei et al,[93] 2004	18 premenopausal women (24–47 y)	PI, GI, PD, and CAL	No statistically significant difference in PI, PD, and CAL across time points; significantly higher GI in OV and PM compared to M
Baser et al,[94] 2009	27 premenopausal women (19–23 y)	BOP, GCF level of IL-1β, and TNF-α	Significant increase in BOP and IL-1β levels (despite optimal plaque control) from first menstruation day to estimated predominant progesterone secretion day
Becerik et al,[95] 2010	50 premenopausal women (20–40 y) divided in 25 periodontally healthy women vs 25 with gingivitis	GCF levels of IL-6, PGE(2), t-PA, PAI-2, PI, and BOP	BOP was significantly higher in M and OV than in PM in gingivitis group, with no difference in periodontally healthy women; significantly higher GCF IL-6 levels in gingivitis group in all menstrual phases; unchanged IL-6, PGE(2), t-PA, and PAI-2 in different menstrual phases in both groups
Markou et al,[96] 2011	18 periodontally healthy premenopausal women (19–25 y)	BOP, PI, GCF levels of IL-1β, IL-6, IL-8, and TNF-α	PI and BOP remained unchanged; IL-6 level significantly increased from OV to progesterone peak; no significant changes in the remaining cytokines

(continued on next page)

Table 2
(continued)

Clinical Studies (Year)	Participants	Periodontal Outcome Measures	Main Findings
Shourie et al,[97] 2012	100 premenopausal women (50 with clinically healthy gingival tissue vs 50 with chronic gingivitis)	PI, GI, PD, ST, PBI, and GCF	No statistically significant changes in periodontal measures in women with clinically healthy gingival tissues; enhanced inflammation in OV and PM as compared to M in women with gingivitis
Khosravisamani et al,[98] 2014	27 periodontally healthy women (18–25 y)	GBI, MGI, IL-1β, TNF-α, and simplified oral health index	GBI and MGI significantly increased during menstrual cycle, and were significantly higher during OV compared to M and PM; no change in simplified oral health index; TNF-α concentration significantly increased during menstrual cycle
Rathore et al,[99] 2015	30 healthy female individuals (18–25 y)	PI, GI, mSBI, and PD	mSBI and GI were higher in PM and OV, compared to M; no difference was seen in PI and PD
Asaad,[100] 2023	25 healthy young female individuals (18–20 y)	PI, GI, and salivary pH	PI and GI were significantly higher during PM and decreased during M; salivary pH decreased slightly during PM; saliva became more alkaline during M
Menopause and postmenopause			
Payne et al,[101] 1999	37 postmenopausal women with a history of periodontitis, divided in bone mineral density vs osteoporosis of lumbar spine	Change in bone density	Women with osteoporosis showed a higher incidence of alveolar bone height loss, crestal and subcrestal density loss compared to women without osteoporosis

Abbreviations: A actinomycetemcomitans, Aggregatibacter actinomycetemcomitans; BOP, bleeding on probing; CAL, clinical attachment loss; CGA, chromogranin A; CRP, C-reactive protein; GBI, gingival bleeding index; GCF, gingival crevicular fluid collection; GI, gingival index; IL-6sr, IL-6 soluble receptor; M, menstruation; MGI, modified gingival index; mSBI, modified sulcular bleeding index; NSPT, nonsurgical periodontal therapy; OV, ovulation; PAI-2, plasminogen activator inhibitor-2; PBI, papillary bleeding index; PD, probing depth; PGE(2), prostaglandin E(2); PI, plaque index; PM, premenstruation; P gingivalis, Porphyromonas gingivalis; P intermedia, Prevotella intermedia; sGP130, soluble glycoprotein 130; sICAM1, soluble intercellular adhesion molecule 1; t-PA, tissue plasminogen activator; 8-iso, 8-isoprostane.

Oral contraceptives Effects of oral contraceptives appeared to be dose-dependent, so much so that modern oral contraceptives (with low-dose estrogens and progestins formulation) do not constitute a risk factor for periodontal disease.[111] Yet, other studies supported greater CRP, gingival inflammation, CAL, and gingival enlargement in women taking oral contraceptives.[112,113] A 5 fold increased implant failure rate was suggested in women on oral contraceptives, which remained significant after controlling for smoking, age, and diabetes.[112]

Pregnancy During pregnancy, increased estrogen levels promote gingivitis and worsen clinical periodontal parameters,[89] which are reversible after childbirth. Gestational diabetes may elevate proinflammatory cytokine levels (IL-6, IL-8, IL-10, TNF-R1/2) compared to nondiabetic pregnancies,[114] while pregnancy hypertension is associated with higher risk of periodontal disease compared to pregnancies without hypertension.[115] Inflammatory periodontal parameters of gingival index (GI) and PD were specifically evident during the second month of pregnancy with a peak during the last trimester.[112] A comparison of healthy pregnant women with those having gingivitis/periodontitis revealed higher levels of IL-17, IL-1βb, and MMP-8 in the latter group.[114,116,117] Interestingly, among pregnant women with gingivitis, ANXA-1 levels were double compared to nonpregnant women with gingivitis, with no variation in IL-1β levels.[114,118] A meta-analysis found that NRPT significantly lowered periodontal parameters of BOP, PD, CAL, gingival inflammatory markers and cytokines (IL-1 and IL-8).[90,119] However, it did not notably decrease serum cytokine levels, which remained elevated until delivery.[120]

Menopause, postmenopausal, and hormone replacement therapy During menopause and postmenopause, estrogen production significantly decreases (from 30–400 to <20 pg/mL) potentially leading to osteoporosis, reduced bone density, and mass in both skeletal bones[121–123] and mandible.[124,125] This decrease in bone density is linked to periodontal attachment loss, tooth loss, and decreased residual ridge height.[101,126–131] Postmenopausal women with estrogen deficiency (<30 pg/mL) had significantly higher gingival crevicular fluid alkaline phosphatase compared to those with normal levels on estrogen supplementation (>30 pg/mL).[132] Conversely, contradictory evidence exists on estrogen's effect on CAL.[133–135] Hormone replacement therapy (HRT) prescribed for menopausal symptoms, including estrogen and progestin or estrogen alone, has been shown to preventing bone loss, reducing gingival inflammation, CAL, and virulence of P gingivalis.[135–139] Estrogen's ability to inhibit various inflammatory mediators (IL-1, IL-6, IL-8, and TNF-α), cellular mechanism (lymphocyte activation and polymorphonuclear leukocytes [PMNs] recruitment), and bone-resorption cytokines, MMP-8 and MMP-13, contribute to these effects.[133,140] Women on HRT showed greater attachment gain at 6 month follow-up after SRPT compared to those without estrogen supplementation.[141] Combining SRP with minocycline microspheres also improved clinical parameters and reduced bacteria in premenopausal and postmenopausal women.[142–145] Yet, other studies questioned HRT's protective impact on clinical periodontal measures.[133] Conflicting results also derived from the impact of HRT on implant survival. Some suggest HRT reduces failure rates in maxillary but not in mandibular implants,[146] linking estrogen deficiency to lower osseointegration and osteoporosis. Conversely, others reported a 2.6 to 5 fold higher implant failure in women on HRT,[147] even after accounting for age, smoking, and diabetes.[112] Additional evidence points to an increased bone loss and reduced bone mineralization around implants.[148] Finally, some studies found no association between HRT and implant success.[149]

Other hormones

Hyposecretion or hypersecretion of hormones influences the periodontal status, predominantly by increasing prevalence and severity of periodontal disease and by altering bone metabolism crucial for implant survival. **Table 3** summarizes the effect of the main hormones on periodontal status.

Inflammatory Bowel Disease

Inflammatory bowel disease (IBD) refers to an inflammatory condition affecting the digestive tract, encompassing Crohn's disease and ulcerative colitis.[201] While the exact cause of IBD remains elusive, host–gut microbiota interactions, altered bone metabolism, and abnormal immune system activations have been proposed.[202,203]

Association between inflammatory bowel disease and periodontal disease

IBD and periodontitis share a similar pathogenesis of dysbiotic microbiota and dysregulated immune-inflammatory reaction,[204–206] including environmental factors (eg, smoking), immunologic traits affecting healing process (eg, increased levels of prostaglandin E2, aMMP8, IL-18 S100A12, and Th17 cell responses),[207–209] change in oral microbiota (eg, *Klebsiella*, *P gingivalis*, and *Fusobacterium nucleatum*),[201,206,207] expression of proinflammatory cytokines at gingival and gut levels,[210] and enhanced activity of macrophages and neutrophils.[201] Individuals with IBD have twice the likelihood of presenting with moderate/severe periodontitis, tooth loss, increased osseous turnover, and decreased bone development rate,[203,204,206,209,211–221] with weak associations between periodontitis and disease severity.[204,212] A higher predisposition toward periodontal disease was also observed in children with IBD, regardless of their hygiene status.[222,223]

Prognosis and outcome of periodontal therapy secondary to inflammatory bowel disease and inflammatory bowel disease medications

Very few studies investigated the effect of IBD and IBD medications on periodontal therapy. However, given that individuals with IBD are commonly treated with medications previously seen for RA (eg, anti-inflammatory drugs, corticosteroids, immunosuppressant drugs, DMARDs, and antibiotics), findings may overlap.

A few studies have suggested that anti-IBD medication regimen may result in postoperative infections or delayed healing process,[224,225] although this conclusion is derived from low-quality evidence.[226] Studies indicate that patients with IBD, especially Crohn's disease, presented early and late implant failure due to altered bone metabolism.[214,227,228] This was attributed to poor nutrition, inflammatory cytokines implicated in bone density and implant osseointegration[206,229] and autoimmune inflammatory process.[214] However, evidence supporting dental implant stability in patients with IBD is limited, requiring further research for a clearer understanding.[214,230,231]

Acquired Immunodeficiency Syndrome and Human Immunodeficiency Virus Infection

Globally, more than 35 million people are affected by HIV infection or acquired immunodeficiency syndrome (AIDS).[232,233]

Association between acquired immunodeficiency syndrome and human immunodeficiency virus infection and periodontal disease

Assessing oral and periodontal issues in patients with HIV is crucial. There is a clear link between oral HIV signs (such as candidiasis, leukoplakia, and ulceration) and

Table 3
Hormonal effects on periodontal health secondary to hormone hyposecretion vs hypersecretion

Hyposecretion	Hypersecretion
PTH	
Decreased PTH are associated with decreased bone capacity due to lower serum calcium levels[150]	PTH stimulates bone formation around implants,[151,152] osseointegration in cancellous bone,[153] and bone turnover[154] Increased tooth mobility leading to tooth loss, malocclusions, tooth spacing, decreased lamina dura, and widened periodontal ligament[155] Teriparatide (a synthetic PTH) reduced PD and increased CAL[156]
Calcitonin	
Low-grade effect of calcitonin hypersecretion on bone mineral density[157]	Increased calcitonin levels in periodontitis patients and negatively correlated with clinical periodontal parameters (GI, PD, and CAL)[158]
T3, T4, and TSH	
Uncontrolled thyroid disease may result in destruction of periodontium[159]	Patients with hyperthyroidism are at higher risk of periodontal disease and progression, due to change in proinflammatory IL-6[160]
Dental implant therapy is not contraindicated in individuals with medically controlled hypothyroidism[161] Thyroid hormone deficiency was found in 25% of patients with dental peri-implantitis[159,163]	Hyperthyroidism did not influence implant survival rates[162]
Hypothalamic-pituitary adrenal axis	
Hyperactivation of the HPA axis and dysregulation of circulating cortisol can increase susceptibility to periodontal disease.[164] Chronically increased cortisol levels contribute to destructive periodontal diseases[164]	
Insulin	
Individuals with uncontrolled Type 1 diabetes due to insulin deficiency had greater PD and more advanced periodontitis compared to controlled diabetes. SRP reversed PD reduction and induced clinical attachment gain[165] Insulin deficiency reduces the contact area between bone and implant.[152] Individuals with diabetes with abnormal insulin metabolism are more susceptible to peri-implantitis[168]	Individuals with hyperglycemia and hyperinsulinemia had more severe periodontitis[166] and greater CAL than nondiabetics[167]
Glucagon	
Patients with periodontitis exhibited impaired glucagon secretion after eating, suggesting dysregulation of glucagon in periodontal disease progression[169]	Glucagon may have anti-inflammatory effects through immune system modulation[170]

(continued on next page)

Table 3
(continued)

Hyposecretion	Hypersecretion
Melatonin	
Low level of melatonin in GF and saliva in subjects with chronic/aggressive periodontitis vs gingivitis[171] and healthy controls[172,173]; difference in plaque-induced gingival inflammation.[171] Lower salivary melatonin levels correlated with worse CPI[174]	Melatonin supplementation following NSPT achieved greater CAL gain and PD reduction,[175–178] improved GI,[177] promotes bone formation around implants,[179] and reduces periodontal severity[180]
GH	
GH deficiency subjects had higher prevalence of periodontal disease than controls[181]	Greater PD in acromegalic female individuals compared to controls; no difference in CAL and tooth loss[182] No difference in periodontal disease, PD, tooth loss and mobility between acromegalic patients vs controls[183] Lower prevalence of advanced chronic periodontitis[184] and lower values of CAL and gingival crevicular fluid volume in acromegalic subjects vs controls[185]
Aldosterone	
N/A	Significantly greater CAL and missing teeth in individuals with hypertension; alveolar crest height and gingival bleeding were not associated after controlling for covariates[186] Greater BOP and PISA with high or uncontrolled BP and with higher systolic BP[187] Association between high/uncontrolled BP and gingival bleeding, unstable periodontitis[188] Significant association between hypertension and gingival bleeding, PD, CAL after adjusting for confounders[189] No significant association between hypertension and periodontal disease, tooth loss, and gingival bleeding[190,191]
Androgens, progesterone, testosterone	
Male individuals with lower bioavailable testosterone levels had higher risk of periodontitis (as measured by CAL and PD)[192]	Male individuals with periodontitis had higher level of testosterone in parotid saliva vs male individuals without periodontitis[193]
Lower testosterone levels were significantly associated with higher GI; testosterone levels did not influence CAL and PD in male individuals with periodontitis; GI and BOP were higher in male individuals with low testosterone[194]	Men with high testosterone had higher odds of exhibiting periodontitis and with more severe presentation[195]

(continued on next page)

Table 3 (continued)	
Hyposecretion	**Hypersecretion**
Men with low testosterone had significantly higher prevalence of missing teeth compared to those without missing teeth[196] Men with androgen deprivation had significantly greater PD, plaque scores and prevalence of periodontal disease, with no effect on bone mineral density[198]	High progesterone in patients with periodontitis[197]
No association between testosterone levels and periodontitis (as measured by CAL and PD),[199] CAL, and tooth loss[200]; no association between sex hormone (testosterone, androgen, dehydroepiandrosterone sulfate, and hormone-binding globulin) levels and periodontal progression (CAL) and tooth loss[200]	
Estradiol	
Low estradiol levels in patients with periodontitis[197]	N/A
No association between estradiol levels and risk of periodontitis in female individuals and male individuals,[192] nor with tooth loss and periodontal disease (as measured by CAL and PD) in male individuals[199]	

Abbreviations: BOP, bleeding on probing; BP, blood pressure; CAL, clinical attachment loss; CPI, community periodontal index; GF, gingival fluid; GH, growth hormone; GI, gingival index; NSPT, nonsurgical periodontal therapy; PD, probing depth; PISA, periodontal inflamed surface area; PTH, parathyroid hormone; T3, triiodothyronine; T4, thyroxinel TSH, thyroid stimulating hormone.

declining CD4 counts. These oral lesions indicate weakened immune function in HIV, highlighting the patient's declining health.[234–240]

Necrotizing ulcerative periodontitis, marked by gingival necrosis and rapid alveolar bone loss, strongly indicates very low CD4 count in HIV-infected individuals.[234,241,242] The resulting immunodeficiency increases patients' vulnerability to severe periodontal diseases like HIV-associated gingivitis, periodontitis, and necrotizing stomatitis.[243]

Prognosis and outcome of periodontal therapy secondary to acquired immunodeficiency syndrome and human immunodeficiency virus infection

The degree of immune suppression and infections such as candidiasis in the oral cavity influence traditional management of periodontal diseases.[234] NSPT can effectively improve periodontal disease in patients with HIV[244] and higher CD4$^+$ counts at baseline were associated to better outcomes from periodontal treatment.[245] Conversely, those with low CD4$^+$ counts were more prone to destructive oral infections.[245] Hence, patient's immune status and HIV stage strongly affect periodontal treatment success.

Human immunodeficiency virus-associated gingivitis. HIV-associated gingivitis (HIVAG; characterized by oral bacteria such as *Candida albicans*, *P gingivalis*, *Bacteroides intermedius*, *Aggregatibacter actinomycetemcomitans* (previously *Actinobacillus actinomycetemcomitans*), *F nucleatum*, and *Wolinella recta*)[243,246,247] manifests as a widespread 2 to 3 mm redness along the gingival margin and nearby tissues. Only a minority of these patients exhibit BOP or spontaneous bleeding. HIVAG does not usually respond to thorough cleaning or improved plaque-control measures alone.[243]

Human immunodeficiency virus-associated periodontitis. In addition to the symptoms listed for HIVAG, HIV-associated periodontitis (HIVAP) is characterized by deep pain, significant gingival bleeding, tissue necrosis, and rapid damage to tooth-supporting structures. While varying in appearance, the lesion of HIVAP progresses and rarely self-resolves. In early stages, there is minimal radiographic bone loss, limited tooth movement, and necrosis confined to the alveolar crest. Moderate cases affect the entire attached gingiva, exposing bone near the gingival margin and increasing tooth movement. Severe cases display extensive radiographic bone loss, tissue and bone necrosis beyond the gingival margin, and severely mobile teeth, risking potential tooth loss.[243]

HIVAP does not improve with standard periodontal treatment and hence may adversely affect prognosis. Treating these lesions typically requires debridement, local antimicrobial treatment, immediate follow-up care, and ongoing maintenance.[243] For severe cases with extensive ulcers and tissue damage, systemic antimicrobial therapy may also be necessary. Gingival necrosis leads to bone exposure and sequestration rather than deep pockets. Debridement and oral hygiene procedures are relatively ineffective, leading to a poorer prognosis, and consequently, tooth extractions have been common therapeutic options.[243] Preventing opportunistic infections (eg, *Pneumocystis carinii*) could help improve prognosis in these patients.[234,241,242] Though limited, evidence suggests dental implants are feasible in patients with HIV, with minimal complications.[248] However, clinicians should consider risks from drug interactions, opportunistic infections, coinfections, and peri-implant disease.

Prognosis and outcome of periodontal therapy secondary to antihuman immunodeficiency virus medications
Understanding the specific highly active antiretroviral therapy (HAART) regimen, viral load status, and CD4 cell count before initiating implant therapy is crucial for effective outcome of implant-supported restorations.[248,249]

Long-term HAART regimen can cause osteoporosis and osteopenia.[249–251] HIV infection is a relative contraindication for dental implant treatment, unless the patient does not have bleeding disorders or severe immunosuppression.[249,252]

Diabetes

Hyperglycemia, a hallmark of diabetes mellitus, has been shown to predispose patients to varied chronic complications, including periodontal disease.[253]

Association between diabetes and periodontal disease
A bidirectional relationship is suggested between diabetes and periodontal disease.[254,255] Individuals with diabetes are more vulnerable to developing periodontal disease, with greater severity in terms of PD and CAL compared to healthy controls, therefore contributing to a poorer prognosis of teeth and restorations.[256] Individuals with uncontrolled diabetes are more prone to severe chronic periodontitis and an increased risk of progressive periodontal deterioration when compared with individuals with controlled diabetes, increasing chances for a poorer periodontal prognosis.[257–260] Overall wound healing is significantly impaired in diabetics and consequently periodontal healing may also be compromised.[261,262]

Health of alveolar bone directly correlates to blood glucose levels.[263,264] Elevated levels of proinflammatory agents (eg, MMPs, IL, TNF-α, and receptor activator of nuclear factor-kappa B ligand/osteoprotegerin ratio) and oxidative stress were observed in individuals with poorly controlled diabetes. All of these contribute to the increased destruction of periodontal structures, thereby adversely affecting prognosis.[264–266]

Elevated blood glucose levels involve a process known as irreversible nonenzymatic glycation, which culminates in the creation of advanced glycation end-products (AGEs). AGEs selectively bind to their designated signaling receptor, receptor for advanced glycation endproducts (RAGE), causing a heightened state of inflammation, intensified oxidative stress, and impairment in the regenerative capacity of bodily tissues. This is particularly impactful for periodontal health. Concurrently, the expression of AGEs is accompanied by markers denoting oxidative stress.[266] AGE proteins were detected in saliva of individuals with diabetes and were associated with greater concentration of dental plaque.[265,267] This cascade of events promotes periodontal degradation and destruction, resulting in poor prognosis of periodontal outcomes.[266] Advanced glycation end product 3 (AGE3) hampers bone cell development and mineralization by binding to RAGE, triggering higher TGF-β levels.[268] Elevated levels of fatty acids in diabetic patients hinder bone cell function and promote osteoclastic activity,[269] leading to complications in bone health and affecting periodontal outcomes.[266,270]

Prognosis and outcome of periodontal therapy secondary to diabetes
Multiple studies have shown that SRP is effective in improving CAL, reducing PD and BOP, in diabetic patients with periodontitis.[271–275] Periodontal treatment in patients with and without diabetes (type 1 and 2) show comparable results with stable healthy periodontium and similar recurrence rates.[276]

Patients with diabetes exhibited significantly increased marginal bone loss, PD, and BOP surrounding dental implants,[277,278] emphasizing the importance of hyperglycemia for peri-implant inflammation control.[277] Likewise, patients with diabetes presented with greater dental implant complication rates and higher PD following immediate loading.[278] However, studies supporting higher peri-implantitis among patients with diabetes appear to have low-to-moderate evidence.[279] On the contrary, other systematic reviews failed to observe any significant increase in implant failure among patients with diabetes as compared to nondiabetic patients.[277,279–281] Further high-quality studies may be needed to determine whether diabetes adversely affects periodontal and implant treatment prognosis.

Cardiovascular Diseases

Cardiovascular diseases (CVDs) are a complex cluster of pathologies encompassing conditions such as ischemic heart disease, stroke, hypertension, rheumatic heart disease, cardiomyopathies, and atrial fibrillation. Altogether, CVDs rank as the foremost contributor to global mortality, constituting as high as 32% of all reported deaths worldwide.[282]

Association between cardiovascular diseases and periodontal disease
The connection between CVDs and bacteria is anchored in the notion of periodontal bacteria infiltrating the circulatory system, precipitating bacteremia, coupled with a systemic inflammation stemming from the persistent presence of periodontitis. A correlation has been established between periodontitis and incipient atherosclerosis.[283–286] Genetic material and viable bacterial entities from periodontal pathogens have been identified within atherothrombotic tissues.[287] Moreover, there is an increased prevalence of subclinical CVDs among individuals with periodontitis.[288] Patients diagnosed with clinically severe periodontitis face a higher risk of experiencing their first coronary event compared to those without periodontitis or with milder forms.[289,290]

586 Sangalli et al

Prognosis and outcome of periodontal therapy in cardiovascular diseases

Periodontal intervention is effective in mitigating low-grade inflammation, as measured through serum CRP and IL-6, while also ameliorating endothelial function in the brachial artery. Furthermore, evidence indicates that periodontal treatment improves arterial blood pressure, diminishing rigidity, and even abating subclinical acute cardiovascular disease markers such as mean carotid intima media thickness.[283,291,292]

Compromised individuals should actively control cardiovascular risk factors, encompassing smoking cessation, physical activity, weight control, blood pressure regulation, lipid and glucose management, in addition to undergoing comprehensive periodontal therapy and scrupulous maintenance. Individuals with both periodontitis and existing CVD should be aware of their augmented vulnerability to subsequent CVD complications.[290]

SUMMARY

It is advisable for treating clinicians to carefully assess medication regimen and systemic conditions of their patients, as these factors may obscure potential effects on periodontal conditions and influence outcomes and prognosis of periodontal treatments.[13,37] An interdisciplinary approach involving medical specialists, general dentists, and periodontists in the management of individuals with systemic condition and periodontal disease is advocated.

CLINICS CARE POINTS

> Pearls
> - Based on the above-mentioned systemic conditions, clinicians performing any periodontal treatment should carefully consider HIV-disease stage, emphasize blood glucose control in patients with diabetes, and communicate the increased vulnerability of CVDs in patients with periodontitis.
> - Systemic medications used to treat RA, IBD, and HIV may influence periodontal outcomes and treatment prognosis.
> - Close monitoring of periodontal status and NSPT are highly recommended.

DISCLOSURE

The authors declare that they have no commercial or financial conflicts of interest.

REFERENCES

1. McGuire MK. Prognosis versus actual outcome: a long-term survey of 100 treated periodontal patients under maintenance care. J Periodontol 1991; 62:51–8.
2. Ioannou AL, Kotsakis GA, Hinrichs JE. Prognostic factors in periodontal therapy and their association with treatment outcomes. World J Clin Cases 2014;2: 822–7.
3. Kwok V, Caton JG. Commentary: prognosis revisited: a system for assigning periodontal prognosis. J Periodontol 2007;78:2063–71.
4. Qin D, Hua F, John MT. Glossary for dental patient-centered outcomes. J Evid-Based Dent Prac 2024;10:19.

5. Thomas DC, Kholi D, Chen N, et al. Orofacial manifestations of rheumatoid arthritis and systemic lupus erythematosus: a narrative review. Quintessence Int 2021;52:454–66.

6. Bartold PM, Lopez-Oliva I. Periodontitis and rheumatoid arthritis: An update 2012-2017. Periodontol 2000 2020;83:189–212.

7. Rodríguez-Lozano B, Gonzalez-Febles J, Garnier-Rodríguez JL, et al. Association between severity of periodontitis and clinical activity in rheumatoid arthritis patients: a case-control study. Arthritis Res Ther 2019;21:27.

8. Kaur S, White S, Bartold PM. Periodontal disease and rheumatoid arthritis: a systematic review. J Dent Res 2013;92:399–408.

9. de Pablo P, Dietrich T, McAlindon TE. Association of periodontal disease and tooth loss with rheumatoid arthritis in the US population. J Rheumatol 2008; 35:70–6.

10. Rahajoe PS, Smit MJ, Kertia N, et al. Cytokines in gingivocrevicular fluid of rheumatoid arthritis patients: A review of the literature. Oral Dis 2019;25:1423–34.

11. Potempa J, Mydel P, Koziel J. The case for periodontitis in the pathogenesis of rheumatoid arthritis. Nat Rev Rheumatol 2017;13:606–20.

12. Krutyhołowa A, Strzelec K, Dziedzic A, et al. Host and bacterial factors linking periodontitis and rheumatoid arthritis. Front Immunol 2022;13:980805.

13. Kobayashi T, Okada M, Ito S, et al. Assessment of interleukin-6 receptor inhibition therapy on periodontal condition in patients with rheumatoid arthritis and chronic periodontitis. J Periodontol 2014;85:57–67.

14. Cetinkaya B, Guzeldemir E, Ogus E, et al. Proinflammatory and anti-inflammatory cytokines in gingival crevicular fluid and serum of patients with rheumatoid arthritis and patients with chronic periodontitis. J Periodontol 2013;84:84–93.

15. Mercado FB, Marshall RI, Bartold PM. Inter-relationships between rheumatoid arthritis and periodontal disease. A review. J Clin Periodontol 2003;30:761–72.

16. Susanto H, Nesse W, Kertia N, et al. Prevalence and severity of periodontitis in Indonesian patients with rheumatoid arthritis. J Periodontol 2013;84:1067–74.

17. Äyräväinen L, Heikkinen AM, Kuuliala A, et al. Inflammatory biomarkers in saliva and serum of patients with rheumatoid arthritis with respect to periodontal status. Ann Med 2018;50:333–44.

18. Biyikoğlu B, Buduneli N, Kardeşler L, et al. Gingival crevicular fluid MMP-8 and -13 and TIMP-1 levels in patients with rheumatoid arthritis and inflammatory periodontal disease. J Periodontol 2009;80:1307–14.

19. Kirchner A, Jager J, Krohn-Grimberghe B, et al. Active matrix metalloproteinase-8 and periodontal bacteria depending on periodontal status in patients with rheumatoid arthritis. J Periodontal Res 2017;52:745–54.

20. Konig MF, Abusieme L, Reinholdt J, et al. Aggregatibacter actinomycetemcomitans-induced hypercitrullination links periodontal infection to autoimmunity in rheumatoid arthritis. Sci Transl Med 2016;8:369ra176.

21. Qiao Y, Wang Z, Li Y, et al. Rheumatoid arthritis risk in periodontitis patients: A systematic review and meta-analysis. Joint Bone Spine 2020;87:556–64.

22. Kim JW, Park J, Yim HW, et al. Rheumatoid arthritis is associated with early tooth loss: results from Korea National Health and Nutrition Examination Survey V to VI. Korean J Intern Med 2019;45:1381–91.

23. Demmer RT, Molitor J, Jacobs DR Jr, et al. Periodontal disease, tooth loss and incident rheumatoid arthritis: results from the First National Health and Nutrition Examination Survey and its epidemiological follow-up study. J Clin Periodontol 2011;38:998–1006.

24. Dissick A, Redman R, Jones M, et al. Association of periodontitis with rheumatoid arthritis: a pilot study. J Periodontol 2010;81:223–30.
25. Mercado FB, Marshall RI, Klestov AC, et al. Relationship between rheumatoid arthritis and periodontitis. J Periodontol 2001;72:779–87.
26. Lee JY, Choi IA, Kim JH, et al. Association between anti-Porphyromonas gingivalis or anti-α-enolase antibody and severity of periodontitis or rheumatoid arthritis (RA) disease activity in RA. BMC Musculoskelet Disord 2015;16:190.
27. Okada M, Kobayashi T, Ito S, et al. Antibody responses to periodontopathic bacteria in relation to rheumatoid arthritis in Japanese adults. J Periodontol 2011;82:1433–41.
28. Shen MT, Shahin B, Chen Z, et al. Unexpected lower level of oral periodontal pathogens in patients with high numbers of systemic diseases. PeerJ 2023; 11:e15502.
29. Gittaboyina S, Kodugant R, Aedula SD, et al. Estimation of pentraxin 3 and porphyromonas gingivalis levels in patients with rheumatoid arthritis and periodontitis- an observational study. J Clin Diagn Res 2017;11:ZC09–12.
30. Bender P, Burgin W, Sculean A, et al. Serum antibody levels against Porphyromonas gingivalis in patients with and without rheumatoid arthritis - a systematic review and meta-analysis. Clin Oral Investig 2017;21:33–42.
31. Ogrendik M, Kokino S, Ozdemir F, et al. Serum antibodies to oral anaerobic bacteria in patients with rheumatoid arthritis. MedGenMed 2005;7:2.
32. Larsen DN, Mikkelsen CE, Kierkegaard M, et al. Citrullinome of porphyromonas gingivalis outer membrane vesicles: confident identification of citrullinated peptides. Mol Cell Proteomics 2020;19:167–80.
33. Corrêa JD, Fernandes GR, Calderaro DC, et al. Oral microbial dysbiosis linked to worsened periodontal condition in rheumatoid arthritis patients. Sci Rep 2019; 9:8379.
34. Vitkov L, Hannig M, Minnich B, et al. Periodontal sources of citrullinated antigens and TLR agonists related to RA. Autoimmunity 2018;51:304–9.
35. Wegner N, Lunderbger K, Kinloch A, et al. Autoimmunity to specific citrullinated proteins gives the first clues to the etiology of rheumatoid arthritis. Immunol Rev 2010;23:34–54.
36. Seegobin SD, Ma MH, Dahanayake C, et al. ACPA-positive and ACPA-negative rheumatoid arthritis differ in their requirements for combination DMARDs and corticosteroids: secondary analysis of a randomized controlled trial. Arthritis Res Ther 2014;16:R13.
37. Patschan S, Bothman L, Patschan D, et al. Association of cytokine patterns and clinical/laboratory parameters, medication and periodontal burden in patients with rheumatoid arthritis (RA). Odontology 2020;108:441–9.
38. Disale PR, Zope S, Suragimath G, et al. Prevalence and severity of periodontitis in patients with established rheumatoid arthritis and osteoarthritis. J Fam Med Prim Care 2020;9:2919–25.
39. Albrecht K, de Pablo P, Eidner T, et al. Association between rheumatoid arthritis disease activity and periodontitis defined by tooth loss: longitudinal and cross-sectional data from two observational studies. Arthritis Care Res (Hoboken) 2021.
40. Schmalz G, Bartl M, Schmickler J, et al. Tooth loss is associated with disease-related parameters in patients with rheumatoid arthritis and ankylosing spondylitis-a cross-sectional study. J Clin Med 2021;10:3052.
41. Hayashi Y, Taylor G, Yoshihara A, et al. Relationship between autoantibody associated with rheumatoid arthritis and tooth loss. Gerodontology 2018.

42. Afilal S, Rkain H, Allaoui A, et al. Oral hygiene status in rheumatoid arthritis patients and related factors. Mediterr J Rheumatol 2021;32:249–55.
43. Kaur G, Mohindra K, Singla S. Autoimmunity-Basics and link with periodontal disease. Autoimmun Rev 2017;16:64–71.
44. Araújo VM, Melo I, Lima V. Relationship between periodontitis and rheumatoid arthritis: review of the literature. Mediators Inflamm 2015;2015:259074.
45. Nair S, Faizuddin M, Dharmapalan J. Role of autoimmune responses in periodontal disease. Autoimmune Dis 2014;2014:596824.
46. Ali J, Pramod K, Tahir MA, et al. Autoimmune responses in periodontal diseases. Autoimmun Rev 2011;10:426–31.
47. Li S, Zhou C, Xu Y, et al. Similarity and potential relation between periimplantitis and rheumatoid arthritis on transcriptomic level: results of a bioinformatics study. Front Immunol 2021;12:702661.
48. Guobis Z, Pacauskiene I, Astramskaite I. General diseases influence on peri-implantitis development: a systematic review. J Oral Maxillofac Res 2016;7:e5.
49. Turri A, Rossetti PH, Canullo L, et al. Prevalence of peri-implantitis in medically compromised patients and smokers: a systematic review. Int J Oral Maxillofac Implants 2016;31:111–8.
50. Krennmair G, Seemann R, Piehslinger E. Dental implants in patients with rheumatoid arthritis: clinical outcome and peri-implant findings. J Clin Periodontol 2010;37:928–36.
51. Esimekara JO, Perez A, Courvoisier DS, et al. Dental implants in patients suffering from autoimmune diseases: a systematic critical review. J Stomatol Oral Maxillofac Surg 2022;123:e464–73.
52. Duttenhoefer F, Fuessinger MA, Beckmann Y, et al. Dental implants in immuno-compromised patients: a systematic review and meta-analysis. Int. J. Implant Dent 2019;5:43.
53. Weinlander M, Krennmair G, Piehslinger E. Implant prosthodontic rehabilitation of patients with rheumatic disorders: a case series report. Int J Prosthodont 2010;23:22–8.
54. Alenazi A. Association between rheumatoid factors and proinflammatory biomarkers with implant health in rheumatoid arthritis patients with dental implants. Eur Rev Med Pharmacol Sci 2021;25:7014–21.
55. de Smit MJ, Westra J, Posthumus MD, et al. Effect of anti-rheumatic treatment on the periodontal condition of rheumatoid arthritis patients. Int J Environ Res Publ Health 2021;17:2529.
56. Mazurek-Mochol M, Brzeska M, Serwin K, et al. IL-18 Gene rs187238 and rs1946518 polymorphisms and expression in gingival tissue in patients with periodontitis. Biomedicine 2022;10:2367.
57. Barnard AR, Regan M, Burke FD, et al. Wound healing with medications for rheumatoid arthritis in hand surgery. ISRN Rheumatol 2012;2012:251962.
58. Brasil-Oliveira R, Cruz ÁA, Sarmento VA, et al. Corticosteroid use and periodontal disease: a systematic review. Eur J Dermatol 2020;14:496–501.
59. Romero-Sanchez C, Rodriguez C, Santos-Moreno P, et al. Is the treatment with biological or non-biological DMARDS a modifier of periodontal condition in patients with rheumatoid arthritis? Curr Rheumatol Rev 2017;13:139–51.
60. Zhang J, Xu C, Gao L, et al. Influence of anti-rheumatic agents on the periodontal condition of patients with rheumatoid arthritis and periodontitis: A systematic review and meta-analysis. J Periodontal Res 2021;56:1099–115.

61. Zamri F, de Vries TJ. Use of TNF inhibitors in rheumatoid arthritis and implications for the periodontal status: for the benefit of both? Front Immunol 2020; 11:591365.

62. Hashimoto H, Hashimoto S, Shimazaki Y. Relationship between tooth loss and the medications used for the treatment of rheumatoid arthritis in japanese patients with rheumatoid arthritis: a cross-sectional study. J Clin Med 2021;10:876.

63. Howell TH. Blocking periodontal disease progression with anti-inflammatory agents. J Periodontol 1993;64(Suppl 8S):828–33.

64. Kobayashi T, Yokoyama T, Ito S, et al. Periodontal and serum protein profiles in patients with rheumatoid arthritis treated with tumor necrosis factor inhibitor adalimumab. J Periodontol 2014;85:1480–8.

65. Pauletto N, Silver JG, Larjava H. Nonsteroidal anti-inflammatory agents: potential modifiers of periodontal disease progression. J Can Dent Assoc 1987;63: 824–9.

66. Howell TH, Williams RC. Nonsteroidal antiinflammatory drugs as inhibitors of periodontal disease progression. Crit Rev Oral Biol Med 1993;4:177–96.

67. Williams RC, Jeffcoat MK, Howell TH, et al. Altering the progression of human alveolar bone loss with the non-steroidal anti-inflammatory drug flurbiprofen. J Periodontol 1989;60:485–90.

68. Altobelli E, Angeletti PM, Piccolo D, et al. Synovial fluid and serum concentrations of inflammatory markers in rheumatoid arthritis, psoriatic arthritis and osteoarthitis: a systematic review. Curr Rheumatol Rev 2017;13:170–9.

69. Äyräväinen L, Heikkinen AM, Kuuliala A, et al. Anti-rheumatic medication and salivary MMP-8, a biomarker for periodontal disease. Oral Dis 2018;24:1562–71.

70. Ziebolz D, Rupprecht A, Schmickler J, et al. Association of different immunosuppressive medications with periodontal condition in patients with rheumatoid arthritis: Results from a cross-sectional study. J Periodontol 2018;89:1310–7.

71. Hobl EL, Mader RM, Erlacher L, et al. The influence of methotrexate on the gene expression of the pro-inflammatory cytokine IL-12A in the therapy of rheumatoid arthritis. Clin Exp Rheumatol 2011;29:963–9.

72. Sung JY, Hong JH, Kang HS, et al. Methotrexate suppresses the interleukin-6 induced generation of reactive oxygen species in the synoviocytes of rheumatoid arthritis. Immunopharmacology 2000;47:35–44.

73. Pers JO, Saraux A, Pierre R, et al. Anti-TNF-alpha immunotherapy is associated with increased gingival inflammation without clinical attachment loss in subjects with rheumatoid arthritis. J Periodontol 2008;79:1645–51.

74. Savioli C, Ribeiro AC, Fabri GM, et al. Persistent periodontal disease hampers anti-tumor necrosis factor treatment response in rheumatoid arthritis. J Clin Rheumatol 2012;18:180–4.

75. Mayer Y, Balbir-Gurman A, Machtei EE. Anti-tumor necrosis factor-alpha therapy and periodontal parameters in patients with rheumatoid arthritis. J Periodontol 2009;80:1414–20.

76. Ortiz P, Bissada NF, Palomo L, et al. Periodontal therapy reduces the severity of active rheumatoid arthritis in patients treated with or without tumor necrosis factor inhibitors. J Periodontol 2009;80:535–40.

77. Mayer Y, Elimelech R, Balbir-Gurman A, et al. Periodontal condition of patients with autoimmune diseases and the effect of anti-tumor necrosis factor-α therapy. J Periodonol 2013;84:136–42.

78. Huang Y, Zhang Z, Zheng Y, et al. Effects of non-surgical periodontal therapy on periodontal clinical data in periodontitis patients with rheumatoid arthritis: a meta-analysis. BMC Oral Health 2021;21:340.

79. Jung GU, Han JY, Hwang KG, et al. Effects of conventional synthetic disease-modifying antirheumatic drugs on response to periodontal treatment in patients with rheumatoid arthritis. BioMed Res Int 2018;2018:1465402.

80. Kurgan Ş, Önder C, Balcı N, et al. Gingival crevicular fluid tissue/blood vessel-type plasminogen activator and plasminogen activator inhibitor-2 levels in patients with rheumatoid arthritis: effects of nonsurgical periodontal therapy. J Periodontal Res 2017;52:574–81.

81. Kaur S, Bright R, Proudman SM, et al. Does periodontal treatment influence clinical and biochemical measures for rheumatoid arthritis? A systematic review and meta-analysis. Semin Arthritis Rheum 2014;44:113–22.

82. Mustufvi Z, Twigg J, Kerry J, et al. Does periodontal treatment improve rheumatoid arthritis disease activity? A systematic review. Rheumatol Adv Pract 2022;6: rkac061.

83. Silva DS, Costa F, Baptista IP, et al. Evidence-based research on effectiveness of periodontal treatment in rheumatoid arthritis patients: a systematic review and meta-analysis. Arthritis Care Res (Hoboken) 2022;74:1723–35.

84. Okada M, Kobayashi T, Ito S, et al. Periodontal treatment decreases levels of antibodies to Porphyromonas gingivalis and citrulline in patients with rheumatoid arthritis and periodontitis. J Periodontol 2013;84:e74–84.

85. Välimaa H, Savolainen S, Soukka T, et al. Estrogen receptor-beta is the predominant estrogen receptor subtype in human oral epithelium and salivary glands. J Endocrinol 2004;180:55–62.

86. Mullally BH, Coulter WA, Hutchinson JD, et al. Current oral contraceptive status and periodontitis in young adults. J Periodontol 2007;78:1031–6.

87. Brusca MI, Rosa A, Albaina O, et al. The impact of oral contraceptives on women's periodontal health and the subgingival occurrence of aggressive periodontopathogens and Candida species. J Periodontol 2010;81:1010–8.

88. Haerian-Ardakani A, Moeintaghavi A, Talebi-Ardakani MR, et al. The association between current low-dose oral contraceptive pills and periodontal health: a matched-case-control study. J Contemp Dent Pract 2010;11:033–40.

89. Offenbacher S, Lin D, Strauss R, et al. Effects of periodontal therapy during pregnancy on periodontal status, biologic parameters, and pregnancy outcomes: a pilot study. J Periodontol 2006;77:2011–24.

90. Khairnar MS, Pawar BR, Marawar PP, et al. Estimation of changes in C-reactive protein level and pregnancy outcome after nonsurgical supportive periodontal therapy in women affected with periodontitis in a rural set up of India. Contemp Clin Dent 2015;6(Suppl 1):S5–11.

91. Penova-Veselinovic B, Keelan JA, Wang CA, et al. Changes in inflammatory mediators in gingival crevicular fluid following periodontal disease treatment in pregnancy: relationship to adverse pregnancy outcome. J Reprod Immunol 2015;112:1–10.

92. Yarkac FU, Gokturk O, Demir O. Effect of non-surgical periodontal therapy on the degree of gingival inflammation and stress markers related to pregnancy. J Appl Oral Sci 2018;26:e20170630.

93. Machtei EE, Mahler D, Sanduri H, et al. The effect of menstrual cycle on periodontal health. J Periodontol 2004;75:408–12.

94. Baser U, Cekici A, Tanrikulu-Kucuk S, et al. Gingival inflammation and interleukin-1 beta and tumor necrosis factor-alpha levels in gingival crevicular fluid during the menstrual cycle. J Periodontol 2009;80:1983–90.

95. Becerik S, Ozcaka O, Nalbantsoy A, et al. Effects of menstrual cycle on periodontal health and gingival crevicular fluid markers. J Periodontol 2010;81: 673–81.

96. Markou E, Boura E, Tsalikis L, et al. The influence of sex hormones on proinflammatory cytokines in gingiva of periodontally healthy premenopausal women. J Periodontal Res 2011;528–32.

97. Shourie V, Dwarakanath CD, Prashanth GV, et al. The effect of menstrual cycle on periodontal health - a clinical and microbiological study. Oral Health Prev Dent 2012;10:185–92.

98. Khosravisamani M, Maliji G, Seyfi S, et al. Effect of the menstrual cycle on inflammatory cytokines in the periodontium. J Periodontal Res 2014;49:770–6.

99. Rathore S, Khuller N, Dev YP, et al. Effects of scaling and root planing on gingival status during menstrual cycle- a cross-sectional analytical study. J Clin Diagn Res 2015;9:ZC35–9.

100. Kamal Asaad N, Abbood HM. Comparing gingival inflammation and salivary acidity to hormonal variation during menstruation. Saudi Dent J 2023;35:251–4.

101. Payne JB, Rreinhardt RA, Nummikoski PV, et al. Longitudinal alveolar bone loss in postmenopausal osteoporotic/osteopenic women. Osteoporos Int 1999;10: 34–40.

102. Darby I, Curtis M. Microbiology of periodontal disease in children and young adults. Periodontol 2000 2001;26:33–53.

103. Mombelli A, Rutar A, Lang NP. Correlation of the periodontal status 6 years after puberty with clinical and microbiological conditions during puberty. J Clin Periodontol 1995;22:300–5.

104. Boyapati R, Cherukuri SA, Bodduru R, et al. Influence of Female Sex Hormones in Different Stages of Women on Periodontium. J Midlife Health 2021;12:263–6.

105. Güncü GN, Tozüm TF, Cağlayan F. Effects of endogenous sex hormones on the periodontium–review of literature. Aust Dent J 2005;50:138–45.

106. Califano JV, Research SaTCAAoP. Position paper: periodontal diseases of children and adolescents. J Periodontol 2003;74:1696–704.

107. Oh TJ, Eber R, Wang HL. Periodontal diseases in the child and adolescent. J Clin Periodontol 2002;29:400–10.

108. Nakagawa S, Fujll H, Machida Y, et al. A longitudinal study from prepuberty to puberty of gingivitis. Correlation between the occurrence of Prevotella intermedia and sex hormones. J Clin Periodontol 1994;21:658–65.

109. Kara C, Demir T, Tezel A. Effectiveness of periodontal therapies on the treatment of different aetiological factors induced gingival overgrowth in puberty. Int J Dent Hyg 2007;5:211–7.

110. Engelsöy U, Svensson MA, Demirel I. Estradiol Alters the Virulence Traits of Uropathogenic Escherichia coli. Front Microbiol 2021;12:682626.

111. Preshaw PM. Oral contraceptives and the periodontium. Periodontol 2000 2013; 61:125–59.

112. Zou MY, Cohen RE, Ursomanno BL, et al. Use of systemic steroids, hormone replacement therapy, or oral contraceptives is associated with decreased implant survival in women. Dent J (Basel) 2023;11:163.

113. Domingues RS, Ferraz BF, Greghi SL, et al. Influence of combined oral contraceptives on the periodontal condition. J Appl Oral Sci 2012;20:253–9.

114. Lieske B, Makarova N, Jagemann B, et al. Inflammatory Response in Oral Biofilm during Pregnancy: A Systematic Review. Nutrients 2022;14:4894.

115. Pralhad S, Thomas B, Kushtagi P. Periodontal disease and pregnancy hypertension: a clinical correlation. J Periodontol 2013;84:1118–25.

116. Yang I, Knight AK, Dunlop AL, et al. Characterizing the Subgingival Microbiome of Pregnant African American Women. J Obstet Gynecol Neonatal Nurs 2019; 48:140–52.
117. Machado V, Mesquita MF, Bernardo MA, et al. IL-6 and TNF-α salivary levels according to the periodontal status in Portuguese pregnant women. PeerJ 2018;6: e4710.
118. Hassan MN, Belibasakis GN, Gumus P, et al. Annexin-1 as a salivary biomarker for gingivitis during pregnancy. J Periodontol 2018;89:875–82.
119. da Silva HEC, Stefani CM, de Santos Melo N, et al. Effect of intra-pregnancy nonsurgical periodontal therapy on inflammatory biomarkers and adverse pregnancy outcomes: a systematic review with meta-analysis. Syst Rev 2017;6:197.
120. Fiorini T, Stefani CM, da Rocha JM, et al. Effect of nonsurgical periodontal therapy on serum and gingival crevicular fluid cytokine levels during pregnancy and postpartum. J Periodontal Res 2013;48:126–33.
121. Guan X, Guan Y, Shi C, et al. Estrogen deficiency aggravates apical periodontitis by regulating NLRP3/caspase-1/IL-1β axis. Am J Transl Res 2020;12: 660–71.
122. Levin VA, Jiang X, Kagan R. Estrogen therapy for osteoporosis in the modern era. Osteoporos Int 2018;29:1049–55.
123. Friedlander AH. The physiology, medical management and oral implications of menopause. J Am Dent Assoc 2002;133:73–81.
124. Jeffcoat MK, Lewis CE, Reddy MS, et al. Post-menopausal bone loss and its relationship to oral bone loss. Periodontol 2000 2000;23:94–102.
125. Jacobs R, Ghyselen J, Koninckx P, et al. Long-term bone mass evaluation of mandible and lumbar spine in a group of women receiving hormone replacement therapy. Eur J Oral Sci 1996;10–6.
126. Preda SA, Comanescu MC, Albulescu DM, et al. Correlations between periodontal indices and osteoporosis. Exp Ther Med 2022;23:254.
127. Brignardello-Petersen R. The magnitude of an association between periodontal attachment loss and osteoporosis or osteopenia is small. J Am Dent Assoc 2017;48:e41.
128. Hernández-Vigueras S, Martinez-Garriga B, Sánchez MC, et al. Oral Microbiota, Periodontal Status, and Osteoporosis in Postmenopausal Females. J Periodontol 2016;87:124–33.
129. Pereira FM, Rodrigues VP, de Oliveira AE, et al. Association between periodontal changes and osteoporosis in postmenopausal women. Climacteric 2015;18:311–5.
130. Yoshihara A, Seida Y, Hanada N, et al. The relationship between bone mineral density and the number of remaining teeth in community-dwelling older adults. J Oral Rehabil 2005;32:735–40.
131. Yoshihara A, Seida Y, Hanada N, et al. A longitudinal study of the relationship between periodontal disease and bone mineral density in community-dwelling older adults. J Clin Periodontol 2004;31:680–4.
132. Daltaban O, Saygun I, Bal B, et al. Gingival crevicular fluid alkaline phosphatase levels in postmenopausal women: effects of phase I periodontal treatment. J Periodontol 2006;77:67–72.
133. Pizzo G, Guiglia R, Licata ME, et al. Effect of hormone replacement therapy (HRT) on periodontal status of postmenopausal women. Med Sci Mon Int Med J Exp Clin Res 2011;17:PH23–7.
134. Ronderos M, Jacobs DR, Himes JH, et al. Associations of periodontal disease with femoral bone mineral density and estrogen replacement therapy: cross-

sectional evaluation of US adults from NHANES III. J Clin Periodontol 2000;27: 778–86.

135. Reinhardt RA, Payne JB, Maze CA, et al. Influence of estrogen and osteopenia/ osteoporosis on clinical periodontitis in postmenopausal women. J Periodontol 1999;70:823–8.

136. Demirel KJ, Guimaraes AN, Demirel I. Effects of estradiol on the virulence traits of Porphyromonas gingivalis. Sci Rep 2022;12:13881.

137. Haas AN, Rosin CK, Oppermann RV, et al. Association among menopause, hormone replacement therapy, and periodontal attachment loss in southern Brazilian women. J Periodontol 2009;80:1380–7.

138. Canderelli R, Leccesse LA, Miller NL, et al. Benefits of hormone replacement therapy in postmenopausal women. J Am Acad Nurse Pract 2007;19:635–41.

139. Norderyd OM, Grossi SG, Machtei EE, et al. Periodontal status of women taking postmenopausal estrogen supplementation. J Periodontol 1993;64:957–62.

140. Ito I, Hayashi T, Yamada K, et al. Physiological concentration of estradiol inhibits polymorphonuclear leukocyte chemotaxis via a receptor mediated system. Life Sci 1995;56:2247–53.

141. Cekici A, Baser U, Isik G, et al. Periodontal treatment outcomes in post menopausal women receiving hormone replacement therapy. J Istanbul Univ Fac Dent 2015;49:39–44.

142. Laza GM, Sufaru IG, Martu MA, et al. Effects of locally delivered minocycline microspheres in postmenopausal female patients with periodontitis: a clinical and microbiological study. Diagnostics (Basel) 2022;12:1310.

143. Prasanna JS, Sumadhura C. Biochemical analysis of three biological fluids and its response to non-surgical periodontal therapy in pre and postmenopausal women with periodontitis. J Menopausal Med 2019;25:149–57.

144. Prasanna JS, Sumadhura C, Karunakar P, et al. Correlative analysis of plasma and urine neopterin levels in the pre- and post-menopausal women with periodontitis, following nonsurgical periodontal therapy. J Indian Soc Periodontol 2017;21:276–84.

145. Prasanna JS, Sumadhura C, Karunakar P, et al. Comparative evaluation of salivary neopterin levels and its effects to periodontal therapy in pre- and post-menopausal women. J Menopausal Med 2017;23:32–41.

146. August M, Chung K, Chang Y, et al. Influence of estrogen status on endosseous implant osseointegration. J Oral Maxillofac Surg 2001;59:1285–9.

147. Moy PK, Medina D, Shetty V, et al. Dental implant failure rates and associated risk factors. Int J Oral Maxillofac Implants 2005;20:569–77.

148. Koszuta P, Grafka A, Koszuta A, et al. Effects of selected factors on the osseointegration of dental implants. Prz Menopauzalny 2015;14:184–7.

149. Minsk L, Polson AM. Dental implant outcomes in postmenopausal women undergoing hormone replacement. Compend Contin Educ Dent 1998;19:859–62.

150. Srirangarajan S, Satyanarayan A, Ravindra S, et al. Dental manifestation of primary idiopathic hypoparathyroidism. J Indian Soc Periodontol 2014;18:524–6.

151. Kuchler U, Luvizuto ER, Tangl S, et al. Short-term teriparatide delivery and osseointegration: a clinical feasibility study. J Dent Res 2011;90:1001–6.

152. Yi M, Yin Y, Sun J, et al. Hormone and implant osseointegration: Elaboration of the relationship among function, preclinical, and clinical practice. Front Mol Biosci 2022;9:965753.

153. Daugaard H, Elmengaard B, Andreassen TT, et al. Systemic intermittent parathyroid hormone treatment improves osseointegration of press-fit inserted implants in cancellous bone. Acta Orthop 2012;83:411–9.

154. Gomes-Ferreira PHS, de Oliveira D, Frigério PB, et al. Teriparatide improves microarchitectural characteristics of peri-implant bone in orchiectomized rats. Osteoporos Int 2020;31:1807–15.
155. Kakade SP, Gogri AA, Umarji HR, et al. Oral manifestations of secondary hyperparathyroidism: A case report. Contemp Clin Dent 2015;6:552–8.
156. Bashutski JD, Eber RM, Kinney JS, et al. Teriparatide and osseous regeneration in the oral cavity. N Engl J Med 2010;363:2396–405.
157. Schneider P, Berger P, Kruse K, et al. Effect of calcitonin deficiency on bone density and bone turnover in totally thyroidectomized patients. J Endocrinol Invest 1991;14:935–42.
158. Wei Y, Ye Q, Tang Z, et al. Calcitonin induces collagen synthesis and osteoblastic differentiation in human periodontal ligament fibroblasts. Arch Oral Biol 2017;74:114–22.
159. Zahid TM, Wang BY, Cohen RE. The effects of thyroid hormone abnormalities on periodontal disease status. J Int Acad Periodontol 2011;13:80–5.
160. Kadhom EH, Radhi NJ. Estimation of Salivary IL-6 Level in relation of Periodontal Status in Patients with Hyperthyroidism. Al-Kindy Coll Med J 2023;19:115–20.
161. Attard NJ, Zarb GA. A study of dental implants in medically treated hypothyroid patients. Clin Implant Dent Relat Res 2002;4:220–31.
162. Torrejon-Moya A, Izquierdo-Gómez K, Pérez-Sayáns M, et al. Patients with Thyroid Disorder, a Contraindication for Dental Implants? A Systematic Review. J Clin Med 2022;11:2399.
163. Shcherbakov MV, Golovina ES, Gil'miiarova FN. [Dental periimplantitis distinctive features diagnostic in cases of minimal thyroid insufficiency]. Stomatologiia (Mosk) 2008;87:50–5.
164. Rosania AE, Low KG, McCormick CM, et al. Stress, depression, cortisol, and periodontal disease. J Periodontol 2009;80:260–6.
165. Novaes AB, Pereira AL, de Moraes N, et al. Manifestations of insulin-dependent diabetes mellitus in the periodontium of young Brazilian patients. J Periodontol 1991;62:116–22.
166. Nesse W, Linde A, Abbas F, et al. Dose-response relationship between periodontal inflamed surface area and HbA1c in type 2 diabetics. J Clin Periodontol 2009;36:295–300.
167. Engebretson SP, Hey-Hadavi J, Ehrhardt FJ, et al. Gingival crevicular fluid levels of interleukin-1beta and glycemic control in patients with chronic periodontitis and type 2 diabetes. J Periodontol 2004;75:1203–8.
168. Ferreira SD, Silva GL, Cortelli JR, et al. Prevalence and risk variables for peri-implant disease in Brazilian subjects. J Clin Periodontol 2006;33:929–35.
169. Komada H, Hirota Y, Sakaguchi K, et al. Impaired glucagon secretion in patients with fulminant type 1 diabetes mellitus. Endocrine 2019;63:476–9.
170. Sunilkumar S, Kimball SR, Dennis MD. Glucagon transiently stimulates mTORC1 by activation of an EPAC/Rap1 signaling axis. Cell Signal 2021;84:110010.
171. Almughrabi OM, Marzouk KM, Hasanato RM, et al. Melatonin levels in periodontal health and disease. J Periodontal Res 2013;48:315–21.
172. Srinath R, Acharya AB, Thakur SL. Salivary and gingival crevicular fluid melatonin in periodontal health and disease. J Periodontol 2010;81:277–83.
173. Balaji TM, Vasanthi HR, Rao SR. Gingival, plasma and salivary levels of melatonin in periodontally healthy individuals and chronic periodontitis patients: a pilot study. J Clin Diagn Res 2015;9:ZC23–5.
174. Cutando A, Galindo P, Gómez-Moreno G, et al. Relationship between salivary melatonin and severity of periodontal disease. J Periodontol 2006;77:1533–8.

175. Tinto M, Sartori M, Pizzi I, et al. Melatonin as host modulating agent supporting nonsurgical periodontal therapy in patients affected by untreated severe periodontitis: A preliminary randomized, triple-blind, placebo-controlled study. J Periodontal Res 2020;55:61–7.

176. El-Sharkawy H, Elmeadawy S, Elshinnawi U, et al. Is dietary melatonin supplementation a viable adjunctive therapy for chronic periodontitis?-A randomized controlled clinical trial. J Periodontal Res 2019;54:190–7.

177. Liu RY, Li L, Zhang ZT, et al. Clinical efficacy of melatonin as adjunctive therapy to non-surgical treatment of periodontitis: a systematic review and meta-analysis. Inflammopharmacology 2022;30:695–704.

178. Balaji TM, Varadarajan S, Jagannathan R, et al. Melatonin as a topical/systemic formulation for the management of periodontitis: a systematic review. Materials (Basel) 2021;14:2417.

179. Gómez-Moreno G, Aguilar-Salvatierra A, Boquete-Castro A, et al. Outcomes of topical applications of melatonin in implant dentistry: a systematic review. Implant Dent 2015;24:25–30.

180. Anton DM, Martu MA, Maris M, et al. Study on the Effects of Melatonin on Glycemic Control and Periodontal Parameters in Patients with Type II Diabetes Mellitus and Periodontal Disease. Medicina (Kaunas) 2021;57:140.

181. Britto IM, Aguiar-Oliveira MH, Oliveira-Neto LA, et al. Periodontal disease in adults with untreated congenital growth hormone deficiency: a case-control study. J Clin Periodontol 2011;38:525–31.

182. Harb AN, Holtfreter B, Friedrich N, et al. Evaluation of the periodontal status in acromegalic patients: a comparative study. ISRN Dent 2012;2012:950486.

183. Lima DL, Montenegro RM Jr, Vieira AP, et al. Absence of periodontitis in acromegalic patients. Clin Oral Investig 2009;13:165–9.

184. Başçıl S, Turhan İyidir Ö, Bayraktar N, et al. Severe chronic periodontitis is not common in Acromegaly: Potential protective role of gingival BMP-2. Turk J Med Sci 2021;51:1172–8.

185. Ozdemir Y, Keceli HG, Helvaci N, et al. The tendency of reduced periodontal destruction in acromegalic patients showing similar inflammatory status with periodontitis patients. Endocrine 2019;66:622–33.

186. Gordon JH, LaMonte MJ, Genco RJ, et al. Association of clinical measures of periodontal disease with blood pressure and hypertension among postmenopausal women. J Periodontol 2018;89:193–1202.

187. Pietropaoli D, Del Pinto R, Ferri C, et al. Association between periodontal inflammation and hypertension using periodontal inflamed surface area and bleeding on probing. J Clin Periodontol 2020;47:160–72.

188. Pietropaoli D, Monaco A, D'Aiuto F, et al. Active gingival inflammation is linked to hypertension. J Hypertens 2020;2018–27.

189. Tsakos G, Sabbah W, Hingorani AD, et al. Is periodontal inflammation associated with raised blood pressure? Evidence from a National US survey. J Hypertens 2010;28:2386–93.

190. Rivas-Tumanyan S, Spiegelman D, Curhan GC, et al. Periodontal disease and incidence of hypertension in the health professionals follow-up study. Am J Hypertens 2012;25:770–6.

191. Iwashima Y, Kokubo Y, Ono T, et al. Additive interaction of oral health disorders on risk of hypertension in a Japanese urban population: the Suita Study. Am J Hypertens 2014;27:710–9.

192. Su X, Jin K, Zhou X, et al. The association between sex hormones and periodontitis among American adults: A cross-sectional study. Front Endocrinol (Lausanne) 2023;14:1125819.
193. Kuraner T, Beksac MS, Kayakirilmaz K, et al. Serum and parotid saliva testosterone, calcium, magnesium, and zinc levels in males, with and without periodontitis. Biol Trace Elem Res 1991;31:43–9.
194. Daltaban O, Saygun I, Bolu E. Periodontal status in men with hypergonadotropic hypogonadism: effects of testosterone deficiency. J Periodontol 2006;77:1179–83.
195. Steffens JP, Wang X, Starr JR, et al. Associations between sex hormone levels and periodontitis in men: results from NHANES III. J Periodontol 2015;86:1116–25.
196. Singh BP, Makker A, Tripathi A, et al. Association of testosterone and bone mineral density with tooth loss in men with chronic periodontitis. J Oral Sci 2011;53:333–9.
197. Vittek J, Kirsch S, Rappaport SC, et al. Salivary concentrations of steroid hormones in males and in cycling and postmenopausal females with and without periodontitis. J Periodontal Res 1984;19:545–55.
198. Famili P, Cauley JA, Greenspan SL. The effect of androgen deprivation therapy on periodontal disease in men with prostate cancer. J Urul 2007;177(3):921–4.
199. Orwoll ES, Chan B, Lambert LC, et al. Sex steroids, periodontal health, and tooth loss in older men. J Dent Res 2009;88:704–8.
200. Samietz S, Holtfreter B, Friedrich N, et al. Prospective association of sex steroid concentrations with periodontal progression and incident tooth loss. J Clin Periodontol 2016;43:10–8.
201. Lira-Junior R, Figueredo CM. Periodontal and inflammatory bowel diseases: Is there evidence of complex pathogenic interactions? World J Gastroenterol 2016;22:7963–72.
202. Shan Y, Lee M, Chang EB. The gut microbiome and inflammatory bowel diseases. Annu Rev Med 2022;73:455–68.
203. Zhang Y, Qiao D, Chen R, et al. The association between periodontitis and inflammatory bowel disease: a systematic review and meta-analysis. BioMed Res Int 2021;2021:6692420.
204. Madsen GR, Bertl K, Pandis N, et al. The impact of periodontitis on inflammatory bowel disease activity. Inflamm Bowel Dis 2023;29:396–404.
205. Byrd KM, Gnanasekaran JM. The "Gum-Gut" axis in inflammatory bowel diseases: a hypothesis-driven review of associations and advances. Front Immunol 2021;12:620124.
206. Vasovic M, Gajovic N, Brajkovic D, et al. The relationship between the immune system and oral manifestations of inflammatory bowel disease: a review. Cent Eur J Immunol 2016;41:302–10.
207. Zhou T, Xu W, Wang Q, et al. The effect of the "Oral-Gut" axis on periodontitis in inflammatory bowel disease: a review of microbe and immune mechanism associations. Front Cell Infect Microbiol 2023;13:1132420.
208. de Mello-Neto JM, Nunes JGR, Tadakamadla SK, et al. Immunological traits of patients with coexistent inflammatory bowel disease and periodontal disease: a systematic review. Int J Environ Res Publ Health 2021;18:8958.
209. Schmidt J, Weigert M, Leuschner C, et al. Active matrix metalloproteinase-8 and periodontal bacteria-interlink between periodontitis and inflammatory bowel disease? J Periodontol 2018;89:699–707.

210. Baima G, Massano A, Squillace E, et al. Shared microbiological and immunological patterns in periodontitis and IBD: A scoping review. Oral Dis 2022;28: 1029–41.

211. Baima G, Muwalla M, Testa G, et al. Periodontitis prevalence and severity in inflammatory bowel disease: A case-control study. J Periodontol 2023;94:313–22.

212. Bertl K, Burisch J, Pandis N, et al. Periodontitis prevalence in patients with ulcerative colitis and Crohn's disease - PPCC: A case-control study. J Clin Periodontol 2022;49:1262–74.

213. Abrol N, Compton SM, Graf D, et al. Inflammatory bowel disease and periodontitis: A retrospective chart analysis. Clin Exp Dent Res 2022;8:1028–34.

214. Voina-Tonea A, Labunet A, Objelean A, et al. A systematic analysis of the available human clinical studies of dental implant failure in patients with inflammatory bowel disease. Medicina (Kaunas) 2022;58:343.

215. Nijakowski K, Gruszczyński D, Surdacka A. Oral health status in patients with inflammatory bowel diseases: a systematic review. Int J Environ Res Publ Health 2021;18:11521.

216. She YY, Kong XB, Ge YP, et al. Periodontitis and inflammatory bowel disease: a meta-analysis. BMC Oral Health 2020;20:67.

217. Zhang L, Gao X, Zhou J, et al. Increased risks of dental caries and periodontal disease in Chinese patients with inflammatory bowel disease. Int Dent J 2020; 70:227–36.

218. Papageorgiou SN, Hagner M, Nogueira AV, et al. Inflammatory bowel disease and oral health: systematic review and a meta-analysis. J Clin Periodontol 2017;44:382–93.

219. Habashneh RA, Khader YS, Alhumouz MK, et al. The association between inflammatory bowel disease and periodontitis among Jordanians: a case-control study. J Periodontal Res 2012;47:293–8.

220. Brito F, de Barros FC, Zaltman C, et al. Prevalence of periodontitis and DMFT index in patients with Crohn's disease and ulcerative colitis. J Clin Periodontol 2008;35:555–60.

221. Grössner-Schreiber B, Fetter T, Hedderich J, et al. Prevalence of dental caries and periodontal disease in patients with inflammatory bowel disease: a case-control study. J Clin Periodontol 2006;33:478–84.

222. Haznedaroglu E, Polat E. Dental caries, dental erosion and periodontal disease in children with inflammatory bowel disease. Int J Med Sci 2023;20:682–8.

223. Koutsochristou V, Zellos A, Dimakou K, et al. Dental caries and periodontal disease in children and adolescents with inflammatory bowel disease: a case-control study. Inflamm Bowel Dis 2015;21:1839–46.

224. Bourgoin A, Agossa K, Seror R, et al. Management of dental care of patients on immunosuppressive drugs for chronic immune-related inflammatory diseases: a survey of French dentists' practices. BMC Oral Health 2023;23:545.

225. Billioud V, Ford AC, Tedesco ED, et al. Preoperative use of anti-TNF therapy and postoperative complications in inflammatory bowel diseases: a meta-analysis. J Crohns Colitis 2013;7:853–67.

226. Law CC, Bell C, Koh D, et al. Risk of postoperative infectious complications from medical therapies in inflammatory bowel disease. Cochrane Database Syst Rev 2020;10:CD013256.

227. Alsaadi G, Quirynen M, Komárek A, et al. Impact of local and systemic factors on the incidence of late oral implant loss. Clin Oral Implants Res 2008;19:670–6.

228. van Steenberghe D, Jacobs R, Desnyder M, et al. The relative impact of local and endogenous patient-related factors on implant failure up to the abutment stage. Clin Oral Implants Res 2002;13:617–22.

229. Ardizzone S, Bollani S, Bettica P, et al. Altered bone metabolism in inflammatory bowel disease: there is a difference between Crohn's disease and ulcerative colitis. J Intern Med 2000;247:63–70.

230. Alsaadi G, Quirynen M, Michiles K, et al. Impact of local and systemic factors on the incidence of failures up to abutment connection with modified surface oral implants. J Clin Periodontol 2008;35:51–7.

231. Bornstein MM, Cionca N, Mombelli A. Systemic conditions and treatments as risks for implant therapy. Int J Oral Maxillofac Implants 2009;24 Suppl:12–27.

232. Ji YLH. Malignancies in HIV-Infected and AIDS Patients. Adv Exp Med Biol 2017;2018:167–79.

233. Shiels MS, Pfeiffer RM, Gail MH, et al. Cancer burden in the HIV-infected population in the United States. J Natl Cancer Inst 2011;103:753–62.

234. Ryder MI. Periodontal management of HIV-infected patients. Periodontol 2000 2000;23:85–93.

235. Smith GL, Felix DH, Wray D. Current classifications of HIV-associated periodontal diseases. Br Dent J 1993;174:102–5.

236. Robinson PG, Winkler JR, Palmer G, et al. The diagnosis of periodontal conditions associated with HIV infection. J Periodontol 1994;65:236–43.

237. Lamster IB, Begg MD, Mitchell-Lewis D, et al. Oral manifestations of HIV infection in homosexual men and intravenous drug users. Study design and relationship of epidemiologic, clinical, and immunologic parameters to oral lesions. Oral Surg Oral Med Oral Pathol 1994;78:163–74.

238. Klein RS, Harris CA, Small CB, et al. Oral candidiasis in high-risk patients as the initial manifestation of the acquired immunodeficiency syndrome. N Engl J Med 1984;311:354–8.

239. Greenspan D, Greenspan JS, Overby G, et al. Risk factors for rapid progression from hairy leukoplakia to AIDS: a nested case-control study. J Acquir Immune Defic Syndr (1988) 1991;4:652–8.

240. Feigal DW, Katz MH, Greenspan D, et al. The prevalence of oral lesions in HIV-infected homosexual and bisexual men: three San Francisco epidemiological cohorts. AIDS 1991;5:519–25.

241. Glick M, Muzyka BC, Lurie D, et al. Oral manifestations associated with HIV-related disease as markers for immune suppression and AIDS. Oral Surg Oral Med Oral Pathol 1994;77:344–9.

242. Glick M, Muzyka BC, Salkin LM, et al. Necrotizing ulcerative periodontitis: a marker for immune deterioration and a predictor for the diagnosis of AIDS. J Periodontol 1994;65:393–7.

243. Winkler JR, Robertson PB. Periodontal disease associated with HIV infection. Oral Surg Oral Med Oral Pathol 1992;73:145–50.

244. Nobre AVV, Pólvora TLS, Ramos Peña DE, et al. Effect of non-surgical periodontal therapy on clinical parameters of periodontitis, oral candida spp. count and lactoferrin and histatin expression in saliva and gingival crevicular fluid of HIV-infected patients. Curr HIV Res 2023;21:27–34.

245. Shintani T, Okada M, Iwata T, et al. Relationship between CD4+ T-cell counts at baseline and initial periodontal treatment efficacy in patients undergoing treatment for HIV infection: A retrospective observational study. J Clin Periodontol 2023;50:1520–9.

246. Murray PA, Grassi M, Winkler JR. The microbiology of HIV-associated periodontal lesions. J Clin Periodontol 1989;16:636–42.

247. Murray PA, Winkler JR, Peros WJ, et al. DNA probe detection of periodontal pathogens in HIV-associated periodontal lesions. Oral Microbiol Immunol 1991;6:34–40.

248. Ata-Ali J, Ata-Ali F, Di-Benedetto N, et al. Does HIV infection have an impact upon dental implant osseointegration? a systematic review. Med Oral Patol Oral Cir Bucal 2015;20:e347–56.

249. Sivakumar I, Arunachalam S, Choudhary S, et al. Does HIV infection affect the survival of dental implants? a systematic review and meta-analysis. J Prosthet Dent 2021;125:862–9.

250. Komatsu A, Ikeda A, Kikuchi A, et al. Osteoporosis-related fractures in HIV-infected patients receiving long-term tenofovir disoproxil fumarate: an observational cohort study. Drug Saf 2018;41:843–8.

251. Hileman CO, Eckard AR, McComsey GA. Bone loss in HIV: a contemporary review. Curr Opin Endocrinol Diabetes Obes 2015;22:446–51.

252. Hwang D, Wang HL. Medical contraindications to implant therapy: Part II: Relative contraindications. Implant Dent 2007;16:13–23.

253. Leite RS, Marlow NM, Fernandes JK, et al. Oral health and type 2 diabetes. Am J Med Sci 2013;345:271–3.

254. Păunică I, Giurgiu M, Dumitriu AS, et al. The bidirectional relationship between periodontal disease and diabetes mellitus-a Review. Diagnostics (Basel) 2023; 13:681.

255. Falcao A, Bullon P. A review of the influence of periodontal treatment in systemic diseases. Periodontol 2000 2019;79:117–28.

256. Ziukaite L, Slot DE, Van der Weijden FA. Prevalence of diabetes mellitus in people clinically diagnosed with periodontitis: a systematic review and meta-analysis of epidemiologic studies. J Clin Periodontol 2018;45:650–62.

257. Genco RJ, Borgnakke WS. Diabetes as a potential risk for periodontitis: association studies. Periodontol 2000 2020;83:40–5.

258. Graves DT, Ding Z, Yang Y. The impact of diabetes on periodontal diseases. Periodontol 2000 2020;82:214–24.

259. Engebretson SP, Hyman LG, Michalowicz BS, et al. The effect of nonsurgical periodontal therapy on hemoglobin A1c levels in persons with type 2 diabetes and chronic periodontitis: a randomized clinical trial. JAMA 2013;310:2523–32.

260. Costa FO, Miranda Cota LO, Pereira Lages EJ, et al. Progression of periodontitis and tooth loss associated with glycemic control in individuals undergoing periodontal maintenance therapy: a 5-year follow-up study. J Periodontol 2013;84: 595–605.

261. Spampinato SF, Caruso GI, De Pasquale R, et al. The treatment of impaired wound healing in diabetes: looking among old drugs. Pharmaceuticals (Basel) 2020;13:60.

262. Wetzler C, Kämpfer H, Stallmeyer B, et al. Large and sustained induction of chemokines during impaired wound healing in the genetically diabetic mouse: prolonged persistence of neutrophils and macrophages during the late phase of repair. J Invest Dermatol 2000;115:245–53.

263. Schacter GI, Leslie WD. Diabetes and bone disease. Endocrinol Metab Clin North Am 2017;46:63–85.

264. Wang X, Wang H, Zhang T, et al. Current knowledge regarding the interaction between oral bone metabolic disorders and diabetes mellitus. Front Endocrinol (Lausanne) 2020;11:536.

265. Polak D, Shapira L. An update on the evidence for pathogenic mechanisms that may link periodontitis and diabetes. J Clin Periodontol 2019;45:150–66.

266. Taylor JJ, Preshaw PM, Lalla E. A review of the evidence for pathogenic mechanisms that may link periodontitis and diabetes. J Clin Periodontol 2013; 40(Suppl 14):S113–34.

267. Yoon MS, Jankowski V, Montag S, et al. Characterisation of advanced glycation endproducts in saliva from patients with diabetes mellitus. Biochem Biophys Res Commun 2014;323:377–81.

268. Notsu M, Yamaguchi T, Okazaki K, et al. Advanced glycation end product 3 (AGE3) suppresses the mineralization of mouse stromal ST2 cells and human mesenchymal stem cells by increasing TGF-β expression and secretion. Endocrinology 2014;155:2402–10.

269. Drosatos-Tampakaki Z, Drosatos K, Siegelin Y, et al. Palmitic acid and DGAT1 deficiency enhance osteoclastogenesis, while oleic acid-induced triglyceride formation prevents it. J Bone Miner Res 2014;29:1183–95.

270. Wu YY, Xiao E, Graves DT. Diabetes mellitus related bone metabolism and periodontal disease. Int J Oral Sci 2015;7:63–72.

271. Santos VR, Lima JA, De Mendonça AC, et al. Effectiveness of full-mouth and partial-mouth scaling and root planing in treating chronic periodontitis in subjects with type 2 diabetes. J Periodontol 2009;80:1237–45.

272. Faria-Almeida R, Navarro A, Bascones A. Clinical and metabolic changes after conventional treatment of type 2 diabetic patients with chronic periodontitis. J Periodontol 2006;77:591–8.

273. Jervøe-Storm PM, Semaan E, AlAhdab H, et al. Clinical outcomes of quadrant root planing versus full-mouth root planing. J Clin Periodontol 2006;33:209–15.

274. Promsudthi A, Pimapansri S, Deerochanawong C, et al. The effect of periodontal therapy on uncontrolled type 2 diabetes mellitus in older subjects. Oral Dis 2005;11:293–8.

275. Apatzidou DA, Kinane DF. Quadrant root planing versus same-day full-mouth root planing. I. Clinical findings. J Clin Periodontol 2004;31:132–40.

276. Westfelt E, Rylander H, Blohmé G, et al. The effect of periodontal therapy in diabetics. Results after 5 years. J Clin Periodontol 1996;23:92–100.

277. Shang R, Gao L. Impact of hyperglycemia on the rate of implant failure and peri-implant parameters in patients with type 2 diabetes mellitus: Systematic review and meta-analysis. J Am Dent Assoc 2021;152:189–201.e181.

278. Jiang X, Zhu Y, Liu Z, et al. Association between diabetes and dental implant complications: a systematic review and meta-analysis. Acta Odontol Scand 2021;79:9–18.

279. Meza Maurício J, Miranda TS, Almeida ML, et al. An umbrella review on the effects of diabetes on implant failure and peri-implant diseases. Braz Oral Res 2019;33(suppl 1):e070.

280. Lu B, Zhang X, Liu B. A systematic review and meta-analysis on influencing factors of failure of oral implant restoration treatment. Ann Palliat Med 2021;10: 12664–77.

281. Chrcanovic BR, Albrektsson T, Wennerberg A. Diabetes and oral implant failure: a systematic review. J Dent Res 2014;93:859–67.

282. Organization WH. Cardiovascular diseases (CVDs). Available at: https://wwwwhoint/news-room/fact-sheets/detail/cardiovascular-diseases-(cvds). Accessed on January 30, 2024. 2021.

283. Herrera D, Sanz M, Shapira L, et al. Association between periodontal diseases and cardiovascular diseases, diabetes and respiratory diseases: Consensus

report of the Joint Workshop by the European Federation of Periodontology (EFP) and the European arm of the World Organization of Family Doctors (WONCA Europe). J Clin Periodontol 2023;50:819–41.

284. Herrera D, Molina A, Buhlin K, et al. Periodontal diseases and association with atherosclerotic disease. Periodontol 2000 2020;83:66–89.

285. Reyes L, Herrera D, Kozarov E, et al. Periodontal bacterial invasion and infection: contribution to atherosclerotic pathology. J Clin Periodontol 2013; 40(Suppl 14):S30–50.

286. Schenkein HA, Loos BG. Inflammatory mechanisms linking periodontal diseases to cardiovascular diseases. J Clin Periodontol 2013;40(Suppl 14):S51–69.

287. Rafferty B, Jönsson D, Kalachikov S, et al. Impact of monocytic cells on recovery of uncultivable bacteria from atherosclerotic lesions. J Intern Med 2011;270: 273–80.

288. Del Pinto R, Pietropaoli D, Munoz-Aguilera E, et al. Periodontitis and Hypertension: Is the Association Causal? High Blood Press Cardiovasc Prev 2020;27: 281–9.

289. Dietrich T, Sharma P, Walter C, et al. The epidemiological evidence behind the association between periodontitis and incident atherosclerotic cardiovascular disease. J Clin Periodontol 2013;40(Suppl 14):S70–84.

290. Sanz M, Marco Del Castillo A, Jepsen S, et al. Periodontitis and cardiovascular diseases: Consensus report. J Clin Periodontol 2020;47:268–88.

291. Orlandi M, Graziani F, D'Aiuto F. Periodontal therapy and cardiovascular risk. Periodontol 2000 2020;83:107–24.

292. Sanz M, Ceriello A, Buysschaert M, et al. Scientific evidence on the links between periodontal diseases and diabetes: Consensus report and guidelines of the joint workshop on periodontal diseases and diabetes by the International diabetes Federation and the European Federation of Periodontology. Diabetes Res Clin Pract 2018;137:231–41.

Systemic Factors Affecting Prognosis in Periodontics

Part II

Priyanka Kodaganallur Pitchumani, BDS, MS[a],
Srishti Parekh, BDS, MDS[b], Rachana Hegde, BDS, MS[c],
Davis C. Thomas, BDS, DDS, MSD, MSc Med, MSc[d],*

KEYWORDS

- Systemic factors • Periodontal prognosis • Periodontal outcomes
- Smoking and periodontitis • Implant prognosis • Implant osseointegration
- Implant failure

KEY POINTS

- An in-depth awareness about systemic factors that could affect prognosis and outcomes is essential for the clinician.
- Suboptimal response to conventional periodontal therapeutic modalities should raise a red flag for the clinician and must prompt further appropriate investigations.
- The clinician should also be cognizant of the importance of referral to the appropriate physician, if a systemic factor modifying treatment prognosis is suspected or proven.

INTRODUCTION

Periodontitis is the sixth most prevalent disease condition, and the number one cause for loss of teeth in the adult population.[1] Tooth loss in patients with periodontitis can be influenced by several variables and may be broadly classified as patient factors, tooth-related factors, systemic factors, and miscellaneous. The patient factors include age, gender, habits, obesity, compliance with oral hygiene, and attitude toward dentistry and dental health, among others.[2,3] Systemic factors include, but not limited to genetics, disease conditions, immunity, nutrition, stress, and medications.[4] Tooth factors include occlusion (trauma from), crown-root ratio, tooth morphology, restorations, force applied on the teeth, position of tooth in the arch, crowding, and anatomic variations.[5] The miscellaneous factors include access to care, health coverage status, and socioeconomic status. All these factors may directly or indirectly enhance or

[a] Department of Periodontics, University of Iowa College of Dentistry and Dental Clinics, Iowa City, IA 52242, USA; [b] Private Practice, Mumbai, India; [c] University of Utah, USA; [d] Department of Diagnostic Sciences, Center for Temporomandibular Disorders and Orofacial Pain, Rutgers School of Dental Medicine, Newark, NJ, USA
* Corresponding author. Department of Diagnostic Sciences, Rutgers School of Dental Medicine, 110 Bergen Street, Newark, NJ 07103.
E-mail address: davisct1@gmail.com

Dent Clin N Am 68 (2024) 603–617
https://doi.org/10.1016/j.cden.2024.07.002   dental.theclinics.com

negate the risk of tooth loss in periodontal disease. In this study, we consider systemic factors including age, hematological disorders, smoking, nutrition, obesity/metabolic syndrome, hypertension (HTN), and sleep. The other systemic factors are discussed in detail elsewhere in the special issue. The reader is reminded that many, if not all, systemic factors can have considerable overlap.

AGE

Older adults with periodontitis were shown to be associated with greater risk of tooth loss in a few studies.[6–11] In patients aged less than 30 years, treating early periodontitis combined with smoking cessation was found to be associated with preventing the disease progression and minimizing further tooth loss.[9] A Swedish study showed that the prevalence of periodontitis increased with age, and in the cohort of the oldest age group, overall oral health was poor despite frequent dental visits.[10] Older individuals had more average bone loss, but least degree of attachment loss.[11] Relatively new scientific terminologies, such as, inflammaging, immunosenescence, and age-related diseases have been introduced into the most recent literature.[12–15] Immunosenescence includes factors such as loss of proteostasis, telomere attrition, mitochondrial dysfunction, oxidative stress, cellular senescence, and epigenetic alterations.[12] Inflammaging includes factors such as increase in proinflammatory mediators, increase in blood pressure, and increased glycosylated hemoglobin (HbA_1C). With regards to the effects of aging on implant survival rate and osseointegration, most published studies favor a general conclusion that aging has no direct deleterious effects on implants.[16,17] However, isolated studies have proposed a possible "incremental positive association" between aging and implant failure.[18]

HYPERTENSION

HTN is thought to affect more than a billion individuals worldwide.[19] The classification of HTN has gone through changes over the last several decades, seemingly indicating an even lower acceptable normal value of blood pressure.[20,21] A number of hypotheses have been proposed as to the exact mechanism of the relationship between HTN and periodontitis, although unclear, it has been thought to be bidirectional.[19] Currently, the link between periodontitis and HTN is described as "plausible." It must be noted that, according to the 2017 World Workshop of Periodontitis, there is an inconclusive association between HTN and periodontitis.[22] A relatively recent cardinal study concluded that aggressive periodontal treatment resulted in short-term inflammation systemically, as well as endothelial dysfunction.[23] The same study showed that endothelial function was improved as a benefit of periodontal treatment in a 6 month timeline. As to the question of the potential for antihypertensive medications affecting periodontal prognosis and treatment outcomes, further succinct studies are necessary.

The direct effect of HTN on implant osseointegration and survival is not clearly understood. However, antihypertensive medications in general,[24] and beta blockers, thiazides, calcium channel blockers and ACE inhibitors in particular, seem to favor osseointegration and increased implant survival rate.[25–28] It must be noted, any conclusive evidence for any of these associations or correlations must be based on future, well-controlled, succinct scientific studies.

SLEEP

A bidirectional relationship has been proposed between sleep quality/duration and disease severity and progression of periodontitis.[29] As with other factors that affect tooth loss in periodontitis, the exact mechanism here is not known. Several hypotheses have been put forward as to how disturbed sleep and sleep disorders can affect tooth loss in periodontitis.[30] Sleep disturbances have been shown to adversely affect the immune system.[31] Both long and short sleep duration have been proposed to be causing immune dysfunction. Long sleep duration not only impairs the immune system[32] but also causes induction of systemic inflammation.[33,34] A short duration of sleep can cause imbalance between the immune system and the microflora of the periodontium.[31] Once again, activation of proinflammatory cytokines by disturbed sleep[35] may contribute mechanistically to immune dysfunction and altered periodontal microflora,[31] thereby worsening periodontitis and eventually enhancing tooth loss.[36]

Inadequate sleep has been hypothesized to be associated with a lower number of teeth present and also with periodontal disease. Obstructive sleep apnea (OSA) has been shown to be a disorder associated with systemic inflammation.[37] A bidirectional relationship has been suggested between OSA and periodontitis, although the exact mechanisms of one entity feeding into the other are yet to be elucidated.[38] Periodontitis has also been shown to have a moderate to significant direct association with OSA.[39,40] It must be noted that there are isolated recent studies that have proposed relatively low evidence of this possible association.[41] Further research and studies in this regard are warranted. The effect on sleep quality and other sleep parameters on dental implant prognosis is not currently clear in the literature. However, the plausible effects of sleep-related conditions such as bruxism on dental implants and restorations have been proposed.[42]

NUTRITION

Role of nutrition in periodontal disease progression and the resultant tooth loss has not been robustly published in the literature. However, there are indicators that deficiency of certain nutritional factors may be associated with increased rate and severity of disease progression, and conceivable tooth loss resulting from it.[43] The current treatment modalities have been aimed at mitigating the bacterial load to control the inflammatory process in the host. However, the role of diet in decreasing the inflammatory response and oxidative stress, has gained some importance.[44]

Vitamin B12 is one of the nutritional factors shown to have an inverse association with periodontal disease progression and risk of tooth loss.[45] Deficiency of the vitamin was shown to be associated with increased probing depth, increased mean clinical attachment loss, and increased risk of tooth loss. Similarly, vitamin D has been suggested as being a protective factor against periodontitis, caries, and tooth loss. A recent study showed that, for every 10 μg per liter increase of serum vitamin D was associated with a reduction in the risk of tooth loss by approximately 15%.[46] Vitamin C is known to have a role in collagen synthesis, immune function, and wound healing. A recent study showed strong suggestive evidence that vitamin C deficiency has association with periodontitis disease severity, and increased C-reactive protein, a marker of inflammation.[47] From the available limited literature, it seems that these nutritional factors are important in predicting a favorable prognosis for periodontal therapy.

There is limited evidence of the role of lipids and fatty acids in periodontal disease progression and its effect on therapy. The lipid content of the cell membrane and the hematological levels of lipoproteins have been linked with susceptibility to oxidative damage.[48] In addition, the host response to bacterial products can also be affected by the cell membrane lipid profile of host.[49] There has been limited evidence to suggest the role of fatty acids in having a positive role in prevention of, and favorable response to, periodontal treatment.[50] Similarly, saturated fat-rich diets increase oxidative stress and in turn increase the inflammatory process.[49] An inverse relationship has been reported between plasma ascorbic acid (vitamin C) levels and the degree of periodontal inflammation, as well as severity in various populations and age groups.[51] Higher vitamin E intake was also associated with a lower number of teeth affected by attachment loss. Conversely, low serum alpha-tocopherol (vitamin E) levels were associated with periodontal disease progression.[52] Similarly, positive effect of higher alpha-tocopherol intake on periodontal healing after subgingival scaling and root planing has been shown.[48,52] The adjunctive intake of vitamin E has been proposed to have some beneficial effects on periodontal parameters as well as antioxidant defense compared to controls; however, further controlled studies are necessary.[52] Low serum calcium–magnesium ratio has been proposed to be associated with an increased attachment loss and the progression of periodontal disease.[52]

A recent systematic review investigated the usefulness of dietary and nutraceutical adjuncts in nonsurgical periodontal therapy.[53] A significant decrease in probing depth and bleeding on probing were found with supplementation of vitamin E, chicory extract, juice powder, green tea, and oolong tea.[53] In summary, there is a lack of robust scientific evidence to prove a causal relationship between nutrition and periodontal prognosis. However, there is increasing evidence to suggest that diets that reduce oxidative stress levels and have anti-inflammatory properties are associated with delayed progression of periodontal disease and better therapy outcomes. The exact role of nutrition, and the effect of nutritional deficiencies on dental implant survival and osseointegration, is not clearly defined in the available literature. Animal studies have yielded mixed results regarding the effect of nutrition on dental implants.[54] The only plausible positive association is for vitamin D, the deficiency of which, seems to favor failure of osseointegration.[54] Also, vitamin D supplementation seems to enhance osseointegration.[55,56]

HEMATOLOGICAL DISORDERS

Some specific hematological disorders have been reported to increase the severity and progression of periodontal attachment loss.[22] Defects in neutrophil migration and function, as well as defects in neutrophil-associated homeostasis, have been significantly associated with periodontal breakdown.[22,57] Periodontitis has been shown to be associated with congenital neutropenia.[22,58,59] Cohen syndrome, a condition associated with neutropenia, was found to be associated with increased, and early periodontal breakdown.[60] Patients with leukocyte adhesion deficiency syndromes have been shown to have recurrent infections, severe gingival inflammations, ulcerations, and early onset rapid bone loss.[61,62] Many of these patients have early loss of primary and permanent dentition.[63] Similarly, patients with congenital neutropenia and cyclic neutropenia are also reported to have increased incidence of recurrent infections, oral ulcerations, and premature loss of dentition.[64–67] Cyclic neutropenia has also been proposed to have an associated increased periodontal bone loss and, conceivably, a poorer prognosis for orthodontic and surgical periodontal treatment.[68] Currently, there is a lack of scientific literature as to the exact mechanistic pathogenesis of how hematological disorders may adversely affect the prognosis and treatment outcomes of periodontal therapy.

Although there is lack of succinct evidence, the limited data available seem to indicate that, provided that the necessary precautions for hemostasis are followed, bleeding disorders may not have a detrimental effect on dental implant osseointegration and implant survival. However, most of the studies that evaluated the effect of bleeding disorders on implants, were derived from information on the effects of tooth extraction and healing after extraction.[69] Early, but limited, data seem to suggest that Von-Willebrand disease may be specifically associated with implant failure upon loading.[70]

SMOKING

Smoking, due to its established detrimental effect on the initiation, progression, and treatment of periodontal disease, has been identified as a "grade modifier" in the new periodontitis classification of 2017.[71,72] The incidence and severity of periodontitis has been shown to increase up to 8 folds depending on the amount of smoking.[73,74] The likeliness of a causal relationship between smoking and tooth loss has been reported in several studies.[73] It is interesting to note that there is published literature on cigarette smoking being a statistically significant risk factor for loss of implants, although the latter does not have a periodontal ligament to be lost. Several systematic reviews and meta-analyses have concluded that cessation of smoking leads to lowering the risk of developing and progression of periodontitis and has a better response to periodontal therapy, to both surgical and nonsurgical interventions.[74–76] It is noteworthy that epidemiologic studies that accounted for nonsmokers that were exposed to second-hand smoking, suggest similar incidence and pathogenesis of oral and periodontal diseases as that of smokers.[77] The reason suggested is that second-hand tobacco smoking leads to exposure of the oral cavity to similar toxins to that of active smoking, resulting in similar harmful effects.[77] A recent systematic review that compared the effects of electronic cigarettes and heat-not-burn tobacco products, concluded that the clinical inflammatory signs of periodontitis may be reduced in e-cigarette users as opposed to traditional tobacco smokers.[78] However, another systematic review shows increased periodontal destruction in patients using e-cigarettes compared to healthy controls.[79] Besides tobacco smoking, smoking of other substances such as cannabis, crack/cocaine, and 3,4-methylenedioxy-methamphetamine has also been shown to have a positive association with the development and progression of periodontal disease.[80]

Numerous clinical studies have explored the effects of various types of periodontal therapy on both smokers and nonsmokers. Smoking has been linked to poorer outcomes across periodontal treatment modalities, with high rates of refractory periodontitis among smokers.[81] Comparatively, nonsmokers tend to show improved outcomes such as reduced probing depths, less bleeding, and enhanced clinical attachment following nonsurgical and surgical interventions.[73,82–84] Similar trends have been observed in regenerative procedures and the treatment of furcation lesions.[73] However, a recent systematic review and meta analyses that studied the effect of smoking on root coverage procedures could not come to a definite conclusion due to scarcity of data.[85]

Although the detrimental effects of smoking on periodontal disease has been established,[86] the exact mechanism remains unknown. The human microbiome can be influenced by smoking through either direct effects or indirect effects.[73,87] It is shown that the pathogenic bacteria are able to colonize shallow pockets in smokers, and there is a significant shift in the balance between the commensals and the pathogens, favoring the latter.[86,88] This could be attributed to the lowered oxygen concentration caused due to smoking that enables the rapid growth of anaerobic bacteria. Bacterial adherence to the epithelial cells is also enhanced, which plays a key role in bacterial aggregation in plaque formation.[87] Several leads in the direction of how smoking limits the response of tissues to periodontal treatment have been published. Nicotine may mediate the specific inflammatory signs and symptoms in smokers.[83,89,90] Nicotine has been shown to be vasoconstrictive and delay wound healing, thereby impairing healing following surgical periodontal therapy. Nicotine also interferes with adhesion molecules of the vascular endothelium such as soluble intercellular adhesion molecule -1 (sICAM-1), and an increased concentration of these molecules in the gingival crevicular fluid (GCF) may be an indicator of increase in destructive enzymes such as elastase.[91,92] It has also been reported that nicotine in association with *Porphyromonas gingivalis* may lead to collagen breakdown and bone resorption.[73,86]

GCF levels of proinflammatory cytokines, tumor necrosis factor alpha (TNF- α), and interleukin (IL)-8 are also increased in smokers,[78] indicating that smoking interferes with the inflammatory defense mechanisms of the periodontium.[93–95] Smoking also inhibits regenerative functions of the periodontium, thereby hampering its chances for renewal.[96–98] In addition to nicotine, other deleterious agents in tobacco smoke may interfere with the healing process.[99–101] Although it is evident that there is robust literature pointing to the possible mechanisms of the deleterious effects of smoking on periodontal tissues, further studies at a cellular and molecular level are essential for establishing the mechanism of a causality of tooth loss in smokers.

OBESITY AND METABOLIC SYNDROME

Metabolic syndrome, sometimes referred to as "Syndrome X"[102,103] is a collection of conditions including central obesity, dyslipidemia, insulin resistance, and arterial HTN that are interconnected. The classic metabolic triad is a combination of hyperglycemia, hyperlipidemia, and HTN. Collectively, these conditions heighten the likelihood of developing cardiovascular diseases and type 2 diabetes mellitus.[103,104] Weight gain and obesity have been identified as risk factors for periodontal disease. A number of systematic reviews and meta-analyses have shown a positive association between overweight individuals and obesity with periodontal disease.[105–107] The mechanism proposed for this association is the affected host immunity, in terms of increase in proinflammatory cytokines such as IL-1β, TNF-α, and IL-6, which are elevated by adipocytes and macrophages in the adipose tissues of people identified as obese, along with T-cell/monocyte/macrophage dysfunction.[108,109] The other postulated mechanism is the systemic oxidative stress causing higher levels of reactive oxygen species (ROS) in turn leading to a heightened inflammatory response. Interference in osteoblast differentiation has also been observed.[110] Certain studies have also shown an increase in the number of periodontal pathogens, such as *Tannerella forsythia*, *Fusobacterium* spp, and *P gingivalis* in the biofilm of the saliva of individuals with obesity.[111–113] It is conceivable, although not yet shown, that metabolic syndrome may be associated with relatively poor periodontal prognosis. It is important to note that though an association has been established, the causality yet needs to be proven.

STRESS

Stress can have direct or indirect effect on the periodontium. The indirect effects are the ones mediated via lifestyle changes that can enhance periodontal destruction.[114] These may include, a compromised oral hygiene, lack of compliance with dental hygiene visits, metabolic abnormalities, and increased habits (smoking, alcohol, and substance use disorder). The direct effects may be mediated by alterations in the composition of the subgingival biofilm and exaggerated inflammatory host response.[115] High financial stress and poor coping skills were reported to be associated with significantly higher loss of alveolar bone, and greater attachment loss than the ones with lower stress levels. This study was adjusted for age, sex, and cigarette smoking.[116] Similar results were found in several other studies.[117–121] There is mounting evidence for a positive association between psychosocial stress and poor periodontal status.

Stress has been shown to activate the hypothalamic-pituitary-adrenal axis, leading to increased secretion of cortisol. This hormone dysregulates the immune system. In addition, autonomic nervous system activation can also impact the immune system[122] and inflammatory response. The blood, saliva, and GCF of patients with periodontitis have shown several stress markers that are positively associated with the extent and severity of periodontitis.[123] Further, these have been shown to mediate the detrimental effects of stress on the periodontal tissues.[122–126] Animal studies have corroborated the link between stress and periodontal disease severity and destruction by virtue of proinflammatory molecules.[127,128] Stress hormones have been shown to favor the growth of periodontal pathogens.[129,130] From the available current literature, it appears that stress, through various proposed mechanisms, enhances periodontal inflammation, increases bone destruction, and, therefore, facilitates tooth loss.

IMMUNODEFICIENCY

The relationship between immune compromise and periodontal disease seems to be bidirectional.[131,132] Factors such as host susceptibility to exogenous and indigenous microorganisms, host response to microbes as well as to periodontal therapy, among others, can influence the relationship between immunity and periodontal disease.[133] Increasing evidence points to factors such as mitochondrial dysfunction acting as a common factor in the pathogenesis of periodontitis as well as systemic diseases such as diabetes.[133] Immune deficiencies can affect periodontal integrity, as well as having other marked effects on the host. Immune deficiency entities can lead to gingival enlargement, impairment of hemostasis, and development of oral lesions secondary to opportunistic infections.[134] This could be true of patients having adverse reactions to medications as well. In immune compromised patients, there is a purported higher risk of local and systemic infections. Consequently, antibiotic prophylaxis may

Table 1
Possible mechanisms of association of increased risk of periodontal disease

Systemic Factor	Possible Mechanisms
Age	Loss of proteostasis, telomere attrition, mitochondrial dysfunction, oxidative stress, cellular senescence, and epigenetic alterations[12]
HTN	Inconclusive; antihypertensives seem to have a positive effect on the implant osseointegration[25–28]
Sleep	Activation of proinflammatory cytokines
Nutrition	Inconclusive
Hematological disorders	Neutrophil dysfunction[22,57]
Smoking	Lowered oxygen concentration,[135] enabling the rapid growth of anaerobic bacteria,[86] increased bacterial adherence to epithelial cells,[87] increase in proinflammatory cytokines IL-8, TNF-α, changes in vascularity,[136] changes in neutrophil function,[136] reduction in immunoglobulin G concentration,[136] increase in periodontal pathogens[136]
Obesity/metabolic syndrome	Affected host immunity, increase in inflammatory cytokines such as IL-6, TNF-α, increase in ROS, T-cell/monocyte/macrophage dysfunction, and increase in periodontal pathogens[108,109]

be necessary either before or after periodontal therapies.[134] The mechanisms by which the systemic diseases discussed in this study increase the risk of periodontal disease is summarized in **Table 1**.

SUMMARY

It is essential that the oral health care provider carefully assesses the systemic history of patients presenting with periodontal disease. A sound knowledge of systemic factors that may affect the prognosis and outcome of periodontal treatment is crucial for an astute clinician. A systematic, multidisciplinary treatment approach may be necessary and of utmost importance in patients with one or more systemic factors, affecting short-term and long-term prognosis. Further succinct studies are required in this regard.

CLINICS CARE POINTS

- The astute clinician should be well-versed with the systemic factors that can affect periodontal prognosis.
- Smoking is one of the key modifying risk factors in significantly adversely affecting periodontal prognosis and treatment outcomes.
- A carefully taken detailed social, and medical history including current and past medications is paramount in predicting the prognosis and outcomes of periodontal treatment.

ACKNOWLEDGMENTS

None

DISCLOSURE

P. Kodaganallur Pitchumani, S. Parekh, R. Hegde, and D.C Thomas declare no conflict of interest. Funding statement: There was no funding for this study. Statement of institutional review board approval or waiver: Institutional review and approval were not necessary for this article.

REFERENCES

1. Balta MG, Papathanasiou E, Blix IJ, et al. Host Modulation and Treatment of Periodontal Disease. J Dent Res 2021;100(8):798–809.
2. El Sayed N, Cosgarea R, Rahim S, et al. Patient-, tooth-, and dentist-related factors influencing long-term tooth retention after resective therapy in an academic setting-a retrospective study. Clin Oral Investig 2020;24(7):2341–9.
3. Koshi E, Rajesh S, Koshi P, et al. Risk assessment for periodontal disease. J Indian Soc Periodontol 2012;16(3):324–8.
4. Genco RJ, Borgnakke WS. Risk factors for periodontal disease. Periodontol 2000. 2013;62(1):59–94.
5. Matthews DC, Tabesh M. Detection of localized tooth-related factors that predispose to periodontal infections. Periodontol 2000 2004;34:136–50.
6. El Sayed N, Rahim-Wöstefeld S, Stocker F, et al. The 2018 classification of periodontal diseases: Its predictive value for tooth loss. J Periodontol 2022;93(4): 560–9.

7. Nilsson H, Sanmartin Berglund J, Renvert S. Longitudinal evaluation of peri-odontitis and tooth loss among older adults. J Clin Periodontol 2019;46(10): 1041–9.

8. Helal O, Göstemeyer G, Krois J, et al. Predictors for tooth loss in periodontitis patients: Systematic review and meta-analysis. J Clin Periodontol 2019;46(7): 699–712.

9. Ramseier CA, Anerud A, Dulac M, et al. Natural history of periodontitis: Disease progression and tooth loss over 40 years. J Clin Periodontol 2017;44(12): 1182–91.

10. Renvert S, Persson RE, Persson GR. Tooth loss and periodontitis in older individ-uals: results from the Swedish National Study on Aging and Care. J Periodontol 2013;84(8):1134–44.

11. Machtei EE, Hausmann E, Dunford R, et al. Longitudinal study of predictive fac-tors for periodontal disease and tooth loss. J Clin Periodontol 1999;26(6): 374–80.

12. Baima G, Romandini M, Citterio F, et al. Periodontitis and Accelerated Biological Aging: A Geroscience Approach. J Dent Res 2022;101(2):125–32.

13. Albuquerque-Souza E, Crump KE, Rattanaprukskul K, et al. TLR9 Mediates Peri-odontal Aging by Fostering Senescence and Inflammaging. J Dent Res 2022; 101(13):1628–36.

14. Aquino-Martinez R. The Emerging Role of Accelerated Cellular Senescence in Periodontitis. J Dent Res 2023;102(8):854–62.

15. Chen S, Zhou D, Liu O, et al. Cellular Senescence and Periodontitis: Mecha-nisms and Therapeutics. Biology (Basel) 2022;11(10). https://doi.org/10.3390/ biology11101419.

16. Schimmel M, Srinivasan M, McKenna G, et al. Effect of advanced age and/or systemic medical conditions on dental implant survival: A systematic review and meta-analysis. Clin Oral Implants Res 2018;29(Suppl 16):311–30.

17. Etöz O, Bertl K, Kukla E, et al. How old is old for implant therapy in terms of implant survival and marginal bone levels after 5-11 years? Clin Oral Implants Res 2021;32(3):337–48.

18. Raikar S, Talukdar P, Kumari S, et al. Factors Affecting the Survival Rate of Dental Implants: A Retrospective Study. J Int Soc Prev Community Dent Nov--Dec 2017;7(6):351–5.

19. Del Pinto R, Pietropaoli D, Munoz-Aguilera E, et al. Periodontitis and Hyperten-sion: Is the Association Causal? High Blood Press Cardiovasc Prev 2020;27(4): 281–9.

20. Whelton PK, Carey RM, Aronow WS, et al. 2017 ACC/AHA/AAPA/ABC/ACPM/ AGS/APhA/ASH/ASPC/NMA/PCNA Guideline for the Prevention, Detection, Evaluation, and Management of High Blood Pressure in Adults: A Report of the American College of Cardiology/American Heart Association Task Force on Clinical Practice Guidelines. Hypertension 2018;71(6):e13–115.

21. Mancia G, Kreutz R, Brunström M, et al. 2023 ESH Guidelines for the manage-ment of arterial hypertension The Task Force for the management of arterial hy-pertension of the European Society of Hypertension: Endorsed by the International Society of Hypertension (ISH) and the European Renal Association (ERA). J Hypertens 2023;41(12):1874–2071.

22. Albandar JM, Susin C, Hughes FJ. Manifestations of systemic diseases and conditions that affect the periodontal attachment apparatus: Case definitions and diagnostic considerations. J Periodontol 2018;89(Suppl 1):S183–203.

23. Tonetti MS, D'Aiuto F, Nibali L, et al. Treatment of periodontitis and endothelial function. N Engl J Med 2007;356(9):911–20.

24. Pierroz DD, Bonnet N, Bianchi EN, et al. Deletion of β-adrenergic receptor 1, 2, or both leads to different bone phenotypes and response to mechanical stimulation. J Bone Miner Res 2012;27(6):1252–62.

25. Al-Subaie AE, Laurenti M, Abdallah MN, et al. Propranolol enhances bone healing and implant osseointegration in rats tibiae. J Clin Periodontol 2016;43(12): 1160–70.

26. Aghaloo T, Pi-Anfruns J, Moshaverinia A, et al. The Effects of Systemic Diseases and Medications on Implant Osseointegration: A Systematic Review. Int J Oral Maxillofac Implants Suppl 2019;34:s35–49.

27. Ghosh M, Majumdar SR. Antihypertensive medications, bone mineral density, and fractures: a review of old cardiac drugs that provides new insights into osteoporosis. Endocrine 2014;46(3):397–405.

28. Wu X, Al-Abedalla K, Eimar H, et al. Antihypertensive Medications and the Survival Rate of Osseointegrated Dental Implants: A Cohort Study. Clin Implant Dent Relat Res 2016;18(6):1171–82.

29. Muniz F, Pola NM, Silva CFE, et al. Are periodontal diseases associated with sleep duration or sleep quality? A systematic review. Arch Oral Biol 2021;129: 105184.

30. Romandini M, Gioco G, Perfetti G, et al. The association between periodontitis and sleep duration. J Clin Periodontol 2017;44(5):490–501.

31. Alhassani AA, Al-Zahrani MS. Is inadequate sleep a potential risk factor for periodontitis? PLoS One 2020;15(6):e0234487.

32. Patel SR, Malhotra A, Gao X, et al. A prospective study of sleep duration and pneumonia risk in women. Sleep 2012;35(1):97–101.

33. Marruganti C, Romandini M, Gaeta C, et al. Healthy lifestyles are associated with a better response to periodontal therapy: A prospective cohort study. J Clin Periodontol 2023;50(8):1089–100.

34. Pink C, Kocher T, Meisel P, et al. Longitudinal effects of systemic inflammation markers on periodontitis. J Clin Periodontol 2015;42(11):988–97.

35. Kapsimalis F, Basta M, Varouchakis G, et al. Cytokines and pathological sleep. Sleep Med 2008;9(6):603–14.

36. Liu M, Wu Y, Song J, et al. Association of Sleep Duration with Tooth Loss and Periodontitis: Insights from the National Health and Nutrition Examination Surveys (2005-2020). Sleep Breath 2023. https://doi.org/10.1007/s11325-023-02966-2.

37. Sanchez-Azofra A, Gu W, Masso-Silva JA, et al. Inflammation biomarkers in OSA, chronic obstructive pulmonary disease, and chronic obstructive pulmonary disease/OSA overlap syndrome. J Clin Sleep Med 2023;19(8):1447–56.

38. Al-Jewair TS, Al-Jasser R, Almas K. Periodontitis and obstructive sleep apnea's bidirectional relationship: a systematic review and meta-analysis. Sleep Breath 2015;19(4):1111–20.

39. Khodadadi N, Khodadadi M, Zamani M. Is periodontitis associated with obstructive sleep apnea? A systematic review and meta-analysis. J Clin Exp Dent 2022;14(4):e359–65.

40. Mukherjee S, Galgali SR. Obstructive sleep apnea and periodontitis: A cross-sectional study. Indian J Dent Res 2021;32(1):44–50.

41. Lembo D, Caroccia F, Lopes C, et al. Obstructive Sleep Apnea and Periodontal Disease: A Systematic Review. Medicina (Kaunas) 2021;57(6). https://doi.org/10.3390/medicina57060640.

42. Thomas DC, Manfredini D, Patel J, et al. Sleep bruxism: The past, the present, and the future-evolution of a concept. J Am Dent Assoc 2024;155(4):329–43.
43. Chapple IL, Bouchard P, Cagetti MG, et al. Interaction of lifestyle, behaviour or systemic diseases with dental caries and periodontal diseases: consensus report of group 2 of the joint EFP/ORCA workshop on the boundaries between caries and periodontal diseases. J Clin Periodontol 2017;44(Suppl 18):S39–51.
44. Najeeb S, Zafar MS, Khurshid Z, et al. The Role of Nutrition in Periodontal Health: An Update. Nutrients 2016;8(9). https://doi.org/10.3390/nu8090530.
45. Zong G, Holtfreter B, Scott AE, et al. Serum vitamin B12 is inversely associated with periodontal progression and risk of tooth loss: a prospective cohort study. J Clin Periodontol 2016;43(1):2–9.
46. Zhan Y, Samietz S, Holtfreter B, et al. Prospective Study of Serum 25-hydroxy Vitamin D and Tooth Loss. J Dent Res 2014;93(7):639–44.
47. Munday MR, Rodricks R, Fitzpatrick M, et al. A Pilot Study Examining Vitamin C Levels in Periodontal Patients. Nutrients 2020;12(8). https://doi.org/10.3390/nu12082255.
48. Neiva RF, Al-Shammari K, Nociti FH Jr, et al. Effects of vitamin-B complex supplementation on periodontal wound healing. J Periodontol 2005;76(7):1084–91.
49. Calder PC. n-3 polyunsaturated fatty acids, inflammation, and inflammatory diseases. Am J Clin Nutr 2006;83(6 Suppl):1505s–19s.
50. Varela-López A, Giampieri F, Bullón P, et al. Role of Lipids in the Onset, Progression and Treatment of Periodontal Disease. A Systematic Review of Studies in Humans. Int J Mol Sci 2016;17(8). https://doi.org/10.3390/ijms17081202.
51. Van der Velden U. Vitamin C and Its Role in Periodontal Diseases - The Past and the Present: A Narrative Review. Oral Health Prev Dent 2020;18:115–24.
52. Shadisvaaran S, Chin KY, Shahida MS, et al. Effect of vitamin E on periodontitis: Evidence and proposed mechanisms of action. J Oral Biosci 2021;63(2):97–103.
53. Woelber JP, Reichenbächer K, Groß T, et al. Dietary and Nutraceutical Interventions as an Adjunct to Non-Surgical Periodontal Therapy-A Systematic Review. Nutrients 2023;15(6). https://doi.org/10.3390/nu15061538.
54. Nastri L, Moretti A, Migliaccio S, et al. Do Dietary Supplements and Nutraceuticals Have Effects on Dental Implant Osseointegration? A Scoping Review. Nutrients 2020;12(1). https://doi.org/10.3390/nu12010268.
55. Werny JG, Sagheb K, Diaz L, et al. Does vitamin D have an effect on osseointegration of dental implants? A systematic review. Int J Implant Dent 2022;8(1):16.
56. Shah A, Singh K, Rao J, et al. Significance of 25(OH) D3 in Early Dental Implant Failure (EDIF) during osseointegration-A systematic review. Natl J Maxillofac Surg 2023;14(3):360–8.
57. Acar B, Cagdas D, Tan Ç, et al. Evaluation of periodontal status and cytokine/chemokine profile of GCF in patients with severe congenital neutropenia. Odontology 2021;109(2):474–82.
58. Ye Y, Carlsson G, Wondimu B, et al. Mutations in the ELANE gene are associated with development of periodontitis in patients with severe congenital neutropenia. J Clin Immunol 2011;31(6):936–45.
59. Hajishengallis E, Hajishengallis G. Neutrophil homeostasis and periodontal health in children and adults. J Dent Res 2014;93(3):231–7.
60. Alaluusua S, Kivitie-Kallio S, Wolf J, et al. Periodontal findings in Cohen syndrome with chronic neutropenia. J Periodontol 1997;68(5):473–8.
61. Hajishengallis G, Moutsopoulos NM. Role of bacteria in leukocyte adhesion deficiency-associated periodontitis. Microb Pathog 2016;94:21–6.

62. Hajishengallis G, Moutsopoulos NM. Etiology of leukocyte adhesion deficiency-associated periodontitis revisited: not a raging infection but a raging inflammatory response. Expert Rev Clin Immunol 2014;10(8):973–5.

63. Spodzieja K, Olczak-Kowalczyk D. Premature Loss of Deciduous Teeth as a Symptom of Systemic Disease: A Narrative Literature Review. Int J Environ Res Public Health 2022;19(6). https://doi.org/10.3390/ijerph19063386.

64. Lu RF, Meng HX. Severe periodontitis in a patient with cyclic neutropenia: a case report of long-term follow-up. Chin J Dent Res 2012;15(2):159–63.

65. Chen Y, Fang L, Yang X. Cyclic neutropenia presenting as recurrent oral ulcers and periodontitis. J Clin Pediatr Dent. Spring 2013;37(3):307–8.

66. da Fonseca MA, Fontes F. Early tooth loss due to cyclic neutropenia: long-term follow-up of one patient. Spec Care Dentist Sep-Oct 2000;20(5):187–90.

67. Zaromb A, Chamberlain D, Schoor R, et al. Periodontitis as a manifestation of chronic benign neutropenia. J Periodontol 2006;77(11):1921–6.

68. Lao Z, Fu J, Wu Z, et al. Case report: Five-year periodontal management of a patient with two novel mutation sites in ELANE-induced cyclic neutropenia. Front Genet 2022;13:972598.

69. Bacci C, Schiazzano C, Zanon E, et al. Bleeding Disorders and Dental Implants: Review and Clinical Indications. J Clin Med 2023;12(14). https://doi.org/10.3390/jcm12144757.

70. Pérez-Fierro M, Castellanos-Cosano L, Hueto-Madrid JA, et al. 2-years retrospective observational case-control study on survival and marginal bone loss of implants in patients with hereditary coagulopathies. Med Oral Patol Oral Cir Bucal 2023;28(6):e572–80.

71. Papapanou PN, Sanz M, Buduneli N, et al. Periodontitis: Consensus report of workgroup 2 of the 2017 World Workshop on the Classification of Periodontal and Peri-Implant Diseases and Conditions. J Clin Periodontol 2018;45(Suppl 20):S162–70.

72. Duarte PM, Nogueira CFP, Silva SM, et al. Impact of Smoking Cessation on Periodontal Tissues. Int Dent J 2022;72(1):31–6.

73. Madi M, Smith S, Alshehri S, et al. Influence of Smoking on Periodontal and Implant Therapy: A Narrative Review. Int J Environ Res Public Health 2023; 20(7). https://doi.org/10.3390/ijerph20075368.

74. Souto MLS, Rovai ES, Villar CC, et al. Effect of smoking cessation on tooth loss: a systematic review with meta-analysis. BMC Oral Health 2019;19(1):245.

75. Leite FRM, Nascimento GG, Baake S, et al. Impact of Smoking Cessation on Periodontitis: A Systematic Review and Meta-analysis of Prospective Longitudinal Observational and Interventional Studies. Nicotine Tob Res 2019;21(12): 1600–8.

76. Caggiano M, Gasparro R, D'Ambrosio F, et al. Smoking Cessation on Periodontal and Peri-Implant Health Status: A Systematic Review. Dent J (Basel) 2022;10(9). https://doi.org/10.3390/dj10090162.

77. Beklen A, Sali N, Yavuz MB. The impact of smoking on periodontal status and dental caries. Tob Induc Dis 2022;20:72.

78. D'Ambrosio F, Pisano M, Amato A, et al. Periodontal and Peri-Implant Health Status in Traditional vs. Heat-Not-Burn Tobacco and Electronic Cigarettes Smokers: A Systematic Review. Dent J (Basel) 2022;10(6). https://doi.org/10.3390/dj10060103.

79. Ralho A, Coelho A, Ribeiro M, et al. Effects of Electronic Cigarettes on Oral Cavity: A Systematic Review. J Evid Based Dent Pract 2019;19(4):101318.

80. Quaranta A, D'Isidoro O, Piattelli A, et al. Illegal drugs and periodontal conditions. Periodontol 2000 2022;90(1):62–87.

81. Hyman JJ, Reid BC. Epidemiologic risk factors for periodontal attachment loss among adults in the United States. J Clin Periodontol 2003;30(3):230–7.
82. Alawaji YN, Alshammari A, Mostafa N, et al. Periodontal disease prevalence, extent, and risk associations in untreated individuals. Clin Exp Dent Res 2022; 8(1):380–94.
83. Bergström J. Tobacco smoking and risk for periodontal disease. J Clin Periodontol 2003;30(2):107–13.
84. Kotsakis GA, Javed F, Hinrichs JE, et al. Impact of cigarette smoking on clinical outcomes of periodontal flap surgical procedures: a systematic review and meta-analysis. J Periodontol 2015;86(2):254–63.
85. Moscowchi A, Moradian-Lotfi S, Koohi H, et al. Levels of smoking and outcome measures of root coverage procedures: a systematic review and meta-analysis. Oral Maxillofac Surg 2023. https://doi.org/10.1007/s10006-023-01172-4.
86. Jiang Y, Zhou X, Cheng L, et al. The Impact of Smoking on Subgingival Microflora: From Periodontal Health to Disease. Front Microbiol 2020;11:66.
87. Buduneli N. Environmental factors and periodontal microbiome. Periodontol 2000 2021;85(1):112–25.
88. Eggert FM, McLeod MH, Flowerdew G. Effects of smoking and treatment status on periodontal bacteria: evidence that smoking influences control of periodontal bacteria at the mucosal surface of the gingival crevice. J Periodontol 2001; 72(9):1210–20.
89. Mavropoulos A, Aars H, Brodin P. Hyperaemic response to cigarette smoking in healthy gingiva. J Clin Periodontol 2003;30(3):214–21.
90. Mosely LH, Finseth F, Goody M. Nicotine and its effect on wound healing. Plast Reconstr Surg 1978;61(4):570–5.
91. Rezavandi K, Palmer RM, Odell EW, et al. Expression of ICAM-1 and E-selectin in gingival tissues of smokers and non-smokers with periodontitis. J Oral Pathol Med 2002;31(1):59–64.
92. Palmer RM, Scott DA, Meekin TN, et al. Potential mechanisms of susceptibility to periodontitis in tobacco smokers. J Periodontal Res 1999;34(7):363–9.
93. Giannopoulou C, Cappuyns I, Mombelli A. Effect of smoking on gingival crevicular fluid cytokine profile during experimental gingivitis. J Clin Periodontol 2003; 30(11):996–1002.
94. Boström L, Linder LE, Bergström J. Clinical expression of TNF-alpha in smoking-associated periodontal disease. J Clin Periodontol 1998;25(10):767–73.
95. Boström L, Linder LE, Bergström J. Influence of smoking on the outcome of periodontal surgery. A 5-year follow-up. J Clin Periodontol 1998;25(3):194–201.
96. Tanur E, McQuade MJ, McPherson JC, et al. Effects of nicotine on the strength of attachment of gingival fibroblasts to glass and non-diseased human root surfaces. J Periodontol 2000;71(5):717–22.
97. James JA, Sayers NM, Drucker DB, et al. Effects of tobacco products on the attachment and growth of periodontal ligament fibroblasts. J Periodontol 1999;70(5):518–25.
98. Giannopoulou C, Geinoz A, Cimasoni G. Effects of nicotine on periodontal ligament fibroblasts in vitro. J Clin Periodontol 1999;26(1):49–55.
99. Poggi P, Rota MT, Boratto R. The volatile fraction of cigarette smoke induces alterations in the human gingival fibroblast cytoskeleton. J Periodontal Res 2002; 37(3):230–5.
100. Cattaneo V, Cetta G, Rota C, et al. Volatile components of cigarette smoke: effect of acrolein and acetaldehyde on human gingival fibroblasts in vitro. J Periodontol 2000;71(3):425–32.

101. Silverstein P. Smoking and wound healing. Am J Med 1992;93(1a):22s–4s.

102. Reaven GM. Banting lecture 1988. Role of insulin resistance in human disease. Diabetes 1988;37(12):1595–607.

103. Aizenbud I, Wilensky A, Almoznino G. Periodontal Disease and Its Association with Metabolic Syndrome-A Comprehensive Review. Int J Mol Sci 2023; 24(16). https://doi.org/10.3390/ijms241613011.

104. Almoznino G, Zini A, Kedem R, et al. Hypertension and Its Associations with Dental Status: Data from the Dental, Oral, Medical Epidemiological (DOME) Nationwide Records-Based Study. J Clin Med 2021;10(2). https://doi.org/10.3390/jcm10020176.

105. Nascimento GG, Leite FR, Do LG, et al. Is weight gain associated with the incidence of periodontitis? A systematic review and meta-analysis. J Clin Periodontol 2015;42(6):495–505.

106. Kim CM, Lee S, Hwang W, et al. Obesity and periodontitis: A systematic review and updated meta-analysis. Front Endocrinol (Lausanne) 2022;13:999455.

107. Nibali L, Tatarakis N, Needleman I, et al. Clinical review: Association between metabolic syndrome and periodontitis: a systematic review and meta-analysis. J Clin Endocrinol Metab 2013;98(3):913–20.

108. Khosravi R, Ka K, Huang T, et al. Tumor necrosis factor-α and interleukin-6: potential interorgan inflammatory mediators contributing to destructive periodontal disease in obesity or metabolic syndrome. Mediators Inflamm 2013;2013: 728987.

109. Martinez-Herrera M, Silvestre-Rangil J, Silvestre FJ. Association between obesity and periodontal disease. A systematic review of epidemiological studies and controlled clinical trials. Med Oral Patol Oral Cir Bucal 2017;22(6):e708–15.

110. Pierce JL, Begun DL, Westendorf JJ, et al. Defining osteoblast and adipocyte lineages in the bone marrow. Bone 2019;118:2–7.

111. Al-Rawi N, Al-Marzooq F. The Relation between Periodontopathogenic Bacterial Levels and Resistin in the Saliva of Obese Type 2 Diabetic Patients. J Diabetes Res 2017;2017:2643079.

112. Maciel SS, Feres M, Gonçalves TE, et al. Does obesity influence the subgingival microbiota composition in periodontal health and disease? J Clin Periodontol 2016;43(12):1003–12.

113. de Andrade DR, Silva PA, Colombo APV, et al. Subgingival microbiota in overweight and obese young adults with no destructive periodontal disease. J Periodontol 2021;92(10):1410–9.

114. Croucher R, Marcenes WS, Torres MC, et al. The relationship between life-events and periodontitis. A case-control study. J Clin Periodontol 1997;24(1): 39–43.

115. Martínez M, Postolache TT, García-Bueno B, et al. The Role of the Oral Microbiota Related to Periodontal Diseases in Anxiety, Mood and Trauma- and Stress-Related Disorders. Front Psychiatr 2021;12:814177.

116. Genco RJ, Ho AW, Grossi SG, et al. Relationship of stress, distress and inadequate coping behaviors to periodontal disease. J Periodontol 1999;70(7): 711–23.

117. Coelho JMF, Miranda SS, da Cruz SS, et al. Is there association between stress and periodontitis? Clin Oral Investig 2020;24(7):2285–94.

118. Wellappulli N, Ekanayake L. Association between psychological distress and chronic periodontitis in Sri Lankan adults. Community Dent Health 2019;36(4): 293–7.

119. Islam MM, Ekuni D, Yoneda T, et al. Influence of Occupational Stress and Coping Style on Periodontitis among Japanese Workers: A Cross-Sectional Study. Int J Environ Res Public Health 2019;16(19). https://doi.org/10.3390/ijerph16193540.
120. Johannsen A, Bjurshammar N, Gustafsson A. The influence of academic stress on gingival inflammation. Int J Dent Hyg 2010;8(1):22–7.
121. Ishisaka A, Ansai T, Soh I, et al. Association of salivary levels of cortisol and dehydroepiandrosterone with periodontitis in older Japanese adults. J Periodontol 2007;78(9):1767–73.
122. Mesa F, Magán-Fernández A, Muñoz R, et al. Catecholamine metabolites in urine, as chronic stress biomarkers, are associated with higher risk of chronic periodontitis in adults. J Periodontol 2014;85(12):1755–62.
123. Cakmak O, Tasdemir Z, Aral CA, et al. Gingival crevicular fluid and saliva stress hormone levels in patients with chronic and aggressive periodontitis. J Clin Periodontol 2016;43(12):1024–31.
124. Decker A, Askar H, Tattan M, et al. The assessment of stress, depression, and inflammation as a collective risk factor for periodontal diseases: a systematic review. Clin Oral Investig 2020;24(1):1–12.
125. Bakri I, Douglas CW, Rawlinson A. The effects of stress on periodontal treatment: a longitudinal investigation using clinical and biological markers. J Clin Periodontol 2013;40(10):955–61.
126. Rai B, Kaur J, Anand SC, et al. Salivary stress markers, stress, and periodontitis: a pilot study. J Periodontol 2011;82(2):287–92.
127. Lu H, Xu M, Wang F, et al. Chronic stress accelerates ligature-induced periodontitis by suppressing glucocorticoid receptor-α signaling. Exp Mol Med 2016;48(3):e223.
128. Gomes EP, Aguiar JC, Fonseca-Silva T, et al. Diazepam reverses the alveolar bone loss and hippocampal interleukin-1beta and interleukin-6 enhanced by conditioned fear stress in ligature-induced periodontal disease in rats. J Periodontal Res 2013;48(2):151–8.
129. Jentsch HF, März D, Krüger M. The effects of stress hormones on growth of selected periodontitis related bacteria. Anaerobe 2013;24:49–54.
130. Roberts A, Matthews JB, Socransky SS, et al. Stress and the periodontal diseases: effects of catecholamines on the growth of periodontal bacteria in vitro. Oral Microbiol Immunol 2002;17(5):296–303.
131. Kapila YL. Oral health's inextricable connection to systemic health: Special populations bring to bear multimodal relationships and factors connecting periodontal disease to systemic diseases and conditions. Periodontol 2000 2021;87(1):11–6.
132. Nagpal R, Yamashiro Y, Izumi Y. The Two-Way Association of Periodontal Infection with Systemic Disorders: An Overview. Mediators Inflamm 2015;2015:793898.
133. Deng Y, Xiao J, Ma L, et al. Mitochondrial Dysfunction in Periodontitis and Associated Systemic Diseases: Implications for Pathomechanisms and Therapeutic Strategies. Int J Mol Sci 2024;25(2). https://doi.org/10.3390/ijms25021024.
134. Holmstrup P, Glick M. Treatment of periodontal disease in the immunodeficient patient. Periodontol 2000 2002;28:190–205.
135. Hanioka T, Tanaka M, Takaya K, et al. Pocket oxygen tension in smokers and non-smokers with periodontal disease. J Periodontol 2000;71(4):550–4.
136. Johnson GK, Hill M. Cigarette smoking and the periodontal patient. J Periodontol 2004;75(2):196–209.

Stress and Hypothalamic–Pituitary–Adrenal Axis
Effect on Prognosis of Dental Treatment

Veronica Iturriaga, DDS, MSc, PhD[a],*, Nicol Velasquez, DDS[a],
Eli Eliav, DMD, PhD[b], Davis C. Thomas, BDS, DDS, MSD, MSc Med, MSc[c]

KEYWORDS

- Stress and dentistry • HPA and dentistry • Stress and dental prognosis
- HPA and dental prognosis

KEY POINTS

- Stress is a process that activates a set of reactions involving behavioral and physiologic responses.
- The stress response involves an efficient and complex system with modulation at different levels of the central nervous system being driven largely by neural mechanisms, including activation of the hypothalamic–pituitary–adrenal (HPA) axis.
- The HPA axis is a neurohormonal system necessary for adaptation, resulting from the interaction among 3 distinct organs, which mediates the secretion of corticotropin-releasing hormone in the hypothalamus, adrenocorticotropic hormone in the pituitary, and glucocorticoid hormone-cortisol in the adrenal cortex.
- Stress and activation of the HPA axis associated with dental care can negatively interfere with the efficacy of dental treatment, affecting adherence and resulting in total treatment interruption or delay of subsequent appointments.

INTRODUCTION

Stress has been a topic of study in various medical specialties for several decades, and to address it, approaches have been made to understand its effects on the different systems of the organism. The response to stressful stimuli is elaborated by a system that integrates a wide diversity of brain structures, which collectively can detect events and interpreting them as real or potential threats.[1,2] The integration of this information

[a] Department of Integral Adult Care Dentistry, Temporomandibular Disorder and Orofacial Pain Program, Sleep & Pain Research Group, Universidad de La Frontera, Temuco, Chile;
[b] Eastman Institute for Oral Health, University of Rochester Medical Center, Rochester, NY, USA;
[c] Department of Diagnostic Sciences, Center for Temporomandibular Disorders and Orofacial Pain, Rutgers School of Dental Medicine, Newark, NJ, USA
* Corresponding author.
E-mail address: veronica.iturriaga@ufrontera.cl

Dent Clin N Am 68 (2024) 619–626
https://doi.org/10.1016/j.cden.2024.07.003
dental.theclinics.com

results in a rapid activation of the hypothalamic–pituitary–adrenal (HPA) axis , being a fundamental component of the stress response.[1,3] On the other hand, people tend to feel stress in association with dental treatment; this can be triggered by restlessness and fear, understanding that this expression is multifactorial and multidimensional, which considers physiologic, behavioral, and cognitive components of the person.[4,5]

Accordingly, the aim of this article is to describe the effect of stress in its interaction with the HPA axis on the prognosis of dental treatment. In the first instance, general aspects related to the stress process and the participation of the HPA axis will be reviewed, to later relate them to the prognosis of dental treatment.

STRESS AS A PROCESS

Understanding the concept of stress and its biologic substrate is fundamental to comprehending its role in different processes. Hans Selye[6] was one of the first to define it from the biologic point of view, considering stress as "a nonspecific response of the body to any demand made on it."[1,2,7] Other definitions consider it as a state of homeostatic alteration, which generates a response in the organism to maintain homeostasis.[2] Stress activates a set of reactions involving behavioral and physiologic responses (neuronal, metabolic, and neuroendocrine) that allow the organism to respond to the stressor in the most adapted way possible.[8] This response ultimately reflects the activation of specific circuits genetically constituted in the individual and constantly modulated by the environment.[2] For this process to be initiated, the organism must perceive a threat, either real or potential, which leads to the release of various types of molecules. The interaction between these molecules with their respective receptors, at the peripheral and central levels, may result in the stress response. This response, through physiologic and behavioral mechanisms, helps restore the body's homeostasis and promote adaptation.[1]

The stress response involves an efficient, evolving, and complex system, with modulation at various levels of the central nervous system (CNS), being driven to a greater extent by neuronal mechanisms, which activate 2 types of circuits in the CNS, and which develop mainly in 2 phases. The first phase begins with the perception of a stressor; when this situation is perceived as a threat, neuronal pathways are recruited in the brain to maintain physiologic integrity, which involves the activation of the first circuit at the level of the spinal cord, particularly the adrenomedullary sympathetic system. In this way, a rapid physiologic adaptation is provided, with a short-duration response, generating a state of alertness, vigilance, and evaluation of the situation to be faced. The second circuit, and with it, the second phase, involves a neurohormonal process, where the interpretation of the information by supraspinal structures is required and refers to the activation of the HPA Axis. This is a slower process, which generates an amplified and prolonged response.[1,2,9]

The neural mechanisms that drive chronic stress responses may be distinct from those that control acute reactions, including the recruitment of new limbic, hypothalamic, and brainstem circuits. It is critical to consider that an individual's response to acute or chronic stress is determined by a variety of factors, including genetics, early life experience, environmental conditions, gender, and age. The context in which the stressors are generated will determine whether the individual's responses are adaptive.[9,10]

Patients in general many a time feel that stress is "bad." However, physiologically speaking, it may not be all that deleterious. Stress is also part of the defensive phenomenon. For example, a mother who loses her toddler child in a crowd does not really sit around waiting for the child just to show up. Her instinctive activation of the acute stress response brings about the rapid response of vigilance and the innate impulse to actively search for her offspring. In general, when stress is not biologic, chronic stress may become pathologic with deleterious effects on the body and mind.

HYPOTHALAMIC–PITUITARY–ADRENAL AXIS

The HPA axis corresponds to a neurohormonal system that integrates the secretion of corticotropin-releasing hormone (CRH) in the hypothalamus, adrenocorticotropic hormone (ACTH) in the anterior pituitary, and cortisol in the adrenal cortex. The HPA axis is therefore initiated in the hypothalamus, particularly in the hypophysiotropic neurons of the parvocellular nucleus (PVN) of the hypothalamus, since it is in this nucleus where information from various areas of the CNS is integrated. These neurons send projections to the median eminence of the brainstem, and when activated, they discharge CRH and other releasing factors into the pituitary portal capillary system. These releasing factors are directed to the anterior pituitary, where they stimulate corticotropes to release ACTH into the systemic circulation. ACTH acts on cells in the zona fasciculars of the adrenal cortex to stimulate the production and secretion of glucocorticoid hormones (GCs) into the general circulation, particularly cortisol in humans, and to a lesser extent mineralocorticoids. Once released into the bloodstream, 75% to 80% of the GCs bind to plasma proteins, and a low fraction remain free exerting their immediate physiologic effect, thus maintaining a constant blood glucose level to nourish the muscles, heart, and brain.[2,3,7,8,10–12]

Under physiologic conditions, the HPA axis presents a circadian regulation, with a low basal activity level that varies with the time of day, in addition to presenting negative feedback mechanisms mediated by GCs. ACTH and GCs levels are highest near the beginning of the waking period and are lowest near the beginning of the inactive period; this rhythm depends on neuronal circuits sensitive to changes in light, including afferents from the suprachiasmatic nucleus to the PVN, which physiologically promotes PVN activation but in stressful situations acts as an inhibitor.[2,7,10–12]

It is important to consider then that the HPA axis response to stress results from the interaction among these 3 distinct organs, each of which has its own intrinsic checkpoints for the regulation of GCs secretion.[7,9]

STRESS: HYPOTHALAMIC–PITUITARY–ADRENAL AXIS INTERACTION AND DENTAL TREATMENT

The regulation of stress reactivity is a fundamental priority for all organisms. Stress responses are critical for survival, but they can also generate effects at the physical as well as the psychological level.[7] As mentioned earlier, stress responds to a real or perceived threat to the organism's homeostasis or well-being, and the HPA axis is necessary for adaptation. The perception of different stressors involves complex activation networks, being dependent on the type of stressor or stressor involved. Reactive responses to homeostatic disruption often involve direct noradrenergic conduction, whereas anticipatory responses use oligosynaptic pathways originating in limbic structures. These brain networks ultimately evoke physiologic responses to stress, including activation of the HPA axis, with consequent release of GCs-cortisol, which act on multiple organ systems to redirect energy resources to meet actual or anticipated demand.[1,9,11] On the other hand, circulating concentrations of GCs-cortisol are maintained within normal limits through negative feedback on hypothalamic–pituitary release of CRH and ACTH.[2,3,8,10] In the hypothalamus, the increase in GCs-cortisol early generates a decrease in the frequency of PVN release; thus, the stimulatory effect of CRH on ACTH secretion is inhibited by the action of GCs-cortisol. Importantly, CRH neurotransmission is not limited to the communication between the PVN and the anterior pituitary, as the existence of extra hypothalamic regulatory mechanisms on PVN function has been observed, since CRH is also expressed in other stress-regulating brain regions, including the central amygdala and the bed nucleus of the stria terminalis,[2,3,7,11] which act as relay centers of the HPA axis, modulating its activity in response to stress.

The purpose of the counter-regulatory mechanism described earlier is to maintain stable basal levels of ACTH and GCs-cortisol. However, repeated or sustained activity of stress responses produces a series of long-term adaptations in these systems, generating changes in gene expression and synaptic plasticity in the stress-regulating brain regions. This situation produces habituation and facilitation phenomena, changes in PVN inputs to favor neuronal excitability, elevated CRH expression, and adrenal hypertrophy, resulting in increased HPA axis excitability with chronic exposure to GCs-cortisol.[2,3,11]

In dentistry, practitioners are aware of the variations that exist in the way patients react to treatment. Maybe small number of people are happy to undergo dental treatment; however, most of them can control themselves sufficiently to accept treatment without excessive signs of stress. However, there is a surprisingly large group of patients in whom stress is more obvious, manifesting itself in a variety of ways and may result in a negative response to treatment. It is estimated that between 10% and 15% of the general population suffers some degree of stress in the face of dental treatment, being perceived as an agonizing experience (**Fig. 1**).[13–15] This is triggered on several occasions by anxiety and fear, with special reference to the expectation of pain, this being one of the main reasons for missing dental appointments. According to the study carried out by Rodriguez and colleagues,[16] approximately 97% of the patients manifest some degree of stress during the execution of their dental treatment.[4,5,13,17,18]

Traditionally dental treatment has been related to pain, where the stress response to pain or even the anticipation of it, initiates the activation of the HPA axis, being a physiologic process that can be expressed in all people.[4] However, the stress generated by dental care causes certain effects in the body in response to the real or perceived threat; these effects include tachycardia, increased blood pressure, hyperglycemia, mydriasis, hyperthermia, nausea, sweating, excessive salivation, and secretion of GCS-cortisol generated by the activation of the HPA axis, which can negatively affect important biologic mechanisms and be a risk factor in the development of certain systemic diseases.[15,18–20] In particular, the immediate period waiting for dental treatment is commonly described as an anxiogenic factor, with prevalence rates ranging from approximately 5% to 20%, being an important factor to consider.[18–22] In reference to the triggers of stress/anxiety in dental treatment, Gale and colleagues[23] reported that the situations that originate high levels of stress/anxiety are in order: the extraction of a tooth, the drilling of a tooth, the dentist's bad opinion about the patient's oral health, and lastly, the action of holding the needle in front of the patient.[24]

From the point of view of dental treatment prognosis, stress and activation of the HPA axis because of dental care influence the efficacy of dental treatment, producing interference in it. It can negatively influence the oral health status of the individual, hinder patient management during care, or also affect subsequent adherence to treatment, which usually results in total interruption or delay in requesting the next appointment, ultimately avoiding subsequent consultations.[14,19–21] Eitnet and colleagues[25] found that dental treatment avoidance is highly correlated with stress/anxiety indices and increased caries morbidity. Yet, when patients with high levels of stress/anxiety attend their consultations, they are highly likely to avoid follow-up appointments to complete their dental treatment. This avoidance results in a higher prevalence of oral pathology, leading to a greater need for and complexity of rehabilitative treatment.[22]

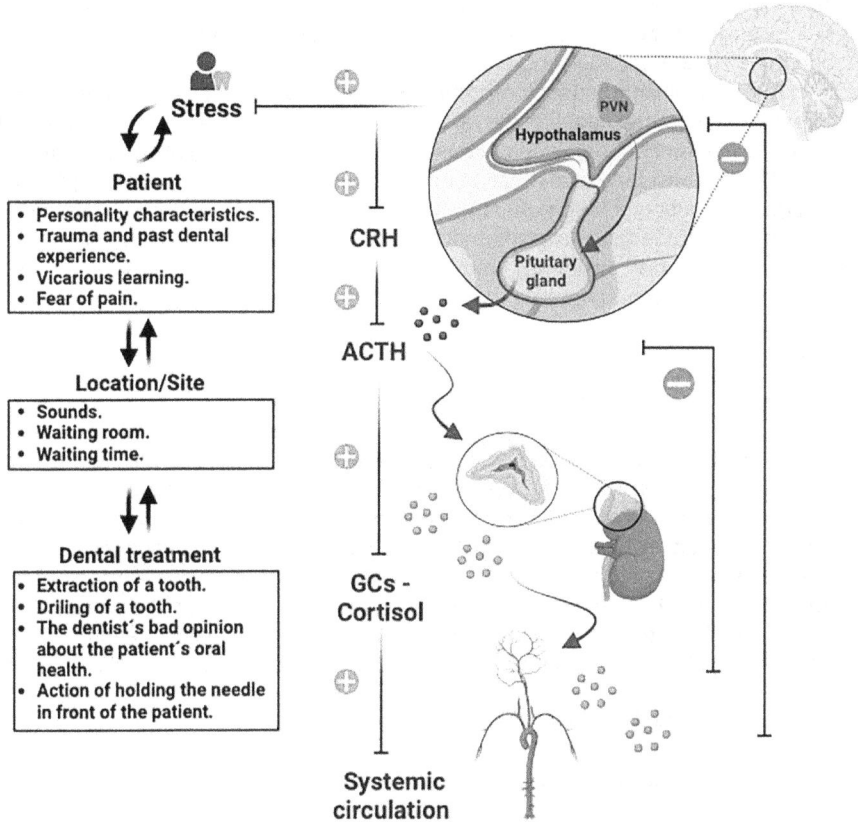

Fig. 1. Schematic representation of HPA axis stimulation. Stress is a complex phenomenon, and its development cannot be due to a single variable. There are a number of factors that have been consistently associated with stress in dentistry, factors that depend on the patient, the site, and the dental treatment. Any one of these factors can initiate the stress response. HPA axis stress responses are initiated by neurons in the PVN, which is the final integrator of the stress response. Neurons in this nucleus produce CRH, which stimulates production in the anterior pituitary of ACTH. ACTH stimulates the production of GCs-cortisol in the adrenal glands. In turn, GCs-cortisol inhibits its own synthesis, inhibiting the synthesis and release of ACTH and CRH, thus self-regulation occurs.

Due to all these factors, there are currently various models of care that seek to help health professionals provide dental care with a view to reducing stress during care and thereby ensure the success of treatment, using affective communication management techniques, relaxation and breathing techniques, music therapy, and even pharmacologic measures such as intravenous sedation, oral sedation, inhalant sedation, and general anesthesia.[13,17,21,24]

CLINICAL IMPLICATIONS IN DENTISTRY

The complexity of the stress response is not limited to neuroanatomy or HPA axis mediators but diverges according to the timing and duration of exposure to the factor, as well as its short-term and/or long-term consequences.[1,2] The stress response, through mediator molecules, promotes alterations in cellular excitability, as well as in neural and synaptic plasticity, leading to transient and/or permanent changes in physiology and behavior, since HPA axis has the capacity to exert generalized effects through the increase of circulating GCs-cortisol.[1,11]

One of the difficulties frequently reported by dentists during dental treatments and with great impact on oral health is the failure to keep appointments and avoidance of the dentist's intervention, because of stress/anxiety before treatment.[24] Furthermore, it is important to consider that in addition to this, there are certain predisposing factors to this type of situation, where patients with low pain thresholds stand out, which increase sensitivity to dental treatment; those patients who present traits of generalized anxiety should also be considered, and, finally, the transmission of unfavorable attitudes toward dental treatment by other people is also recognized.[17,19,24]

SUMMARY

Considering all of the above, it is essential to understand that the regulation of stress reactivity and HPA axis is a fundamental priority of all organisms, and that this response is controlled by emotional, behavioral, and physiologic components, generating an effect in the short and long term. The knowledge of such organization should allow the dentist a better understanding of the process and the consequences associated with stress and its HPA axis interaction, bearing in mind that one of the main consequences is the interference with dental treatment, which will usually generate the interruption of the treatment and the avoidance of subsequent appointments, negatively affecting the prognosis in these patients. Thus, there is a new challenge for future dentists in the search for new tools and models of care to reduce the levels of stress/anxiety during dental treatment.

CLINICS CARE POINTS

- The response to stressful stimuli is elaborated by a system that integrates a wide diversity of anatomic systems and structures.
- Repeated or sustained activity of stress responses produces a series of long-term adaptations, generating changes in gene expression and synaptic plasticity, with associated habituation and facilitation phenomena in stress-regulating brain regions.
- The interaction between stress and HPA axis in dental treatment can interfere in the prognosis of the treatment, negatively influencing the oral health status of individuals, hindering patient management during care, or affecting subsequent adherence to treatment.

DISCLOSURES

V. Iturriaga and N. Velasquez contributed to the conception and design and wrote the initial draft and figure preparation. D.C. Thomas and E. Eliav contributed to the manuscript by critically revising important intellectual content. All authors gave final approval and agreed to be accountable for all aspects of this work. The study was financed by Project DI20-0018 and the Temporomandibular Disorder and Orofacial Pain Program, Universidad de La Frontera, Chile. The authors declare that they have no conflict of interest.

REFERENCES

1. Godoy LD, Rossignoli MT, Delfino-Pereira P, et al. A Comprehensive Overview on Stress Neurobiology: Basic Concepts and Clinical Implications. Front Behav Neurosci 2018;12:127.

2. Rodríguez-Fernández J, García-Acero M, Franco P. Neurobiología del estrés agudo y crónico: su efecto en el eje hipotálamo-hipófisis-adrenal y la Memoria. Rev Ecuat Neurol 2012;21:1–3.

3. Karaca Z, Grossman A, Kelestimur F. Investigation of the Hypothalamo-pituitary-adrenal (HPA) axis: a contemporary synthesis. Rev Endocr Metab Disord 2021; 22(2):179–204.

4. Dušková M, Vašáková J, Dušková J, et al. The role of stress hormones in dental management behavior problems. Physiol Res 2017;66(3):317–22.

5. Umemori S, Noritake K, Tonami KI, et al. The Effects of Providing Advance Notice and Stress-Coping Traits on Physiological Stress of Patients during Dental Treatment. Int J Environ Res Public Health 2022;19(5):2540.

6. Selye H. The stress concept. Can Med Assoc J 1976;115:718.

7. Herman JP, Nawreen N, Smail MA, et al. Brain mechanisms of HPA axis regulation: neurocircuitry and feedback in context Richard Kvetnansky lecture. Stress 2020;23(6):617–32.

8. Duval F, González F, Rabia H. Neurobiology of stress. Rev Chil Neuro-Psiquiat. 2010;48(4):307–18.

9. Herman JP, McKlveen JM, Ghosal S, et al. Regulation of the Hypothalamic-Pituitary-Adrenocortical Stress Response. Compr Physiol 2016;6(2):603–21.

10. Panagiotakopoulos L, Neigh GN. Development of the HPA axis: where and when do sex differences manifest? Front Neuroendocrinol 2014;35(3):285–302.

11. Packard AE, Egan AE, Ulrich-Lai YM. HPA Axis Interactions with Behavioral Systems. Compr Physiol 2016;6(4):1897–934.

12. Vélez-Palacio A, Balthazar-González V, Campuzano-Maya G. Evaluation of hypothalamic-pituitary-adrenal axis function in children treated with steroids. Med Lab 2013;19:111–25.

13. Bancarali L, Oliva P. Music Therapy Effect on Stress Levels of Internal Users of the Dental clinic of universidad del desarrollo. Int J Odontostomat 2012;6(2): 189–93.

14. Lima M, Casanova Y. Fear, Anxiety and phobia to dentistry treatment. Rev Hum Med 2006;6(1):1–21.

15. Messer JG. Stress in dental patients undergoing routine procedures. J Dent Res 1977;56(4):362–7.

16. Rodríguez O. Prevalencia de ansiedad dental en los estudiantes de la UPAO, Trujillo. 2015. Available at: https://hdl.handle.net/20.500.12759/1055. [Accessed 12 April 2024].

17. Aravena PC, Almonacid C, Mancilla MI. Effect of music at 432 Hz and 440 Hz on dental anxiety and salivary cortisol levels in patients undergoing tooth extraction: a randomized clinical trial. J Appl Oral Sci 2020;28:e20190601.

18. Cohen SM, Fiske J, Newton JT. The impact of dental anxiety on daily living. Br Dent J 2000;189(7):385–90.

19. Mejía-Rubalcava C, Alanís-Tavira J, Mendieta-Zerón H, et al. Changes induced by music therapy to physiologic parameters in patients with dental anxiety. Complement Ther Clin Pract 2015;21(4):282–6.

20. Barreiro-Vera CL, Armijos-Moreta JF, Gavilánez-Villamarín SM. La ansiedad dental en pacientes durante un tratamiento odontológico. Rev Cienc Med (Lourenco Marques) 2023;27:e6010.

21. Ríos M, Herrera A, Rojas G. Dental anxiety: Assessment and treatment. Av Odontoestomatol 2014;30(1):39–46.

22. Hmud R, Walsh LJ. Ansiedad dental: causas, complicaciones y métodos de manejo. J Minim Interv Dent 2009;2(1):237–48.

23. Gale EN. Fears of the dental situation. J Dent Res 1972;51(4):964–6.
24. Caycedo C, Cortés F, Gama R, et al. Ansiedad al tratamiento odontológico: características y diferencias de género. Suma Psicol 2008;15(1):259–78.
25. Eitner S, Wichmann M, Paulsen A, et al. Dental anxiety - an epidemiological study on its clinical correlation and effects on oral health. J Oral Rehabil 2006;33: 588–93.

The Effect of Coronavirus Disease 2019 and Other Emerging Infections on Dentistry

Ramesh Balasubramaniam OAM, BSc, BDSc (UWA), MS, Cert Orofacial Pain
(UK), Cert Oral Medicine (Penn), MRACDS (OralMed), ABOP, FOMAA[a],*,
Jaimin Patel, BDS, MDS[b],
Karpagavalli Shanmugasundaram, BDS, MDS[c],
Steven R. Singer, DDS[d]

KEYWORDS

- COVID-19 • Pandemic • SARS-CoV-2 • Infection • Dental care • Telehealth
- Teledentistry

KEY POINTS

- Coronavirus disease 2019 (COVID-19) and other emerging infections have impacted dentistry, considering the risk of transmission in dental settings.
- Patients may be screened through teledentistry during an outbreak of a novel or re-emerging infection to triage the needed dental care.
- The complete impact of delayed dental care during the COVID-19 lockdown is yet to be determined.

INTRODUCTION

The emergence of coronavirus disease 2019 (COVID-19) and other recent infectious disease outbreaks has significantly impacted the delivery of health care, including dentistry. The pandemic has posed unique challenges, necessitating significant adaptations in dental settings. COVID-19 has prompted a reassessment of infection control strategies and the implementation of special precautions in dental settings to mitigate the risk of virus transmission. The pandemic has highlighted the need for enhanced

[a] The University of Western Australia Dental School, The University of Western Australia, 17 Monash Avenue, Nedlands, Western Australia 6009, Australia; [b] 32 PEARLS: Multispeciality Dental Clinics & Implant Center, 311, 312, Shanti Arcade, Near Jaymangal BRTS stop, 132 Feet Ring Road, Naranpura, Ahmedabad-13, Gujarat, India; [c] Department of Oral Medicine and Radiology, Seema Dental College and Hospital, Virbhadra Road, Pashulok post, Rishikesh-249203, Uttarakhand, India; [d] Department of Diagnostic Sciences, Rutgers School of Dental Medicine, 110 Bergen Street, | P.O. Box 1709, Newark, NJ, 07101-1709 USA
* Corresponding author.
E-mail address: ramesh.balasubramaniam@uwa.edu.au

Dent Clin N Am 68 (2024) 627–646
https://doi.org/10.1016/j.cden.2024.07.007
0011-8532/24/© 2024 Elsevier Inc. All rights reserved, including those for text and data mining, AI training, and similar technologies.

knowledge and preparedness among dental professionals, particularly in the context of managing infectious diseases and anticipating the specter of future pandemics.[1] This article primarily explores the effects of the COVID-19 pandemic on dentistry, highlighting changes in dental practice parameters especially infection control measures. Understanding the effects of COVID-19, as well as other emerging infections, is crucial for dentistry to adapt to new challenges and ensure the safety of patients, staff, and the community.

CORONAVIRUS DISEASE 2019 PANDEMIC AND OTHER EMERGING INFECTIONS

The COVID-19 pandemic was a major global health care crisis caused by the severe acute respiratory syndrome coronavirus 2 (SARS-CoV-2).[2] Initial reports suggested COVID-19 was a novel pneumonia of unknown etiology that was first recognized in December 2019 in Wuhan, China, and subsequently spread rapidly worldwide.[3] Various theories regarding its origin were proposed, including zoonotic transmission from bat coronaviruses. In fact, its exact origin and transmission remains an enigma and subject to ongoing scientific scrutiny.[4]

The early identification of the diverse clinical presentation of COVID-19 was crucial for isolation and treatment of infected individuals. The most common symptoms were fever, cough, dyspnea, fatigue, lymphopenia, and shortness of breath,[5] among other systemic signs and symptoms. Gastrointestinal manifestations included vomiting and diarrhea.[6,7] Keratoconjunctivitis was a known early sign of ocular manifestation.[8] Further, there were reports of neurologic manifestations of abnormal smell and taste.[9] Less typical signs and symptoms, even in mild cases, included delirium, anxiety, depression, and supraglottitis with vocal cord hypomobility.[10–12] Of interest, acute COVID-19 infection was not reported in all SARS-CoV-2 detections and coinfection of SARS-CoV-2 and the influenza viruses was common.[13,14]

The estimated overall death rate was 0.66% (7.8% in those aged >80 years and 0.0016% in those aged <9 years).[15] Mortality was strongly associated with comorbidities such as tuberculosis, hypertension, human immunodeficiency virus/acquired immunodeficiency syndrome (HIV/AIDS), alcohol misuse, and diabetes.[16] Of note, the 3 most common causes of COVID-19 mortality were multiple organ failure, circulatory failure, and respiratory failure.[17]

Given the risk for morbidity associated with contracting COVID-19, preventive strategies aimed at preventing the spread of the virus were critical. Adherence to preventive strategies is associated with socioeconomic status, access to public health education and awareness, favorable attitude, trust in science, and stigma related to being infected. Preventive measures against transmission include hand hygiene such as hand washing with soap and water, alcohol-based hand rub, social distancing, masking, screening (SARS-CoV-2 antigen tests kits or polymerase chain reaction at screening centers), avoiding hand contact with eyes, and vaccination.[18–20] Of note, unvaccinated individuals were 5 times more likely to be infected and 29 times more likely to be hospitalized than those vaccinated.[21] Once an individual is infected, secondary transmission occurs with prolong contact among individuals, typically within a household. As such, timely notification of unknown close contacts, and subsequent pre-emptive isolation and quarantine if infected significantly reduces the risk for further transmission of SARS-CoV-2.[22]

The spectrum in the clinical presentation of individuals infected by SARS-CoV-2 varies from asymptomatic to symptoms of viral pneumonia. In select cases, this virus can be lethal. Severity of clinical presentation and urgency of treatment are related to underlying risk factors such as diabetes, hypertension, immune response, and chronic pulmonary obstructive disease.[23] Also, individuals with certain conditions such as Down's syndrome, recent organ transplant, renal disease, multiple sclerosis, motor neuron disease, Huntington's disease, myasthenia gravis, sickle cell disease, and certain cancers are at a greater risk for morbidity and mortality.[24]

For hospitalized individuals with hypoxic acute respiratory distress syndrome, mechanical respiratory support is necessary. The need for pharmacotherapeutic intervention is based on clinical presentation and guidelines for treatments are available but continue to evolve based on scientific evidence. These include antivirals such as nirmatrelvir and ritonavir (antivirals acting on the viral RNA polymerase), sotrovimab (monoclonal antibodies targeting the viral spike protein), corticosteroids such as dexamethasone (for immunosuppressed individuals), casirivimab and imdevimab (inpatient use only), tocilizumab, baricitinib (inpatient use only), and antibiotics (only for cases of bacterial coinfection).[25]

Over the past few decades (and prior to the emergence of COVID-19), there have been several emerging and re-emerging infectious disease outbreaks globally. These infectious diseases were primarily zoonotic, and correlated to socioeconomic, environmental, ecological, globalization, and mobility factors.[26] Generally, the public health response in managing these infectious outbreaks has been largely similar and aims to prevent geographic spread and manage the potential morbidity and mortality associated with the disease. These strategies include education and public health campaigns, personal protection processes such as hygiene and vaccination, social distancing, and quarantine measures.[27] **Table 1** is an overview of these emerging and re-emerging infectious diseases.

EFFECTS OF LOCKDOWN ON DENTAL TREATMENT PROGNOSIS

The lockdowns imposed during the COVID-19 outbreaks severely affected health care systems, which was challenging for patients who required urgent care. During lockdowns, dental care was largely inaccessible,[44] as dental providers were vulnerable to contracting COVID-19 and other respiratory infections while providing dental care. Aerosol-generating procedures in particular posed a significant risk for dental personnel, as well as infection from patients and their companions during COVID-19 outbreaks.[45]

In the initial phase of the COVID-19 pandemic and during the lockdown period, there was significant risk for patients, dentists, and auxiliary staff, owing to the scarcity of PPE. These challenges were amplified in medically complex and special care patients. For example, patients with neurocognitive deficits struggled to comply with new guidelines, including aseptic clinical environments.[46] A significant challenge faced by dental providers during the COVID-19 pandemic was the need to stratify the priority of patients at high risk of transmitting SARS-CoV-2 during dental care. Dental providers were required to make decisions to provide necessary dental treatment (and delay elective procedures), which was weighed against the need to protect their own health and that of their staff and family members. Understandably, in the early stages of the COVID-19 pandemic, definitive universal guidelines were unavailable. This issue was further complicated by the many varied and contradictory guidelines from local, national, and international authorities. Months after the first outbreak of COVID-19, information regarding the SARS-CoV-2 infection was accessible and more consistent guidelines from the relevant authorities were available. Screening modalities were routinely adopted by private dental practices, public dental clinics, and dental hospitals to identify patients who were possibly infected with SARS-CoV-2. Screening instruments were developed that include screening questions, teledentistry

Table 1
Origins of emerging and re-emerging infections and their dental considerations

Infection	Dental Considerations
Middle east respiratory syndrome coronavirus (MERS-CoV) • Dromedary camels in Middle East (2012)[28]	• MERS-CoV may spread between dental providers and patients through aerosol generation during dental procedures • There are no reported cases of spread of MERS-CoV at dental settings[29] • Appropriate use of personal protective equipment (PPE) • Use appropriate infection control strategies
Ebola virus disease • Belongs to family Filoviridae, order Mononegavirales • 5 species of the genus (4 cause Ebola virus disease in humans: Zaire ebolavirus, Sudan ebolavirus, Bundibugyo ebolavirus, and Taï Forest ebolavirus; Reston ebolavirus is asymptomatic) • First identified in 1976 in southern Sudan (may have been in Democratic Republic of Congo in 1972) • Two recent re-emergence: 2014 in West Africa and Democratic Republic of Congo in 2018 • Animal borne likely bats or primates[30,31]	• Ebola virus spread through direct contact with bodily fluids • Half-life in aerosol has been calculated to be 15 min, with a decay rate of 3.06% per minute[31] • Dental providers are at risk during the dental procedures
H_1N_1 influenza (swine flu) • The 2009 outbreak strain in Mexico had origins from swine, avian, and human influenza viruses • Found in pigs in North America and Europe[32]	• H_1N_1 may be transmitted via blood, oral or respiratory secretions • Aerosols generated during dental procedures significantly increases the risk for spread of H_1N_1[33]
Measles • Highly contagious viral infection caused by wild-type measles virus transmitted by aerosolized droplets and direct contact with infected individuals[34] • Resurgence in 2018 in the Americas related to Venezuela migration crisis[35] • Similar increase in Europe was noted in 2018–2019 related to migration and vaccine hesitancy[36]	• Small Koplik's spots of the buccal mucosa (pathognomonic) • Koplik's spots may appear on the buccal mucosa, labial mucosa, and soft palate • Oral manifestations candidiasis, necrotizing ulcerative gingivitis, necrotizing stomatitis (in severe malnutrition), and enlarged lingual and pharyngeal tonsils • Pitted enamel hypoplasia of developing permanent dentition in severe childhood measles[37]
Mpox (formerly known as monkeypox) • A zoonotic disease caused by the Mpox virus[38] • First identified in 1958 among colonies of monkeys housed for research in Democratic Republic of Congo[39] • African rodents, prairie dogs, and nonhuman primates were hosts to the virus and transmitted it to humans • Resurgence in the United Kingdom in 2019 when transmitted by 2 separate travelers[40]	• Presence of the virus in saliva droplets and contaminated surfaces from aerosols and subsequent transmission is possible • The Mpox virus may be transmitted via oral mucosa • Oral and pharyngeal lesions are known clinical presentation of the Mpox virus including confluent ulcerated lesions of the dorsal surface of the tongue; ulcerated lesions with raised margin of the labial mucosa; and enlarged, erythematous, and ulcerated tonsils

(continued on next page)

Table 1 (*continued*)	
Infection	**Dental Considerations**
	• Elective dental procedures should be delayed where possible for possible or confirmed cases • Emergency dental procedures may be performed with appropriate PPE but ideally aerosol-generating procedures should be avoided[41]
Zika • Originally identified in Zika Forest of Uganda in 1947 • A flavivirus carried by the *Aedes aegypti* mosquito, with associated congenital disease • Potential for sexual transmission[42] • Outbreak in the Americas was declared in January 2016	• Presence of virus in bodily fluids such as saliva and urine increase the risk for transmission in dental settings • Newborn with congenital Zika syndrome present with microcephaly (smaller than 32 cm occipitofrontal head circumference) and neurologic and functional disturbances • Orofacial presentation of congenital Zika syndrome include periodontal disease, malocclusion (incomplete primary dentition and narrow palate), enamel defects, hypersalivation, bruxism, micrognathia, ankyloglossia, short labial frenum, hypertonic muscles of mastication, and dysphagia[43]

appointments prior to in-office appointments, and use of temperature monitoring devices to exclude actively infected patients from visiting the health care facility.[47]

The lockdown imposed by relevant authorities and consequent isolation from activities of daily living affected the quality of life and mental health of dental patients across the world.[48] The impact of the COVID-19 lockdowns on the psychological and social well-being of dental patients is well documented. Of note, a close association was found among COVID-19, mental health, and oral health. Most common manifestations were increase in depression and anxiety over unaddressed oral health conditions due to the lack of access to dental care in affected patients.[47]

The COVID-19 lockdown had also adversely affected the financial stability of dental providers and their facilities. There was a significant decline in the number of patients accessing dental care. Elective dental procedures were especially affected. This negatively impacted the income generated by dental providers, which also affected the auxiliary staff and administrative employees, as their work hours were cut back. While teledentistry was able to serve as an emergency consultation service, most dental diagnosis and treatment require in-person office visits.[49]

Considering the possibility of lockdowns and restrictions in response to future novel and re-emerging infections, guidelines and the establishment of protocols to access emergency, preventive, and restorative dental services for patients during lockdowns are necessary.[44]

Emergency Dental Care During the Coronavirus Disease 2019 Pandemic

Routine dental care, by nature, is associated with unavoidable contact with saliva. Potentially contaminated aerosol is often produced during diagnostic and treatment procedures in a setting where the patient, dental provider, and dental assistant are in close proximity. Hence, dental personnel, patients, and accompanying companions are at highest risk of cross infection with aerosol-borne infection, including SARS-CoV-2.[50] Although there exists a high risk of cross infection during the pandemic, dental health, especially involving nonelective treatments, cannot be delayed due to the significant impact of dental health on general health.[51,52] Lockdown conditions evolved frequently and dramatically during the pandemic. Dental providers were advised to follow COVID-19 guidelines of their respective countries and authorities and execute them in the best possible manner so as to reduce the risk for transmission to ensure safety of dental personnel and the community.

During the pandemic and especially when there were restrictions on travel and lockdowns, triaging of dental patients and treatments was routine practice.[53] Preclinical communication with patients, in form of teledentistry, was often carried out to triage patients with regard to screening for COVID-19 symptoms and to determine the urgency of the dental care prior to a face-to-face dental visit.[54–57] As part of the teledentistry consultation to triage patients, patients who are identified as high-risk should be managed through teledentistry where feasible. All elective dental care should be postponed; however, patients may be provided with pain medication and antibiotics as indicated to manage their dental condition until such time they are able to attend the dental office. However, vulnerable patients requiring urgent care, such as those with disabilities, pregnancy, or malignancy must be given priority and dental care must be provided.[51,56–61] During the diagnostic aspects of dental care, intraoral radiographs should be limited due to their propensity to initiate a gag reflex and generate aerosol.[62] If possible, extraoral radiographs are preferable if the diagnosis or treatment is not compromised as they are less likely to generate aerosols.[63,64] Ideally, digital radiographs should be utilized if possible to minimize the possibility of cross-contamination.[62]

It is critical to recognize that the purpose of the teledentistry triage process is to limit the spread of the SARS-CoV-2 infection by minimizing unnecessary close contact. The decision to delay care should be made individually in the context of the patient's overall health.[53] In general, routine dental care was avoided or postponed by many during the pandemic out of fear of contracting the SARS-CoV-2 infection. While it may be postulated that the incidence of common dental diseases such as dental caries and periodontal disease has likely increased postpandemic, the true impact of the pandemic on dental health especially aggressive lesions, such as oral cancer, is yet to be determined both in the short term and long term.

Effect of Telehealth on Dental Treatment Prognosis

Given the risk for the transmission of the COVID-19 infection, teledentistry (telehealth in dentistry) was soon recognized as an effective modality to facilitate remote communication between the patient and the dental provider, either via telephone consultation (audio) or videoconference.[44] While some patients found it challenging to adapt to these innovative communication processes involving technology, the vast majority of patients embraced these changes. Patients were able to transmit digital images or videos of their dental conditions or were able present for a remote examination via videoconferencing, enabling the dental provider to remotely assess the patient. Teledentistry facilitates remote diagnosis and treatment recommendations, including prescription of medications and determining the need for face-to-face dental care, remote palliation (eg, analgesics and antibiotics) or referral for specialist care.[65] Challenges to teledentistry include Internet connection quality, limitations of smartphone cameras to produce an image of adequate quality, patients' lack of familiarity with technology, and lack of dexterity to produce adequate quality images of the relevant sites of the oral cavity and extraoral tissues, and the secure storage of patient data. Patients who found the teledentistry process challenging may have the option of receiving support from a next of kin, family member, or caregiver. Teledentistry was also utilized for conferencing among dental providers, especially to discuss complex cases with relevant specialists.

DELAYED TREATMENT AND LONG-TERM TREATMENT OUTCOMES

In addition to the short-term sequelae to long-term limited access to dental care, long-term treatment plans requiring many visits, possibly over the course of several years, were also affected by the COVID-19 pandemic. The American Dental Association recommendations in March of 2020 stated, "postponement of all but urgent or emergency procedures."[66] This recommendation expired at the end of April 2020 and was not extended.[67] From this point, both general dentists and specialists began to return to their offices and provide care, albeit in a heavily modified manner.

It rapidly became apparent that, while not all dental treatment can be categorized as emergent, timely treatment often leads to improved outcomes for care, reduced progression of disease, lowered cost, and overall improved oral health for patients. These factors must be weighed in terms of the risk presented by the COVID-19 infection to all parties involved in the direct provision of dental care. This includes the dental team, patients, and others who may come in to contact with the SARS-CoV-2 , such as laboratory technicians and ultimately its consequence on the community.

Fortunately, treatment-specific recommendations and documentation of treatment modifications rapidly found their way into the literature, allowing both general dentists and specialists worldwide to share techniques for maintaining office safety for dental providers, staff, and patients, while providing timely high-quality care. While some of the article address general methods for reducing the transmission of the SARS-CoV-2, others discuss the impact of COVID-19 pandemic on dental specialty practice.

Orthodontics

Numerous authors have written about the effects of the COVID-19 pandemic on orthodontic treatment. It was recommended, during times when patient visits are restricted, that "an in-depth analysis of every patient of record be performed." Patients who have the greatest potential for harm should be given priority for in-office follow-up for adjustment to treatment and direct monitoring.[68]

Orthodontic treatment is of particular concern for the following reasons:

i. Patients are often minors who require parents or guardians to make treatment decisions.
ii. Orthodontics can be more effective when treatment is timed to coincide with growth and maturation of the patient.
iii. Orthodontic treatment requires consistent monitoring for treatment progress, interim goals, maintenance of treatment appliances, and oral hygiene.

Of note, when orthodontic office visits are not possible or are delayed, there are potential harms to the patient such as unsupervised mechanics for tooth movement, harm related to incomplete treatment, psychological harm to patients such as anxiety over treatment outcome, and harm to the teeth and periodontium.[66,69]

One study assessed the outcomes of 50 cases that were completed prior to the COVID-19 pandemic, along with a second set of 50 cases which were completed subsequent to the pandemic onset. The results revealed differences in certain treatment, such as the number of visits and canceled visits; however, treatment duration and outcomes were acceptable for cases in both groups.[70] Similarly, another study found an increase in treatment time, commensurate with the time period that offices were closed during the lockdowns was noted. Of interest, when assessed according to the objective Peer Assessment Rating score, both the COVID-19-affected group and the nonaffected group demonstrated adequate outcomes.[71]

Prosthodontics

Prosthodontic practices faced similar challenges during the COVID-19 pandemic. These include aerosol sprays from handpieces, contaminated material particles from adjustments of prosthetics, and contact with saliva. Recommendation for alterations in practice include the use of telehealth previsits to screen for patients who are displaying symptoms of COVID-19 infection, or for whom treatment could otherwise be manages remotely, use of PPE, as well as high velocity evacuation, and rubber dam to decrease the spread of potentially contaminated salvia and limiting treatment to urgent or emergent issues. Further, visitors and persons accompanying the patient should be requested to remain outside of the office whenever possible. Four-handed dentistry is advised, when possible, for effect suctioning, as well as limiting the contamination of surfaces and objects in the operatory.[72]

Endodontics

Endodontic practices also faced specific challenges and were severely impacted by COVID-19. A cross-sectional study of endodontic specialists in Brazil collected data via an online questionnaire on treatment modifications during COVID-19. An interesting finding was that the use of "minimally adequate PPE" was dependent on "area of residence and the marital status of participants." Clearly, at the time of writing, access to PPE and modern equipment was still of great concern for the respondents to the survey.[73]

Periodontics

A cross-sectional study of members of the British Society of Periodontology and Implant Dentistry practicing in the United Kingdom months into the pandemic noted that while periodontists were "generally worried" by the COVID-19 pandemic, they reportedly had the capability and motivation to make the necessary changes to their practices to adapt to challenges posed by the pandemic.[74] Of relevance, the use "bio-inspired systems" as an adjuvant to nonsurgical periodontal therapy to reduce the risk of bacteremia and aerosol generation may be useful; however, more research is needed to assess their validity.[75]

Oral and Maxillofacial Radiology

Changes to oral and maxillofacial radiology practice include employing, whenever possible, extraoral imaging techniques, including panoramic, extraoral bitewings, and cone-beam computed tomography. The primary concept is to avoid or limit intraoral radiographic procedures due to their propensity to initiate a gag reflex, potentially broadcasting contaminated respiratory droplets on the operator and surrounding surfaces.[62] While the line pair resolution of extraoral imaging is indeed somewhat lower than that of intraoral periapical and bitewing radiographs, it is often adequate for most diagnostic tasks, as per As Low As Diagnostically Acceptable being Indication-oriented and Patient-specific (ALADA-IP).[71] Further, it is recommended that "hard copies" of radiographs be eliminated, with radiographs, acquired, viewed, stored, and transmitted electronically to minimize possibility of cross-contamination.[62]

In Brazil, where oral and maxillofacial radiologists more often practice in stand-alone oral and maxillofacial radiology clinics, a survey found that in addition to upgraded infection control processes, more extraoral examinations were being performed than before the onset of the pandemic in March of 2020. Further, fewer patients overall were being seen in these oral and maxillofacial radiology clinics.[63]

In the event that more invasive radiographic procedures are indicated and substitution with an extraoral procedure is not possible, in these scenarios, it is imperative that PPE and meticulous infection control procedures are adhered to. Extraoral radiographic procedures are preferable in cases where diagnosis or treatment will not be compromised.[64]

OPPORTUNISTIC COINFECTION AND SUPERINFECTION IN PATIENTS WITH CORONAVIRUS DISEASE 2019

Throughout the COVID-19 pandemic, an increase in bacterial, viral, and fungal coinfection and superinfection was noted. Coinfection occurs simultaneously with the primary infection (SARS-CoV-2), while superinfection implies that infection with the secondary infectious agent occurs later.[76] Based on time and place of diagnosis, coinfections are considered community-acquired, and superinfection, hospital-acquired.[77] These opportunistic infectious agents cause an increase in morbidity and mortality in patients with COVID-19. A list of more than 30 bacterial, viral, and fungal coinfections has been reported.[78] Bacterial copathogens are seen in conjunction with respiratory tract infections, especially, in severely ill patients with COVID-19.[79] Superinfection with *Mycobacterium tuberculosis* and *Klebsiella pneumoniae* was reported in a Columbian study.[78] Different parts of the world may face different challenges in identifying and treating COVID-19 coinfections. For example, dengue is more common in tropical countries. Further, dengue and COVID-19 share a number of symptoms, making diagnosis of this coinfection more challenging.[78] Serology, as well as appropriate blood studies are indicated where coinfection is suspected. An indicator of coinfection may be the severity of the symptoms.[80]

Rhinoviruses and enteroviruses have been identified as causing common viral coinfection with COVID-19.[78,81] Individuals living with HIV/AIDS (caused by a retrovirus) who have low CD4 T-cell counts are reported to have worse outcomes from COVID-19 than those without the infection.[82] Also, patients with severe COVID-19 infections requiring prolonged hospitalization may be at risk for acquiring fungal infections.[83] Risk factors include broad-spectrum antibiotics and medical devices.[84] Mucormycosis, a fungal condition, has been associated with immunocompromised individuals, as well as patients with uncontrolled diabetes and glucocorticosteroid use and pulmonary alterations from SARS-CoV-2.[85] Careful diagnosis includes clinical, radiological, histopathological, and culture assessments. Treatment typically involves surgical debridement and antifungal drugs like liposomal amphotericin B, isavuconazole, or posaconazole, with early detection and intensive care management pivotal for favorable outcomes.[86] Mucormycosis infections seem to be centered in the nose and paranasal sinuses and may extend to the surrounding structures, including presenting as ophthalmologic symptoms. Extreme mucormycosis infections have been reported to cause death, via brain abscesses and infarction. During the COVID-19 pandemic, an increased number of mucormycosis patients have been reported, with many of the cases located in India. Patients who have received COVID-19 vaccines have a lower reported infection rate,[87] suggesting association, possibly, related to immunosuppression. Symptoms of mucormycosis include facial pain, discharge, edema, bleeding, paresthesia, and sudden loss of vision.[88]

In addition to mucormycosis, aspergillosis has been found in patients with COVID-19. It has been hypothesized that the increase in aspergillosis during the third wave of COVID-19 may be due to the antiviral therapy aimed specifically at mucormycosis during the second wave.[76,81] Invasive pulmonary aspergillosis is reported to be lethal in immunocompromised patients; however, COVID-19 did not worsen risk or outcome.[89] Increase in the abundance of *Candida albicans* has also been found in the upper respiratory tract of patients with COVID-19.[90] This may predispose the patient to oral candidiasis. Oral candidiasis has been linked to aspiration pneumonia, gastrointestinal infection, pleural infection, and bacterial endocarditis, in addition to the effects on the oral mucosa, such as denture stomatitis.[91]

The risk of opportunistic coinfection and superinfection should not be minimized, as it can worsen the course of the primary disease process, such as COVID-19, as well as adversely impact outcomes.

ORAL MUCOSAL DISEASES AND ORAL CANCER CONSIDERATIONS RELATED TO CORONAVIRUS DISEASE 2019

Over 70% of COVID-19 disease cases were noted to have oral manifestations, presenting 4 days before and up to 12 weeks after systemic symptoms, without gender predilection and symptomatic in 68% of cases. Based on real-time polymerase chain reaction testing for the diagnosis of SARS-CoV-2 infection, 13% of cases developed oral lesions before their positive result.[92] Oral manifestations include ulceration (most common; >50%), erosion, bulla, vesicle, pustule, fissured and/or depapillated tongue, macule, papule, plaque, pigmentation, hemorrhagic crust, necrosis, petechiae, swelling, erythema, and spontaneous bleeding. They may occur in any part of the oral cavity but typically on the tongue (38%), labial mucosa (26%), palate (22%), gingiva (8%), and buccal mucosa (5%).[93] The pathogenesis has been subject of much debate with several hypothesis presented. The interaction between SARS-CoV-2 and angiotensin converting enzyme-2 expressing epithelial cells is postulated to disrupt the integrity of the oral mucosa resulting in oral ulceration. Other plausible explanations for oral lesions may be related to thrombocytopenia, disseminated intravascular coagulation, anticoagulant therapy, systemic inflammation, and primary or secondary vascular inflammation associated with COVID-19, generalized or localized immunosuppression, oral microbiome dysbiosis, and drug therapies (antimicrobials and corticosteroids) utilized for the treatment of COVID-19.[94]

The most common clinical diagnoses of for oral manifestations of COVID-19 were aphthous-like lesions, herpetiform lesions, candidiasis, and oral lesions of Kawasaki-like disease. Predictive factors for oral diseases (and greater severity) of COVID-19 include age, severe of SARS-CoV-2 infection (hyperinflammatory response), poor oral hygiene, opportunistic infections, stress, immunosuppression, and trauma (secondary to intubation).[93] Similarly, among children with COVID-19, common oral manifestations include oral lesions, taste and smell disorders, oral candidiasis, hemorrhagic crust, tongue discoloration, lip and tongue fissuring, gingivitis, and salivary gland inflammation. These oral manifestations may present more frequently in either multisystem inflammatory syndrome in children or Kawasaki disease.[95] Current consensuses favor the likelihood that oral manifestations in SARS-CoV-2 infections are related to disease-associated immune impairment and/or the adverse effects of pharmacotherapeutics.[94]

Community concerns about SARS-CoV-2 vaccine safety and consequently vaccine hesitancy was partly related to potential adverse effects including adverse oral effects.

An Australian study on adverse oral effects after COVID-19 vaccination reported oral paresthesia to be most common (75.28 out of 10,000 reports). Other adverse oral effects included dysgeusia, swollen tongue and lip, ageusia, dry mouth, oral ulceration, oral hypoesthesia, and oral herpes simplex virus infection. Most of these adverse oral effects occur in both the COVID-19 and influenza vaccines; however, the taste disorders, dry mouth, and oral herpes simplex virus infection were significantly more common after COVID-19 vaccination, especially in female individuals and mRNA vaccine recipients.[96] Multiple cases of life-threatening autoimmune mucocutaneous blistering diseases after SARS-CoV-2 vaccination including bullous pemphigoid, mucous membrane pemphigoid, linear immunoglobulin A bullous dermatosis, pemphigus vulgaris, and pemphigus foliaceus have been reported.[97,98] However, to keep these reports in perspective, a systematic review of oral lesions as a side effect of SARS-CoV-2 vaccine administration reported only 16 cases (rare), which included lichen planus, erythema multiforme, pemphigus vulgaris, Stevens–Johnson syndrome, angular cheilitis, and aphthous-like ulcers.[99] Future research is necessary to elucidate the physiopathology of oral manifestations after the SARS-CoV-2 vaccination.

The effect of the COVID-19 pandemic on the diagnosis and progression of oral cancer remains unclear. Despite mandatory lockdown and shutdown of nonessential services, the maintenance of an efficient emergent care pathway for patients with oral cancer was achieved in some, but not all, regions around the world.[100,101] Tumor, Node, Metastasis (TNM) staging at level 4a and above for oral cancer staging had increased to 68% during the COVID-19 pandemic compared to 48% the year prior.[102] These findings were supported by another study, which reported the stage and depth of invasion of tongue cancer was higher during the COVID-19 outbreak.[103]

While the incidence rate of oral cavity and pharyngeal cancers had declined during the first year of the COVID-19 pandemic,[104] there was logical concern that an increase in advanced-stage oral cancer diagnoses will likely result at a later stage due to postponement of routine dental care and consequentially delays in diagnosis, which has now evidently transpired.[105] Another possible explanation for the occurrence of advanced-stage oral cancer could be that the exposure to the COVID-19 infection is an independent influencing factor for higher expression of Ki-67 and cyclin D1 in oral squamous cell carcinoma, which is associated with more invasive malignant behavior of cancer cells.[106]

BRUXISM AND TEMPOROMANDIBULAR DISORDERS

The immediate impact of the COVID-19 pandemic on temporomandibular disorders (TMDs) and on both awake and sleep bruxism has been established. A questionnaire study of medical students during the social isolation period of the pandemic found the prevalence of TMD symptoms, self-reported awake bruxism, and self-reported sleep bruxism to be 77%, 48%, and 59%, respectively.[107] Comparably, the odds of dental patients diagnosed with painful TMDs was 3.3 times higher compared to prepandemic levels. Similarly, the odds for self-reported sleep bruxism and self-reported awake bruxism among these patients were 2.7 times and 3.2 times higher, respectively, as compared to prepandemic levels.[108] It is postulated that the increase in TMDs, which was more profound among female individuals, is influenced by worry, anxiety, and depression and the associated upregulation of the hypothalamic-pituitary-adrenal axis during the pandemic.[109,110] Similarly, the increase in awake bruxism and other parafunctional oral activities can be viewed as an adaptive coping response to stressors associated with the pandemic.[111] A study at the early stages of the pandemic reported 54% and 65% of individuals had difficulty falling asleep and disturbed or restless sleep, respectively, which potentially reduces the threshold for the development of sleep bruxism, awake bruxism, TMDs, and headache.[112]

OROFACIAL CONSIDERATIONS RELATED TO OLFACTORY AND TASTE DYSFUNCTION

As previously stated, olfactory and taste dysfunction are not uncommon symptoms of the COVID-19 infection. These are typically transitory neurologic presentations that vary in severity from minor anosmia to total anosmia and varying taste dysfunctions including hypogeusia, dysgeusia, and ageusia. Of interest, chemosensory dysfunction may present as prodromal symptoms of COVID-19 infection.[113] There appears to be a variable pattern of olfactory dysfunction associated with COVID-19 infection across the world, whereby anosmia and dysgeusia were noted in over 70% ambulatory and hospitalized patients in mild-to-severe infection. In the United States, Europe, and Iran, it was noted that olfactory and gustatory symptoms preceded COVID-19 symptoms.[114] Approximately 85% of cases of COVID-19 infection during the first wave reported chemosensory dysfunction,[115,116] typically presenting as sudden onset of anosmia or hyposmia, dysgeusia, and loss of chemesthesis (cold, hot, and irritation from the trigeminal nerve in the eyes, nose, and mouth).[117,118] It is of significance that approximately 15 million cases worldwide report persistent smell dysfunction post-COVID-19 infection, aptly referred to as "smell long-haulers," and over 7 million of these cases represent persistent parosmia typically noted as bad smells.[119]

Damage to the olfactory bulb and other early olfactory areas by the SARS-CoV-2 virus likely occurs via the transcribriform route, through the olfactory nerve fascicles, cerebrospinal fluid, or terminal nerve and also via the sensory epithelium vasculature in the nose and the olfactory bulb. The virus causes olfactory bulb inflammation, microvascular damage, and reduced volume of the olfactory bulb and reduced volume of cortical areas connected to the olfactory system. This damage may explain the persistent hyposmia and parosmia noted in post-COVID-19 infection cases.[120]

Most symptoms of taste and smell alterations with COVID-19 infection are self-limiting and typically subside most within 2 weeks.[121] In cases of persistent olfactory dysfunction (loss of smell/anosmia), 43% report relief of their symptoms with the combination of nasal budesonide irrigation and olfactory training.[122] For patients with anosmia treatment includes saline irrigation, nasal corticosteroids, decongestants, and vitamins.[115] Dysgeusia associated with COVID-19 infection may respond to clonazepam 0.5 to 1 mg taken once daily, or L-carnitine and vitamins.[115,123]

SUMMARY

It can be concluded from the literature that the COVID-19 pandemic compelled dental providers and dental practices to drastically change many aspects in the direct delivery of dental care. While some of the more draconian changes have not persisted beyond the original wave of the SARS-CoV-2, the dental profession has upgraded infection control, improved the delivery of safe care, and has incorporated innovations into routine practice. Of significance, the emergence of novel infections and the re-emergence of infections pose a risk for future pandemics. Therefore, dentistry must remain vigilant to the possibility of future disruptions to the provision of dental care. Dentistry may be once again called upon to rapidly learn to adapt patient care practices in the interest of the safety of dental providers, office staff, patients and their families, and the community at large.

CLINICS CARE POINTS

- Given the risk for emerging and reemerging infections on dentistry, dentists should be prepared to implement established protocols to rapidly adapt to infectious disease outbreaks. This may include vaccination, screening questions and temperature monitoring devices to exclude infected patients, utilization of teledentistry, enhanced personal protective equipment for dentists and support staff, air filtration systems, and modification of dental service delivery to minimize the risk for infectious disease transmission.

- Teledentistry may be utilized to triage patients to determine urgency of care and need for in-office appointments to limit the spread of infection by minimizing unnecessary close contact.

- Teledentistry may be utilized for remote communication between the patient and the dental provider for diagnosis and treatment recommendations such as prescription of medications, remote palliation, and referral for specialist care.

- Guidelines for the provision of safe dental care including for specialist services during an infection disease outbreak should be implemented to ensure timely treatment to improved outcomes, reduced progression of disease, lowered cost, and overall improved oral health for patients.

- Early diagnosis and treatment of opportunistic coinfections and superinfections especially related to the oral cavity is necessary.

- Oral manifestations of an infection disease and side effects of vaccination should be diagnosed and treated early.

REFERENCES

1. Arora S, Abullais Saquib S, Attar N, et al. Evaluation of knowledge and preparedness among indian dentists during the current COVID-19 pandemic: a cross-sectional study. J Multidiscip Healthc 2020;13:841–54.
2. Nalbandian A, Sehgal K, Gupta A, et al. Post-acute COVID-19 syndrome. Nat Med 2021;27(4):601–15.
3. Andersen KG, Rambaut A, Lipkin WI, et al. The proximal origin of SARS-CoV-2. Nat Med 2020;26(4):450–2.
4. Lau SKP, Luk HKH, Wong ACP, et al. Possible bat origin of severe acute respiratory syndrome coronavirus 2. Emerg Infect Dis 2020;26(7):1542–7.
5. Ye G, Pan Z, Pan Y, et al. Clinical characteristics of severe acute respiratory syndrome coronavirus 2 reactivation. J Infect 2020;80(5):e14–7.
6. Nobel YR, Phipps M, Zucker J, et al. Gastrointestinal symptoms and coronavirus disease 2019: a case-control study from the United States. Gastroenterology 2020;159(1):373–375 e372.
7. Pan L, Mu M, Yang P, et al. Clinical characteristics of COVID-19 patients with digestive symptoms in hubei, china: a descriptive, cross-sectional, multicenter study. Am J Gastroenterol 2020;115(5):766–73.
8. Cheema M, Aghazadeh H, Nazarali S, et al. Keratoconjunctivitis as the initial medical presentation of the novel coronavirus disease 2019 (COVID-19). Can J Ophthalmol 2020;55(4):e125–9.
9. Ellul MA, Benjamin L, Singh B, et al. Neurological associations of COVID-19. Lancet Neurol 2020;19(9):767–83.
10. Alkeridy WA, Almaghlouth I, Alrashed R, et al. A unique presentation of delirium in a patient with otherwise asymptomatic COVID-19. J Am Geriatr Soc 2020; 68(7):1382–4.

11. Dassie-Leite AP, Gueths TP, Ribeiro VV, et al. Vocal signs and symptoms related to COVID-19 and risk factors for their persistence. J Voice 2024;38(1):189–94.

12. Sung S, Kim SH, Lee C, et al. The association of acute signs and symptoms of COVID-19 and exacerbation of depression and anxiety in patients with clinically mild COVID-19: retrospective observational study. JMIR Public Health Surveill 2023;9:e43003.

13. Tsai J, Traub E, Aoki K, et al. Incidentally detected SARS-COV-2 among hospitalized patients in Los Angeles County, August to October 2020. J Hosp Med 2021;16(8):480–3.

14. Yue H, Zhang M, Xing L, et al. The epidemiology and clinical characteristics of co-infection of SARS-CoV-2 and influenza viruses in patients during COVID-19 outbreak. J Med Virol 2020;92(11):2870–3.

15. Verity R, Okell LC, Dorigatti I, et al. Estimates of the severity of coronavirus disease 2019: a model-based analysis. Lancet Infect Dis 2020;20(6):669–77.

16. Mwananyanda L, Gill CJ, MacLeod W, et al. Covid-19 deaths in Africa: prospective systematic postmortem surveillance study. BMJ 2021;372:n334.

17. Sun YJ, Feng YJ, Chen J, et al. Clinical features of fatalities in patients with COVID-19. Disaster Med Public Health Prep 2021;15(2):e9–11.

18. Bante A, Mersha A, Tesfaye A, et al. Adherence with COVID-19 preventive measures and associated factors among residents of Dirashe District, Southern Ethiopia. Patient Prefer Adherence 2021;15:237–49.

19. Matthias J, Patrick S, Wiringa A, et al. Epidemiologically linked COVID-19 outbreaks at a youth camp and men's conference — Illinois, June–July 2021. MMWR (Morb Mortal Wkly Rep) 2021;70(35):1223–7.

20. Zelka MA, Jimma MS, Wondashu PJ, et al. Practice of people towards COVID-19 infection prevention strategies in Benishangul Gumuz Region, North-West Ethiopia: Multilevel analysis. PLoS One 2022;17(2):e0263572.

21. Griffin JB, Haddix M, Danza P, et al. SARS-CoV-2 infections and hospitalizations among persons aged ≥16 years,by vaccination status — Los Angeles County, California, May 1–July 25, 2021. MMWR (Morb Mortal Wkly Rep) 2021;70: 1170–6.

22. Luo L, Liu D, Liao X, et al. Contact settings and risk for transmission in 3410 close contacts of patients with COVID-19 in Guangzhou, China : A Prospective Cohort Study. Ann Intern Med 2020;173(11):879–87.

23. Fricke-Galindo I, Falfan-Valencia R. Genetics insight for COVID-19 susceptibility and severity: a review. Front Immunol 2021;12:622176.

24. Blann AD, Heitmar R. SARS-CoV-2 and COVID-19: a narrative review. Br J Biomed Sci 2022;79:10426.

25. COVID-19 rapid guideline: managing COVID-19. London: National Institute for Health and Care Excellence (NICE); 2022. PMID: 34181371.

26. Jones KE, Patel NG, Levy MA, et al. Global trends in emerging infectious diseases. Nature 2008;451(7181):990–3.

27. Vaidya R, Herten-Crabb A, Spencer J, et al. Travel restrictions and infectious disease outbreaks. J Travel Med 2020;27(3):taaa050.

28. Memish ZA, Al-Tawfiq JA, Alhakeem RF, et al. Middle East respiratory syndrome coronavirus (MERS-CoV): a cluster analysis with implications for global management of suspected cases. Travel Med Infect Dis 2015;13(4):311–4.

29. Al-Sehaibany FS. Middle East respiratory syndrome in children. dental considerations. Saudi Med J 2017;38(4):339–43.

30. Saeed M, Ashraf A, Sabir B, et al. In-silico screening of origanum vulgare phytocompounds as potential drug agents against Vp35 protein of the ebola virus. bioRxiv 2023. 2023-03.

31. Vetter P, Fischer WA 2nd, Schibler M, et al. Ebola virus shedding and transmission: review of current evidence. J Infect Dis 2016;214(suppl 3):S177–84.

32. Brockwell-Staats C, Webster RG, Webby RJ. Diversity of influenza viruses in swine and the emergence of a novel human pandemic influenza A (H1N1). Influenza Other Respir Viruses 2009;3(5):207–13.

33. Kshatriya RM, Khara NV, Ganjiwale J, et al. Lessons learnt from the Indian H1N1 (swine flu) epidemic: predictors of outcome based on epidemiological and clinical profile. J Family Med Prim Care 2018;7(6):1506–9.

34. Ludlow M, Rennick LJ, Sarlang S, et al. Wild-type measles virus infection of primary epithelial cells occurs via the basolateral surface without syncytium formation or release of infectious virus. J Gen Virol 2010;91(Pt 4):971–9.

35. Torres JR, Castro JS. Venezuela's migration crisis: a growing health threat to the region requiring immediate attention. J Travel Med 2019;26(2):tay141.

36. Mahase E. Measles cases rise 300% globally in first few months of 2019. BMJ 2019;365:l1810.

37. Gordon SC, MacDonald NE, Osap TSDV. Managing measles in dental practice: a forgotten foe makes a comeback. J Am Dent Assoc 2015;146(7):558–60.

38. Alakunle E, Moens U, Nchinda G, et al. Monkeypox Virus in Nigeria: infection biology, epidemiology, and evolution. Viruses 2020;12(11):1257.

39. Sharma A, Priyanka, Fahrni ML, Choudhary OP. Monkeypox outbreak: new zoonotic alert after the COVID-19 pandemic. Int J Surg 2022;104:106812.

40. Petersen E, Abubakar I, Ihekweazu C, et al. Monkeypox - Enhancing public health preparedness for an emerging lethal human zoonotic epidemic threat in the wake of the smallpox post-eradication era. Int J Infect Dis 2019;78:78–84.

41. Zemouri C, Beltran EO, Holliday R, et al. Monkeypox: what do dental professionals need to know? Br Dent J 2022;233(7):569–74.

42. Lustig Y, Mendelson E, Paran N, et al. Detection of Zika virus RNA in whole blood of imported Zika virus disease cases up to 2 months after symptom onset, Israel, December 2015 to April 2016. Euro Surveill 2016;21(26). https://doi.org/10.2807/1560-7917.ES.2016.21.26.30269. PMID: 27386894.

43. Barbosa MR, de Farias Martorelli SB, Diniz DA, et al. Orofacial changes of patients with congenital Zika syndrome in Northeast Brazil: an integrative literature review. Clin Lab Res Dent 2021;1–9.

44. Mac Giolla Phadraig C, van Harten MT, Diniz-Freitas M, et al. The impact of COVID-19 on access to dental care for people with disabilities: a global survey during the COVID-19 first wave lockdown. Med Oral Patol Oral Cir Bucal 2021;26(6):e770–7.

45. Mattos FF, Pordeus IA. COVID-19: a new turning point for dental practice. Braz Oral Res 2020;34:e085.

46. Picciani BLS, Bausen AG, Michalski dos Santos B, et al. The challenges of dental care provision in patients with learning disabilities and special requirements during COVID-19 pandemic. Spec Care Dent 2020;40(5):525–7.

47. Isaila OM, Drima E, Hostiuc S. An ethical analysis regarding the COVID-19 pandemic impact on oral healthcare in patients with mental disorders. Healthcare (Basel) 2023;11(18):2585.

48. Al-Hourani Z, Almhdawi K, AlBakri I, et al. Health and quality of life of individuals with dental conditions during COVID-19 lockdown in Jordan. Oral Health Prev Dent 2022;20(1):449–55.

49. Witton R, Plessas A, Wheat H, et al. The future of dentistry post-COVID-19: perspectives from urgent dental care centre staff in England. Br Dent J 2021;1–5.

50. Chmielewski M, Zalachowska O, Rybakowska W, et al. COVID-19 in dental care: what do we know? J Oral Microbiol 2021;13(1):1957351.

51. Gurzawska-Comis K, Becker K, Brunello G, et al. Recommendations for dental care during COVID-19 pandemic. J Clin Med 2020;9(6):1833.

52. Pan Y, Liu H, Chu C, et al. Transmission routes of SARS-CoV-2 and protective measures in dental clinics during the COVID-19 pandemic. Am J Dent 2020; 33(3):129–34.

53. Shamsoddin E, DeTora LM, Tovani-Palone MR, et al. Dental care in times of the COVID-19 pandemic: a review. Med Sci 2021;9(1):13.

54. Janakiram C, Nayar S, Varma B, et al. Dental Care Implications in Coronavirus Disease-19 Scenario: Perspectives. J Contemp Dent Pract 2020;21(8):935–41.

55. Al-Halabi M, Salami A, Alnuaimi E, et al. Assessment of paediatric dental guidelines and caries management alternatives in the post COVID-19 period. A critical review and clinical recommendations. Eur Arch Paediatr Dent 2020;21(5): 543–56.

56. Izzetti R, Nisi M, Gabriele M, et al. COVID-19 transmission in dental practice: brief review of preventive measures in Italy. J Dent Res 2020;99(9):1030–8.

57. Mahdi SS, Ahmed Z, Allana R, et al. Pivoting dental practice management during the COVID-19 pandemic-a systematic review. Medicina (Kaunas) 2020; 56(12):644.

58. Dacic SD, Miljkovic MN, Jovanovic MC. Dental care during the Covid-19 pandemic - to treat or not to treat? J Infect Dev Ctries 2020;14(10):1111–6.

59. Melo P, Manarte-Monteiro P, Veiga N, et al. COVID-19 management in clinical dental care part III: patients and the dental office. Int Dent J 2021;71(3):271–7.

60. Ostrc T, Pavlovic K, Fidler A. Urgent dental care on a national level during the COVID-19 epidemic. Clin Exp Dent Res 2021;7(3):271–8.

61. Rutkowski JL, Camm DP, Chaar EE. AAID white paper: management of the dental implant patient during the COVID-19 pandemic and beyond. J Oral Implantol 2020;46(5):454–66.

62. Soltani P, Isola G, Patini R. Oral and maxillofacial radiology in the era of COVID-19: what needs to be done? Oral Radiol 2021;37(2):352–3.

63. Sampaio-Oliveira M, de Lima MPM, Doriguetto PVT, et al. Impacts of the COVID-19 pandemic on the routine of Brazilian oral radiologists. Oral Radiol 2023;39(3): 570–5.

64. Hamedani S, Farshidfar N. The practice of oral and maxillofacial radiology during COVID-19 outbreak. Oral Radiol 2020;36(4):400–3.

65. Nuvvula S, Mallineni SK. Remote management of dental problems in children during and post the COVID-19 pandemic outbreak: A teledentistry approach. Dent Med Probl 2021;58(2):237–41.

66. (ADA), A. D. A. ADA recommending dentists postpone elective procedures. 2020. Available at: https://www.ada.org/en/about/press-releases/2020-archives/ ada-calls-upon-dentists-to-postpone-elective-procedures. [Accessed 13 February 2024].

67. (ADA), A. D. A. As dental practices resume operations, ADA offers continued guidance. 2020. Available at: https://www.ada.org/about/press-releases/2020-archives/as-dental-practices-resume-operations-ada-offers-continued-guidance.

68. Jerrold L. Exceptional circumstances. Am J Orthod Dentofacial Orthop 2020; 157(6):852–5.

69. Abed Al Jawad F, Alhashimi N. Orthodontic treatment pause during COVID-19 outbreak: are we overlooking potential harms to our patients and their treatment outcomes? Dental Press J Orthod 2021;26(2):e21ins2.

70. Meric P, Naoumova J. Did the coronavirus disease 2019 pandemic affect orthodontic treatment outcomes? a clinical evaluation using the objective grading system and Peer Assessment Rating index. Am J Orthod Dentofacial Orthop 2022;162(1):e44–51.

71. Jopson JL, Ellis PE, Jerreat AS, et al. Patient reported experiences and treatment outcomes of orthodontic patients treated within secondary care settings in the South West of England during the COVID-19 pandemic. J Orthod 2022; 49(1):39–47.

72. Batista AUD, Silva P, Melo LA, et al. Prosthodontic practice during the COVID-19 pandemic: prevention and implications. Braz Oral Res 2021;35:e049.

73. Gomes FDA, Malhão EC, Maniglia-Ferreira C, et al. Endodontic treatment during the COVID-19 pandemic – perception and behaviour of dental professionals. Acta Odontol Latinoam 2021;34:63–70.

74. Nibali L, Ide M, Ng D, et al. The perceived impact of Covid-19 on periodontal practice in the United Kingdom: a questionnaire study. J Dent 2020;102:103481.

75. Butera A, Maiorani C, Natoli V, et al. Bio-inspired systems in nonsurgical periodontal therapy to reduce contaminated aerosol during COVID-19: a comprehensive and bibliometric review. J Clin Med 2020;9(12):3914.

76. Del Pozo JL. Respiratory co-and superinfections in COVID-19. Rev Esp Quimioter 2021;34(Suppl1):69–71.

77. Garcia-Vidal C, Sanjuan G, Moreno-Garcia E, et al. Incidence of co-infections and superinfections in hospitalized patients with COVID-19: a retrospective cohort study. Clin Microbiol Infect 2021;27(1):83–8.

78. Duenas D, Daza J, Liscano Y. Coinfections and superinfections associated with COVID-19 in Colombia: a narrative review. Medicina (Kaunas) 2023;59(7):1336.

79. Sysiak-Slawecka J, Wichowska O, Piwowarczyk P, et al. The impact of bacterial superinfections on the outcome of critically ill patients with COVID-19 associated acute respiratory distress syndrome (ARDS) - a single-centre, observational cohort study. Anaesthesiol Intensive Ther 2023;55(3):163–7.

80. Agudelo Rojas OL, Tello-Cajiao ME, Rosso F. Challenges of dengue and coronavirus disease 2019 coinfection: two case reports. J Med Case Rep 2021; 15(1):439.

81. Garg P, Ranjan V, Avnisha, Hembrom S, et al. The changing trend of fungal infection in invasive rhinosinusitis in the COVID era. J Family Med Prim Care 2024;13(4):1428–33.

82. Ortiz-Martinez Y, Mogollon-Vargas JM, Lopez-Rodriguez M, et al. A fatal case of triple coinfection: COVID-19, HIV and Tuberculosis. Travel Med Infect Dis 2021; 43:102129.

83. Chaudhari V, Vairagade V, Thakkar A, et al. Nanotechnology-based fungal detection and treatment: current status and future perspective. Naunyn-Schmiedeberg's Arch Pharmacol 2024;397(1):77–97.

84. Arastehfar A, Carvalho A, Nguyen MH, et al. COVID-19-associated candidiasis (CAC): an underestimated complication in the absence of immunological predispositions? J Fungi (Basel) 2020;6(4):211.

85. Kusumesh R, Singh V, Sinha S, et al. Risk factors and clinical presentation of rhino-orbital mucormycosis: lesson learnt during Covid pandemic. J Family Med Prim Care 2024;13(4):1354–61.

86. Shah NN, Khan Z, Ahad H, et al. Mucormycosis an added burden to Covid-19 patients: an in-depth systematic review. J Infect Public Health 2022;15(11): 1299–314.

87. Lakshmi JN, Sai Kalyan JB, Priya TG, et al. Retrospective study of patient characteristics and treatment for mucormycosis in post COVID-19 population in a tertiary care hospital. Eur J Hosp Pharm Sci Pract 2024. ejhpharm-2024-004127.

88. Honavar SG. Code mucor: guidelines for the diagnosis, staging and management of rhino-orbito-cerebral mucormycosis in the setting of COVID-19. Indian J Ophthalmol 2021;69(6):1361–5.

89. Trapaga MR, Poester VR, Basso RP, et al. Aspergillosis in critically Ill patients with and without COVID-19 in a tertiary hospital in Southern Brazil. Mycopathologia 2024;189(3):48.

90. Zhang X, Nurxat N, Aili J, et al. The characteristics of microbiome in the upper respiratory tract of COVID-19 patients. BMC Microbiol 2024;24(1):138.

91. Ali MO, Alva B, Nagaral S, et al. Association between candida albicans and COVID-19 in complete denture wearers: an observational study. Cureus 2023; 15(10):e47777.

92. Pergolini D, Graniero F, Magnifico L, et al. COVID-19 and oral mucosal lesions: a systematic review. Clin Ter 2023;174(6):550–63.

93. Iranmanesh B, Khalili M, Amiri R, et al. Oral manifestations of COVID-19 disease: a review article. Dermatol Ther 2021;34(1):e14578.

94. Fakhruddin KS, Samaranayake LP, Buranawat B, et al. Oro-facial mucocutaneous manifestations of coronavirus disease-2019 (COVID-19): a systematic review. PLoS One 2022;17(6):e0265531.

95. Nasiri K, Tehrani S, Mohammadikhah M, et al. Oral manifestations of COVID-19 and its management in pediatric patients: a systematic review and practical guideline. Clin Exp Dent Res 2023;9(5):922–34.

96. Riad A, Issa J, Attia S, et al. Oral adverse events following COVID-19 and influenza vaccination in Australia. Hum Vaccin Immunother 2023;19(2):2253589.

97. Calabria E, Canfora F, Mascolo M, et al. Autoimmune mucocutaneous blistering diseases after SARS-Cov-2 vaccination: a case report of pemphigus vulgaris and a literature review. Pathol Res Pract 2022;232:153834.

98. Calabria E, Antonelli A, Lavecchia A, et al. Oral mucous membrane pemphigoid after SARS-CoV-2 vaccination. Oral Dis 2024;30(2):782–3.

99. Di Spirito F, Amato A, Di Palo MP, et al. Oral lesions following anti-SARS-CoV-2 vaccination: a systematic review. Int J Environ Res Public Health 2022;19(16): 10228.

100. Cwintal M, Shih H, Idrissi Janati A, et al. The effect of the COVID-19 pandemic on the diagnosis and progression of oral cancer. Int J Oral Maxillofac Surg 2024; 53(8):629–34.

101. Koyama S, Morishima T, Saito MK, et al. Faster surgery initiation in oral cancer patients during the COVID-19 pandemic in Osaka, Japan. Oral Dis 2024;30(2): 307–12.

102. Lopez J, Mumtaz S, Amini A. Did the COVID-19 pandemic have an effect on oral cancer staging? a single-centre retrospective observational study. Br Dent J 2024. https://doi.org/10.1038/s41415-024-7056-x. Epub ahead of print. PMID: 38326460.

103. Akbari M, Ahadi S, Karimi E, et al. Increasing stage and depth of invasion (DOI) in patients with tongue cancer during the COVID-19 pandemic: a time series study. Health Sci Rep 2024;7(1):e1832.

104. Semprini J, Pagedar NA, Boakye EA, et al. Head and neck cancer incidence in the United States before and during the COVID-19 pandemic. JAMA Otolaryngol Head Neck Surg 2024;150(3):193–200.

105. Remschmidt B, Gaessler J, Brcic L, et al. The impact of COVID-19 on oral squamous cell carcinoma's diagnostic stage-a retrospective study. Oral Dis 2024; 30(2):216–22.

106. Hua Y, Ma P, Li C, et al. Association between COVID 19 exposure and expression of malignant pathological features in oral squamous cell carcinoma: a retrospective cohort study. Oral Oncol 2024;151:106740.

107. Saczuk K, Lapinska B, Wawrzynkiewicz A, et al. Temporomandibular disorders, bruxism, perceived stress, and coping strategies among Medical University Students in Times of social isolation during outbreak of COVID-19 pandemic. Healthcare (Basel) 2022;10(4).

108. Shalev-Antsel T, Winocur-Arias O, Friedman-Rubin P, et al. The continuous adverse impact of COVID-19 on temporomandibular disorders and bruxism: comparison of pre- during- and post-pandemic time periods. BMC Oral Health 2023;23(1):716.

109. Winocur-Arias O, Winocur E, Shalev-Antsel T, et al. Painful temporomandibular disorders, bruxism and oral parafunctions before and during the COVID-19 pandemic era: a sex comparison among dental patients. J Clin Med 2022; 11(3):589.

110. Emodi-Perlman A, Eli I, Smardz J, et al. Temporomandibular disorders and bruxism outbreak as a possible factor of orofacial pain worsening during the COVID-19 pandemic-concomitant research in two countries. J Clin Med 2020; 9(10):3250.

111. Soto-Goni XA, Alen F, Buiza-Gonzalez L, et al. Adaptive stress coping in awake bruxism. Front Neurol 2020;11:564431.

112. Colonna A, Guarda-Nardini L, Ferrari M, et al. COVID-19 pandemic and the psyche, bruxism, temporomandibular disorders triangle. Cranio 2024;42(4):429–34.

113. Thomas DC, Baddireddy SM, Kohli D. Anosmia: a review in the context of coronavirus disease 2019 and orofacial pain. J Am Dent Assoc 2020;151(9): 696–702.

114. Samaranayake LP, Fakhruddin KS, Panduwawala C. Sudden onset, acute loss of taste and smell in coronavirus disease 2019 (COVID-19): a systematic review. Acta Odontol Scand 2020;78(6):467–73.

115. Lechien JR, Chiesa-Estomba CM, De Siati DR, et al. Olfactory and gustatory dysfunctions as a clinical presentation of mild-to-moderate forms of the coronavirus disease (COVID-19): a multicenter European study. Eur Arch Oto-Rhino-Laryngol 2020;277(8):2251–61.

116. Parma V, Ohla K, Veldhuizen MG, et al. More than smell-COVID-19 is associated with severe impairment of smell, taste, and chemesthesis. Chem Senses 2020; 45(7):609–22.

117. Hannum ME, Koch RJ, Ramirez VA, et al. Taste loss as a distinct symptom of COVID-19: a systematic review and meta-analysis. Chem Senses 2023;48: bjad043.

118. Hannum ME, Ramirez VA, Lipson SJ, et al. Objective sensory testing methods reveal a higher prevalence of olfactory loss in COVID-19-positive patients compared to subjective methods: a systematic review and meta-analysis. Chem Senses 2020;45(9):865–74.

119. Ohla K, Veldhuizen MG, Green T, et al. A follow-up on quantitative and qualitative olfactory dysfunction and other symptoms in patients recovering from COVID-19 smell loss. Rhinology 2022;60(3):207–17.

120. Kay LM. COVID-19 and olfactory dysfunction: a looming wave of dementia? J Neurophysiol 2022;128(2):436–44.

121. Krishnakumar HN, Momtaz DA, Sherwani A, et al. Pathogenesis and progression of anosmia and dysgeusia during the COVID-19 pandemic. Eur Arch Oto-Rhino-Laryngol 2023;280(2):505–9.

122. Santos REA, da Silva MG, do Monte Silva MCB, et al. Onset and duration of symptoms of loss of smell/taste in patients with COVID-19: a systematic review. Am J Otolaryngol 2021;42(2):102889.

123. Hoffman HJ, Rawal S, Li CM, et al. New chemosensory component in the U.S. National Health and Nutrition Examination Survey (NHANES): first-year results for measured olfactory dysfunction. Rev Endocr Metab Disord 2016;17(2): 221–40.

Sleep Disorders Affecting Prognosis of Dental Treatment

Anna Colonna, DDS, MSC[a],*,
Davis C. Thomas, BDS, DDS, MSD, MSc Med, MSc[b],
Thao Thi Do, DDS, MSc, PhD[c], Daniele Manfredini, DDS, MSc, PhD[a]

KEYWORDS

- Sleep disorders • Bruxism • Obstructive sleep apnea
- Gastroesophageal reflux disease • Dental treatment • Sleep bruxism
- Orofacial pain • Temporomandibular disorders

KEY POINTS

- The main dental sleep disorders and conditions (sleep bruxism, obstructive sleep apnea, and gastroesophageal reflux disease) have a non-negligible prevalence and may be interconnected.
- Such conditions may have consequences of dental interest, ranging from tooth wear and intraoral complications to orofacial pains.
- Dental practitioners have the twofold role of sentinels and potential caregivers in the diagnosis and management of the main sleep disorders and conditions of dental interest.

INTRODUCTION

Among the main sleep-related disorders and conditions that are of interest for dentists, sleep bruxism (SB), obstructive sleep apnea (OSA), gastroesophageal reflux disease (GERD), xerostomia, hypersalivation, and the effect of orofacial pain (OFP) on sleep quality must be taken into consideration.[1] It is interesting to note that the Australasian Academy of Dental Sleep Medicine also introduced OFP and temporomandibular disorders (TMDs) as dental sleep-related conditions[2]; on the other hand, the American Academy of Orofacial Pain introduced sleep in their mandate.[3]

These changes indicate an ongoing evolution in the dental world, as they highlight that dental sleep medicine (DSM) embraces more than snoring and OSA. For this reason, a group of DSM experts[4] stressed that the management and treatment of

[a] Department of Medical Biotechnologies, School of Dentistry, University of Siena, Siena, Italy; [b] Department of Diagnostic Sciences, Center for Temporomandibular Disorders and Orofacial Pain, Rutgers School of Dental Medicine, Newark, NJ, USA; [c] Faculty of Odonto-Stomatology, Can Tho University of Medicine and Pharmacy, Can Tho, Vietnam
* Corresponding author.
E-mail address: dr.annacolonna@gmail.com

Dent Clin N Am 68 (2024) 647–657
https://doi.org/10.1016/j.cden.2024.05.002
0011-8532/24/© 2024 Elsevier Inc. All rights reserved, including those for text and data mining, AI training, and similar technologies.
dental.theclinics.com

this type of patients require collaboration between dentist and physicians. In particular, dentists can play a significant role in the prevention and/or assessment and/or management of patients with certain sleep-related disorders by observing the clinical consequences in the mouth and teeth and by identifying possible risk factors; on the other hand, it is fundamental to stress that physicians are responsible for the diagnosis and treatment of sleep-related disorders.

Within this scenario, several studies reported that dental sleep-related conditions frequently coexist and constitute a complex multimorbidity network. For instance, some studies discussed the existence of a possible correlation between SB and OSA,[5–7] while others suggest that patients with OSA experience more temporomandibular pain than otherwise healthy individuals.[8] In addition, a recent study shows that effective mandibular advancement device (MAD) therapy significantly reduces jaw-closing muscle activities that are time related to respiratory arousals in patients with OSA.[9] Concerning SB and GERD, it was found that they are temporally associated with each other, with bruxism episodes often occurring after reflux events.[10,11]

This study discusses the main sleep disorders and conditions (ie, SB, OSA, and GERD) affecting prognosis of dental treatment and examines the role that dentist can play in the assessment and management of these conditions.

Sleep Bruxism

Bruxism is a much debated oromandibular condition that interests several disciplines, such as dentistry, neurology, psychology, and sleep medicine, in both clinical and research settings. This condition is characterized by different activities of the jaw muscles (ie, grinding or clenching of the teeth and/or thrusting or bracing of the mandible) and 2 distinct circadian manifestations, viz., SB and awake bruxism.[12,13]

In 2018, an expert consensus provided the following definition for SB: *"SB is a masticatory muscle activity (MMA) during sleep that is characterized as rhythmic (phasic) or nonrhythmic (tonic) and is not a movement disorder or a sleep disorder in otherwise healthy individuals."*[13] It is noteworthy that the definition begins with MMA, to emphasize the concept that bruxism would not be considered a disorder per se in otherwise healthy individuals, but it might be viewed as a protective and/or a risk factor for some clinical consequences independently on any specific neurologic correlates.[12–17]

The potential negative clinical consequences in the dental field include intrinsic mechanical tooth wear (attrition),[18,19] repeated fractures of teeth, dental restorations and implants,[20] masticatory muscle and temporomandibular joint pain,[21,22] and finally temporomandibular disc displacements.[23] On the other hand, some potential protective effects have also been considered, such as an increased upper airway patency that would aid in the prevention of the airway collapse leading to OSA[5,6] or a reduced risk of detrimental chemical tooth wear by increasing salivation in case of GERD.[11] These specific aspects will be discussed in the following paragraphs.

Current knowledge on the epidemiology of SB reflects the adoption of different evaluation strategies, since the literature reports wide ranges of prevalence for both adults and children/adolescents. The prevalence rates for SB in adults range from 8% to 16%, even if a comprehensive scoping review cautioned about the interpretation of results due to the poor methodological quality and inconsistency of the reviewed studies.[24]

In the attempt to provide homogeneity to the evaluation, a Standardized Tool for the Assessment of Bruxism has been recently proposed by an international expert panel.[25,26] The document highlights the need to evaluate not only the presence or absence of MMA (ie, bruxism status), but also the potential risk factors and comorbid conditions as well as the potential clinical consequences.[25,26] The assessment relies on a combination of self-reported, clinical, and instrumental strategies. As for self-reported information, it can be obtained from questionnaires and history taking, and in the case of SB, also multiple informants can be interviewed (ie, bed partner or, in the case of children, their parents).[12–14] This approach can be useful to recruit large samples and to screen for the possible presence of bruxism at the individual level, without prejudice to the well-known limitations. The instrumental measurement of electromyographic (EMG) activity in the natural environment during sleep is the most appropriate approach available to collect information on SB behaviors.[27] In recent years, several home EMG recording devices have been introduced to detect SB episodes[28–30] as alternatives to the more technically demanding polysomnography (PSG). On the other hand, it is necessary to underline how these devices, in order to be used routinely in a clinical setting, must necessarily be improved both in terms of software and hardware.

As regards management, in the clinical setting it is necessary to underline that the association of bruxism with occlusal features is negligible, if at all present[14,31–34] and for this reason, performing irreversible occlusal changes with the aim to decrease pain symptoms in the jaw muscles and/or the temporomandibular joints (TMJ) or to reduce bruxism activities is not recommendable. Clinicians must keep in mind that since bruxism should not be considered a disorder but rather a muscle behavior that can be harmless, harmful, or even protective with respect to several health outcomes the treatment, where applicable, must be conservative referring to the so-called "Multiple-P" approach as the standard of reference[34]:

- Pep talk (counseling)
- Psychology (cognitive behavioral strategies)
- Physiotherapy (exercises of the jaw muscles)
- Plates (oral appliances)
- Pills (drugs)

In this scenario, the dentist represents the main figure for diagnosing and managing bruxism, but he/she should treat the disorder only if it results in negative clinical consequences for the patient (ie, TMD pain or severe tooth wear) and, importantly, by trying to address the causes of SB, which is often just an epiphenomenon of some underlying conditions that disrupt sleep. In addition, it must be pointed out that since SB appears to be associated with other sleep-related disorders (ie, periodic leg movements in sleep,[35] rapid eye movement sleep behavior disorder,[36] and insomnia,[37]), in more severe cases the diagnosis and treatment can be carried out together with medical specialists.[38]

Obstructive Sleep Apnea

OSA is a sleep-related breathing disorder characterized by repetitive episodes of a complete (apnea) or partial collapse (hypopnea) of the upper airway with an associated decrease in blood oxygen saturation, with oxygen levels falling as much as 40% or more in severe cases, or arousal from sleep; this pattern can occur hundreds of times in one night.[39]

The obstructive events (apneas or hypopneas) cause a progressive asphyxia that increasingly stimulates breathing efforts against the collapsed airway, typically until the person is awakened. It occurs when the muscles relax during sleep, causing soft tissue in the back of the throat to collapse and block the upper airway, leading to partial reductions (hypopneas) and complete interruption (apneas) in breathing that lasts at least 10 seconds during sleep. For this reason, this disturbance results in fragmented, nonrestorative sleep that often produces an excessive level of daytime sleepiness.[40]

A common measurement of sleep apnea is the apnea–hypopnea index. This index is the combined average number of apneas and hypopneas that occur per hour of sleep. According to the American Academy of Sleep Medicine, it is categorized into mild (5–15 events/hour), moderate (15–30 events/hr), and severe (>30 events/hr).[40] Other indices, such as the oxygen desaturation index, are also emerging as important predictors for clinical impact.

It is interesting to note that from an epidemiologic point of view, OSA is a common condition that affects almost 1 billion people globally,[41] with 425 million adults aged 30 to 69 years having moderate-to-severe OSA (15 or more events/h).[42] Prevalence increases with age and is more frequent in men than in women, with a 2:1 ratio that tends to equalize over the age of 50 years.[43] Prevalence rates seem to increase following the rise in obesity rates; this could be explained by the fact that obesity appears to be part of the genetically (and phenotypically) determined characteristics of the apneic patients along with upper airway soft tissue structure.[44] As an important remark, it must be borne in mind that despite the potential severe clinical consequences, approximately 80% to 90% of adults with OSA remain undiagnosed.[45]

The pathophysiology of OSA is complex and involves an interaction between unfavorable pharyngeal anatomy and ventilatory control instability[46]; for this reason, anatomic features associated with a small upper airway volume (eg, retrognathia, maxillary hypoplasia, tonsillar and lingual hypertrophy, excess adipose tissue around the airway lumen) may facilitate collapse during sleep when muscle compensation is absent.[47,48] Large neck circumference, cervical soft tissue, vessels, and bony structures are among the anatomic factors that promote pharyngeal narrowing. Many of these factors promote pharyngeal collapsibility by decreasing the caliber of the upper airway or by increasing the upper airway surrounding pressure.[48]

The primary role of a dental clinician as far as OSA is concerned is to act as a sentinel.[49] The suspicion of OSA is based on the presence of clinical symptoms, such as daytime sleepiness, excessive tiredness, witnessed apneas, choking or gasping at night, nocturia, and loud snoring with periods of silence when airflow is reduced or blocked.[50] The majority of these signs and symptoms are easy to intercept through the use of simple and reliable self-report questionnaires (ie, the Epworth Sleepiness Scale[51] and the STOP-Bang questionnaire[52]) and clinical examination. Regarding the latter, the dental practitioner has the role of identifying physical characteristics that potentially predispose to OSA, such as mandibular retrognathia, maxillary micrognathia, arched palate and signs of nasal obstruction (ie, polyps, septal deviation, turbinate hypertrophy, significant congestion), and soft tissue hypertrophy (ie, tonsillar hypertrophy, macroglossia, enlarged or elongated uvula).[53] The early recognition of predisposing factors has a considerable importance, as it reduces the risk of long-term pathologic consequences of OSA (ie, systemic hypertension, cardiovascular, neuropsychological, and metabolic consequences).[54]

The definite diagnosis is made with PSG, which allows for measurement of the number of apnea/hypopnea as well as oxygen desaturation events to rate the condition's severity.[55] PSG is always recommended when clinical examination and history taking suggest the possible presence of OSA.[56] On the other hand, it is important to underline that PSG does not reveal the specific obstruction site, nor does it provide any differential diagnostic information as far as the potential relationship between the site of obstruction and OSA severity is concerned.[57] For this reason, drug-induced sleep endoscopy (DISE) is the standard of reference to evaluate the anatomic features of the upper airway, the number and location of the sites of collapse and the degree and configuration of collapse. In addition, from a clinical point of view, this type of evaluation can guide the treatment choice, also including the predictability of MADs.[58]

Treatment of OSA patients' needs a multidisciplinary approach and it is classified into behavioral, medical, and surgical. The aims are to relieve symptoms such as loud snoring and daytime sleepiness and to restore normal breathing during sleep.

Behavioral therapy is always recommended when needed, but in the majority of cases, a combination with surgical medical or medical treatment is necessary. Continuous positive airway pressure (PAP) is considered the gold standard treatment for any symptomatic individual with OSA. In the cases of primary snoring, mild-moderate OSA, and those cases where PAP is not tolerated, a therapy with MAD is recommended and dentist can play a crucial role.[59] MADs are oral appliances that maintain the mandible in a protruded position with respect the normal relationship, resulting in an enlarged upper airway volume and, consequently, reduced obstruction.[60] Dental clinicians must take into consideration that patients with high loop gain and/or with multiple obstruction sites identified at DISE show poor response to MAD; on the contrary, young age, female gender, retrognathia, short soft palate, absence of severe obesity, tongue base collapse, and high collapsibility are predictors of positive response to MAD.[61,62] Concerning the surgical approach, the aim is to prevent collapse by modifying upper airway anatomic abnormalities. Multiple interventions have been described, involving different nose and throat specialist (ENT) and maxillofacial surgery techniques, which must be considered mainly in selected patients after noninvasive treatments have been unsuccessful.

As highlighted in the previous paragraphs, the role of the dental specialist is 2 fold, possibly acting both as a sentinel in identifying the pathology and a caregiver/management provider with the use of MADs.

Gastroesophageal Reflux Disease

GERD is a chronic gastrointestinal disorder characterized by the regurgitation of gastric contents into the esophagus.[63] It affects approximately 20% of the adult population in high-income countries, and in the United States, the prevalence of GERD is between 18.1% and 27.8%.[64]

The etiology of GERD is caused by multiple mechanisms leading to the disruption of the esophagogastric junction barrier, resulting in exposure of the esophagus to acidic gastric contents.

The pathophysiology of GERD is multifactorial, including the presence of a hiatal hernia, the influence of the tone of the lower esophageal sphincter, esophageal motility, and esophageal mucosal defense against the refluxate.[65]

Clinically, GERD typically manifests with symptoms of heartburn and regurgitation. It can also be present in an atypical fashion with extra-esophageal symptoms such as chest pain, dental erosions, chronic cough, laryngitis, or asthma.[66] Concerning dental erosion, several papers described a strong association between GERD and intrinsic chemical tooth wear. In addition, the severity of GERD symptoms seems to be associated with the severity of the tooth wear.[18,67] In addition, oral lesions, mucositis,[68] and burning mouth syndrome[69–71] were associated with GERD. Furthermore, symptomatic GERD is associated with chronic, painful TMD[72] and the increased TMD in patients with GERD.[73] There was an increased risk of postoperative complications of dentoalveolar treatment in patients with GERD.[74]

The diagnosis of GERD is made solely based on symptoms or in combination with other factors such as responsiveness to antisecretory therapy, esophagogastroduodenoscopy, and ambulatory reflux monitoring.[63] From a therapeutic point of view, the treatment options from the least invasive to the most invasive include lifestyle modifications, medical management with antacids and antisecretory agents, surgical therapies, and endoluminal therapies, with the aims to address the resolution of symptoms and prevent complications such as esophageal adenocarcinoma and esophagitis.[75]

Since the complications of GERD should be promptly recognized, also dentists can play a determinant role in the diagnosis by recognizing complications at the dental level (eg, dental erosion), also because it can cause erosive (chemical) tooth wear, resulting in sensitive teeth. Consequently, the restorative dentist has a major role in this field.

INTERRELATION OF SLEEP BRUXISM, GASTROESOPHAGEAL REFLUX DISEASE, AND OBSTRUCTIVE SLEEP APNEA

The interrelation between SB, OSA, and GERD has raised a lot of interest in the fields of dental and medical research.[1,76] More than 30 years ago, Lavigne and colleagues defined DSM as a new discipline that focuses on several sleep-related disorders (viz., SB, OSA, xerostomia, hypersalivation, OFP, and GERD) that are of interest to dental clinicians.[77] Successive definitions have followed thereafter, in parallel with the increasing attention.

Concerning the correlation between SB and GERD, some investigations suggested that the 2 phenomena are temporally associated[10,11,78,79]: importantly, when the onset of a GERD event precedes the onset of an SB event, more tooth wear can be expected due to the fact that grinding on teeth covered by acid saliva may accelerate the amount of hard tissue loss by the SB activities.[10] On the other hand, to date, several studies investigated the existence of association between SB and OSA reported inconsistent and often conflicting results.[5–7,80] Thus, despite the many speculations, currently there is not enough scientific evidence yet to define a clear temporal relationship, if any, between SB and respiratory events during sleep.[5–7,80] Finally, GERD is also considered a factor that is associated with potential worsening of snoring and OSA, even if the evidence of a clear pathophysiology is still lacking.[81]

It is important to underline that most of the phenomena that fall into the category of DSM are disorders (ie, OSA, GERD) that have adverse consequences on the patient and should therefore be diagnosed and, if necessary, treated with immediacy. The only exception is SB, which is considered a muscular activity and therefore does not always occur to harm the patient; for this reason, a cautious approach to its pathogenesis is recommended before jumping to speculations on treatment, as is often typical of dentists.

In light of the available data, it can be suggested that dental sleep-related conditions are rarely found in isolation, while they frequently coexist and constitute a complex network.[82] In addition, these phenomena (ie, SB, OSA, GERD) have in common the capacity of potentially affecting the dental practice: SB may cause intrinsic mechanical tooth wear,[18,19] fractures of teeth, restorations, and implants[20]; GERD may cause dental erosion; and finally, the use of oral appliances in case of SB must be carefully valued to avoid possible worsening of respiratory pathology. For these reasons, dental practitioners play a relevant role in the prevention, assessment, and management of OSA, SB, and sleep-related gastroesophageal reflux condition.

SUMMARY

Sleep-related disorders have attracted a growing interest among dental practitioners for a twofold reason: (1) for the possible clinical consequences to which they can lead and (2) for the potential role of the dentist in the screening and early recognition of individuals with sleep-related conditions.

The knowledge and the ability to identify signs and symptoms, risk factors and consequences of SB, OSA, GERD as well as their mutual relationships can be helpful to recognize other conditions and avoid their possible negative consequences at a systemic and oral level.

CLINICS CARE POINTS

- Sleep bruxism, obstructive sleep apnea and gastroesophageal reflux disease, also defined as sleep-related disorders and conditions, have a non negligible prevalence in the population, can often be found in association and, finally, may have consequences of dental interest.

- Clinicians must thus be aware of the fact that management of patients with these conditions may require a thorough evaluation and in this scenario they can play a key role in the diagnosis and treatment of these pathologies.

DISCLOSURE

The authors declare that they have no known competing financial interests or personal relationships that could have appeared to influence the work reported in this article.

REFERENCES

1. Huang Z, Zhou N, Lobbezoo F, et al. Dental sleep-related conditions and the role of oral healthcare providers: A scoping review. Sleep Med Rev 2023;67:101721.
2. Australasian Academy of Dental Sleep Medicine. Available at: https://www.aadsm.com.au/.
3. American Academy of Orofacial Pain. Available at: https://aaop.org/.
4. Lobbezoo F, Lavigne GJ, Kato T, et al. The face of dental sleep medicine in the 21st century. J Oral Rehabil 2020;47:1579e89.
5. Manfredini D, Guarda-Nardini L, Marchese-Ragona R, et al. Theories on possible temporal relationships between sleep bruxism and obstructive sleep apnea events. An expert opinion. Sleep Breath 2015;19:1459–65.
6. Colonna A, Cerritelli L, Lombardo L, et al. Temporal relationship between sleep-time masseter muscle activity and apnea-hypopnea events: A pilot study. J Oral Rehabil 2022;49:47–53.
7. Saito M, Yamaguchi T, Mikami S, et al. Temporal association between sleep apnea-hypopnea and sleep bruxism events. J Sleep Res 2014;23:196–203.
8. Alessandri-Bonetti A, Scarano E, Fiorita A, et al. Prevalence of signs and symptoms of temporo-mandibular disorder in patients with sleep apnea. Sleep Breath 2021;25:2001e6.
9. Aarab G, Arcache P, Lavigne GJ, et al. The effects of mandibular advancement appliance therapy on jaw-closing muscle activity during sleep in patients with obstructive sleep apnea: a 3-6 months followup. J Clin Sleep Med 2020;16:1545e53.
10. Miyawaki S, Tanimoto Y, Araki Y, et al. Association between nocturnal bruxism and gastroesophageal reflux. Sleep 2003;26:888e92.
11. Ohmure H, Oikawa K, Kanematsu K, et al. Influence of experimental esophageal acidification on sleep bruxism: a randomized trial. J Dent Res 2011;90:665e71.

12. Lobbezoo F, Ahlberg J, Glaros AG, et al. Bruxism defined and graded: an international consensus. J Oral Rehabil 2013;40:2–4.

13. Lobbezoo F, Ahlberg J, Raphael KG, et al. International consensus on the assessment of bruxism: Report of a work in progress. J Oral Rehabil 2018;45:837–44.

14. Manfredini D, Colonna A, Bracci A, et al. Bruxism: a summary of current knowledge on aetiology, assessment and management. Oral surgery 2019. https://doi.org/10.1111/ors.12454.

15. Manfredini D, De Laat A, Winocur E, et al. Why not stop looking at bruxism as a black/white condition? Aetiology could be unrelated to clinical consequences. J Oral Rehabil 2016;43:799–801.

16. Manfredini D, Ahlberg J, Lavigne GJ, et al. Five years after the 2018 consensus definitions of sleep and awake bruxism: An explanatory note. J Oral Rehabil 2024;51(3):623–4.

17. Lobbezoo F, Ahlberg J, Manfredini D. The advancement of a discipline: The past, present and future of bruxism research. J Oral Rehabil 2024;51(1):1–4.

18. Wetselaar P, Lobbezoo F. The tooth Wear evaluation system (TWES): a modular clinical guideline for the diagnosis and management planning of worn dentitions. J Oral Rehabil 2016;43:69–80.

19. Manfredini D, Lombardo L, Visentin A, et al. Correlation between sleep-time masseter muscle activity and tooth wear: an electromyographic study. J Oral Facial Pain Headache 2019;33:199–204.

20. Manfredini D, Poggio CE, Lobbezoo F. Is bruxism a risk factor for dental implants? A systematic review of the literature. Clin Implant Dent Relat Res 2014;16:460–9.

21. Manfredini D, Cantini E, Romagnoli M, et al. Prevalence of bruxism in patients with different research diagnostic criteria for temporomandibular disorders (RDC/TMD) diagnoses. Cranio 2003;21(4):279–85.

22. Manfredini D, Lobbezoo F. Sleep bruxism and temporomandibular disorders: a scoping review of the literature. J Dent 2021;111:103711.

23. Kalaykova SI, Lobbezoo F, Naeije M. Effect of chewing upon disc reduction in the temporomandibular joint. J Orofac Pain 2011;25:49–55.

24. Manfredini D, Winocur E, Guarda-Nardini L, et al. Epidemiology of bruxism in adults: a systematic review of the literature. J Orofac Pain 2013;27:99–110.

25. Manfredini D, Ahlberg J, Aarab G, et al. Towards a standardised tool for the assessment of bruxism (STAB) - Overview and general remarks of a multidimensional bruxism evaluation system. J Oral Rehabil 2020;47:549–56.

26. Manfredini D, Ahlberg J, Aarab G, et al. Standardised tool for the assessment of bruxism. J Oral Rehabil 2024;51(1):29–58.

27. Manfredini D, Ahlberg J, Wetselaar P, et al. The bruxism construct: from cut-off points to a continuum spectrum. J Oral Rehabil 2019;46:991–7.

28. Colonna A, Noveri L, Ferrari M, et al. Electromyographic assessment of masseter muscle activity: a proposal for a 24 h recording device with preliminary data. J Clin Med 2022;12:247.

29. Mainieri VC, Saueressig AC, Pattussi MP, et al. Validation of the Bitestrip versus polysomnography in the diagnosis of patients with a clinical history of sleep bruxism. Oral Surg Oral Med Oral Pathol Oral Radiol 2012;113:612–7.

30. Colonna A, Segù M, Lombardo L, et al. Frequency of sleep bruxism behaviors in healthy young adults over a four-night recording span in the home environment. Appl Sci 2021;11:195.

31. Manfredini D, Serra-Negra J, Carboncini F. LobbezooF. Current concepts of bruxism. Int J Prosthodont (IJP) 2017;30:437–8.

32. Thomas DC, Singer SR, Markman S. temporomandibular disorders and dental occlusion: what do we know so far? Dent Clin North Am 2023;67(2):299–308.
33. Thomas DC, Manfredini D, Patel J, et al. Sleep bruxism: The past, the present, and the future-evolution of a concept. J Am Dent Assoc 2024;16. S0002-S8177(23)00759-6.
34. Manfredini D, Ahlberg J, Winocur E, et al. Management of sleep bruxism in adults: a qualitative systematic literature review. J Oral Rehabil 2015;42:862–74.
35. van der Zaag J, Naeije M, Wicks DJ, et al. Time-linked concurrence of sleep bruxism, periodic limb movements, and EEG arousals in sleep bruxers and healthy controls. Clin Oral Invest 2014;18:507–13.
36. Abe S, Gagnon JF, Montplaisir JY, et al. Sleep bruxism and oromandibular myoclonus in rapid eye movement sleep behavior disorder: a preliminary report. Sleep Med 2013;14:1024–30.
37. Maluly M, Andersen ML, Dal-Fabbro C, et al. Polysomnographic study of the prevalence of sleep bruxism in a population sample. J Dent Res 2013;92(7 Suppl):97S–103S.
38. Mungia R, Lobbezoo F, Funkhouser E, et al, National Practice-Based Research Network Collaborator Group. Dental practitioner approaches to bruxism: Preliminary findings from the national dental practice-based research network. Cranio 2023;4:1–9.
39. Sankri-Tarbichi AG. Obstructive sleep apnea-hypopnea syndrome: etiology and diagnosis. Avicenna J Med 2012;2(1):3–8.
40. Berry RB, Budhiraja R, Gottlieb DJ, et al. Rules for scoring respiratory events in sleep: update of the 2007 AASM Manual for the Scoring of Sleep and Associated Events—Deliberations of the Sleep Apnea Definitions Task Force of the American Academy of Sleep Medicine. J Clin Sleep Med 2012;8:597–619.
41. Malhotra A, Ayappa I, Ayas N, et al. Metrics of sleep apnea severity: beyond the apnea-hypopnea index. Sleep 2021;44(7).
42. Benjafield AV, Ayas NT, Eastwood PR, et al. Estimation of the global prevalence and burden of obstructive sleep apnoea: a literature-based analysis. Lancet Respir Med 2019;7(8):687–98.
43. Peppard PE, Young T, Barnet JH, et al. Increased prevalence of sleep-disordered breathing in adults. Am J Epidemiol 2013;177(9):1006–14, 01.
44. Garvey JF, Pengo MF, Drakatos P, et al. Epidemiological aspects of obstructive sleep apnea. J Thorac Dis 2015;7:920–9.
45. Lee W, Nagubadi S, Kryger MH, et al. Epidemiology of obstructive sleep apnea: a population-based perspective. Expet Rev Respir Med 2008;1(2):349–64.
46. Wang X, Jia L, Xu X, et al. The relationship between aerodynamic characteristics of the upper airway and severity of obstructive sleep apnea in adults. Cranio 2023;19:1–8.
47. Eckert DJ. Phenotypic approaches to obstructive sleep apnoea—New pathways for the targeted therapy. Sleep Med Rev 2018;37:45–59.
48. Isono S, Remmers JE, Tanaka A, et al. Anatomy of pharynx in patients with obstructive sleep apnea and in normal subjects. J Appl Physiol 1997;82:1319–26.
49. Manfredini D. The evolution of a field: A challenge and an opportunity. Cranio 2024;26:1–2.
50. Mannarino MR, Di Filippo F, Pirro M. Obstructive sleep apnea syndrome. Eur J Intern Med 2012;23:586–93.
51. Johns MW. A new method for measuring daytime sleepiness: the Epworth sleepiness scale. Sleep 1991;14:540–5.

52. Tripathi A, Gupta A, Rai P, et al. Reliability of STOP-Bang questionnaire and pulse oximetry as predictors of OSA - a retrospective study. Cranio 2022;26:1–5.

53. Nair DJ, Varma SNK, Ghosh P, et al. Reliability of Friedman Staging System and Modified Mallampati Scoring as clinical assessment methods for Obstructive Sleep Apnea - A cross sectional study. Cranio 2023;22:1–8.

54. Kaneko Y, Hajek VE, Zivanovic V, et al. Relationship of sleep apnea to functional capacity and length of hospitalization following stroke. Sleep 2003;26:293–7.

55. Sommermeyer D, Zou D, Grote L, et al. Detection of sleep disordered breathing and its central/obstructive character using nasal cannula and finger pulse oximeter. J Clin Sleep Med 2012;8:527–33.

56. Gottlieb DJ, Punjabi NM. Diagnosis and management of obstructive sleep apnea: a review. JAMA 2020;14(323):1389–400.

57. Pollis M, Lobbezoo F, Aarab G, et al. Correlation between apnea severity and sagittal cephalometric features in a population of patients with polysomnographically diagnosed obstructive sleep apnea. J Clin Med 2022;11(15):4572.

58. Viana A, Estevão D, Zhao C. The clinical application progress and potential of drug-induced sleep endoscopy in obstructive sleep apnea. Ann Med 2022;54: 2909–20.

59. Marchese-Ragona R, Manfredini D, Mion M, et al. Oral appliances for the treatment of obstructive sleep apnea in patients with low C-PAP compliance: a long-term case series. Cranio 2014;32(4):254–9.

60. Marklund M, Braem MJA, Verbraecken J. Update on oral appliance therapy. Eur Respir Rev 2019;28(153):190083.

61. Guarda-Nardini L, Manfredini D, Mion M, et al. Anatomically based outcome predictors of treatment for obstructive sleep apnea with intraoral splint devices: a systematic review of cephalometric studies. J Clin Sleep Med 2015;11(11): 1327–34.

62. Chen H, Eckert DJ, van der Stelt PF, et al. Phenotypes of responders to mandibular advancement device therapy in obstructive sleep apnea patients: A systematic review and meta-analysis. Sleep Med Rev 2020;49:101229.

63. Vakil N, van Zanten SV, Kahrilas P, et al, Global Consensus Group. The Montreal definition and classification of gastroesophageal reflux disease: a global evidence-based consensus. Am J Gastroenterol 2006;101:1900–20 ; quiz 1943.

64. Dent J, El-Serag HB, Wallander MA, et al. Epidemiology of gastro-oesophageal reflux disease: a systematic review. Gut 2005;54:710–7.

65. De Giorgi F, Palmiero M, Esposito I, et al. Pathophysiology of gastro-oesophageal reflux disease. Acta Otorhinolaryngol Ital 2006;26:241–6.

66. Hom C, Vaezi MF. Extraesophageal manifestations of gastroesophageal reflux disease. Gastroenterol Clin N Am 2013;42:71–91.

67. Pace F, Pallotta S, Tonini M, et al. Systematic review: gastro-oesophageal reflux disease and dental lesions. Aliment Pharmacol Ther 2008;27:1179–86.

68. Shu L, Tong X. Exploring the causal relationship between gastroesophageal reflux and oral lesions: A mendelian randomization study. Front Genet 2022;13: 1046989.

69. Russo M, Crafa P, Franceschi M, et al. Burning mouth syndrome and reflux disease: Relationship and clinical implications. Acta Biomed 2022;93(6):e2022329.

70. Li L, Wu S, Noma N, et al. Relationship between burning mouth disorder and gastroesophageal reflux disease: A scoping review. Oral Dis 2023.

71. Lechien JR, Hans S, De Marrez LG, et al. Prevalence and features of laryngopharyngeal reflux in patients with primary burning mouth syndrome. Laryngoscope 2021;131(10): E2627–e2633.

72. Li Y, Fang M, Niu L, et al. Associations among gastroesophageal reflux disease, mental disorders, sleep and chronic temporomandibular disorder: A case-control study. CMAJ (Can Med Assoc J) 2019;191(33):E909–e915.
73. Gharaibeh TM, Jadallah K, Jadayel FA. Prevalence of temporomandibular disorders in patients with gastroesophageal reflux disease: A case-controlled study. J Oral Maxillofac Surg 2010;68(7):1560–4.
74. Lens C, Berne JV, Politis C. The impact of gastrointestinal diseases on oral and maxillofacial surgery outcomes. Oral Surg, Oral Med, Oral Pathol Oral Radiol 2023;136(5):577–83.
75. Katz PO, Gerson LB, Vela MF. Guidelines for the diagnosis and management of gastroesophageal reflux disease. Am J Gastroenterol 2013;108(3):308–28, quiz 329.
76. Lavigne G, Kato T, Herrero Babiloni A, et al. Research routes on improved sleep bruxism metrics: Toward a standardised approach. J Sleep Res 2021;30(5): e13320.
77. Lavigne GJ, Goulet JP, Zuconni M, et al. Sleep disorders and the dental patient: an overview. Oral Surg Oral Med Oral Pathol Oral Radiol Endod 1999;88:257–72.
78. Miyawaki S, Tanimoto Y, Araki Y, et al. Relationships among nocturnal jaw muscle activities, decreased esophageal pH, and sleep positions. Am J Orthod Dentofacial Orthop 2004;126:615–9.
79. Mengatto CM, da Dalberto S, Scheeren B, et al. Association between sleep bruxism and gastroesophageal reflux disease. J Prosthet Dent 2013;110:349–55.
80. Da Costa Lopes AJ, Cunha TCA, Monteiro MCM, et al. Is there an association between sleep bruxism and obstructive sleep apnea syndrome? A systematic review. Sleep Breath 2020;24:913–21.
81. Lim KG, Morgenthaler TI, Katzka DA. Sleep and nocturnal gastroesophageal reflux: an update. Chest 2018;154:963–71.
82. Manfredini D, Thomas DC, Lobbezoo F. Temporomandibular disorders within the context of sleep disorders. Dent Clin North Am 2023;67:323–34.

Genetics Affecting the Prognosis of Dental Treatments

Olga A. Korczeniewska, PhD[a],
Janani Dakshinamoorthy, MTech, PhD[b],*,
Vaishnavi Prabhakar, BDS, MDS[c], Upasana Lingaiah, BDS, MDS[d]

KEYWORDS

- Dental disorders • Oral cancer • Dental pathology • Dental implant • Dental caries
- Genetic predisposition • Pharmacogenomics • Treatment prognosis

KEY POINTS

- Understanding about the genetic predisposition in dental pathologies can help us to pre-determine the treatment prognosis.
- Precise dental treatment protocol can be planned in more complex dental procedures to achieve favorable treatment outcomes.
- The prevention and further destruction of dental caries can be avoided and practiced with the help of genetic screening.
- Understanding the role of genomics in disease etiology paves way for further research to develop better diagnostic and treatment protocols with maximum efficiency.

INTRODUCTION

Dental health is influenced by a multitude of factors, including oral hygiene, dietary habits, environmental factors, and genetics. While the role of traditional factors such as oral hygiene and diet is well established in dental fields,[1–3] the role of genetics in dental health and the prognosis of dental treatments is emerging and has gained significant attention in recent years. Genetic factors can affect how an individual

[a] Department of Diagnostic Sciences, Center for Orofacial Pain and Temporomandibular Disorders, Rutgers School of Dental Medicine, Rutgers, The State University of New Jersey, 110 Bergen Street, Room D-880, Newark, NJ 07101, USA; [b] GeneAura Pvt. Ltd, AP1166, 4th street, Anna Nagar, Thendral Colony, Chennai 600040, India; [c] Department of Dental Sciences Dr. M.G. R. Educational And Research Institute Periyar E.V.R. High Road, (NH 4 Highway) Maduravoyal, Chennai 600095, India; [d] Upasana Lingaiah, Department of Oral Medicine and Radiology, V S Dental College and Hospital, Room number 1, K R Road, V V Puram, Bengaluru, Karnataka 560004, India
* Corresponding author.
E-mail address: jmoortybiotech1990@gmail.com

Dent Clin N Am 68 (2024) 659–692
https://doi.org/10.1016/j.cden.2024.05.003
0011-8532/24/© 2024 Elsevier Inc. All rights reserved, including those for text and data mining, AI training, and similar technologies.

dental.theclinics.com

responds to various dental procedures and treatments and therefore can influence the prognosis of dental treatments. Examples of how genetic factors may affect the prognosis of dental treatments include genetic contributions to dental caries,[4–6] saliva flow, and composition as well as periodontal disease and inflammation[7,8]; individuals with genetic predisposition to gum disease may have less favorable prognosis for dental treatments related to gum health, such as periodontal surgery or root planning. Furthermore, genetic factors can affect an individual's inflammatory response and ability to heal and regenerate oral tissues after dental procedures. Some individuals heal fast without complications, while others may heal more slowly and be prone to complications with excessive inflammation leading to discomfort. Additionally, genetic factors may affect an individual's sensitivity and perception of pain as well as response to medications with some individuals requiring higher doses of local anesthetic to achieve the same level of pain relief. Wide interindividual differences in pain perception and analgesia have been reported.[9–12] Finally, interindividual variations in drug metabolism can impact the efficacy and side effects of drugs including antibiotics and analgesics prescribed after dental treatments.

Many factors can affect the success of dental procedures and genetics is just one component of a multifaceted approach to dental health. Understanding of the genetic factors affecting dental health and prognosis of treatments will allow for the development of personalized treatment plans ultimately improving the overall quality of dental care. However, at present, genetic testing is not a standard practice in dentistry. While genetic testing holds potential for clinical applications in the future, clinical measurements including the patient's medical history, oral health status, and lifestyle factors remain the best approach for the assessment and treatment planning of dental conditions. Advances in personalized medicine and genetic testing may provide insights into individual patient profiles allowing for more tailored treatment approaches in the future.

Restorative Dentistry

Caries and dental restorations

Dental caries, commonly known as tooth decay, is one of the most prevalent dental conditions with an estimated 2 billion people suffering from caries of permanent teeth and 514 million children suffering from caries of primary teeth worldwide.[13] The etiology of dental caries is complex and multifactorial with multiple environmental, behavioral, and genetic factors as well as their interactions being implicated.[4] While it is well known that oral hygiene and dietary choices are crucial in maintaining good oral health, the discovery of a direct role of individual gene variants in the etiology of dental caries has proven challenging and produced inconsistent results. Twin studies of dental caries suggested partial genetic control ranging between 20%[14,15] and 85%.[15–17] Understanding the genetic bases of susceptibility to dental caries is essential for personalized dental care and preventive strategies.

Several genes have been associated with an increased risk of dental caries including those involved in enamel formation, the defense mechanisms of the oral cavity, and saliva composition. In this section, the authors will briefly review some of the genes involved in enamel development, saliva composition, including its ability to break down carbohydrate, and defense mechanisms, all of which may contribute to the development of dental caries. For a more complete list of genes that have been associated with delta caries, please refer to **Table 1**.

Genes affecting enamel and dentin resistance

Amelogenin (AMELX), enamelin (ENAM), and tuftelin (TUFT1) genes are involved in enamel development and mineralization. Variations in these genes can impact enamel

Table 1
Genes implicated in the etiology of dental caries

Group	Gene	Role	Associated Disease
Enamel development & structure	Ameloblastin (AMBN)	Enamel matrix	Caries[36-39]
	Amelogenin (AMELX)	Tooth mineralization	Amelogenesis imperfecta,[40] caries[20,37,41-44]; Molar incisor hypomineralization[45,46]
	Enamelin (ENAM)	Enamel matrix	Amelogenesis imperfecta,[40] molar incisor hypomineralization,[46] caries[23,42,44,47-50]
	Estrogen-related receptor beta (ESRRB)	Enamel hardness	Caries[51-53]
	Tuftelin 1 (TUFT1)	Enamel matrix	Caries[24,36,44,54]
	Tuftelin-interacting protein 11 (TFIP11)	Enamel matrix	Caries[37,54,55]
	Kallikrein 4 (KLK4)	Enamel matrix strengthening	Hypomaturation amelogenesis imperfecta,[56,57] caries susceptibility[20,39]
	Matrix metalloproteinase 20 (MMP20)	Early stages of tooth development	Caries[39,58,59] (possibly protective in some populations)[60]
Saliva composition & production	Alpha-amylase 1 (AMY1)	Salivary starch digestion	Obesity, caries (high copy number protective)[28,61,62]
	Aquaporin 5 (AQP5)	Saliva production	Caries[52]
	Carbonic anhydrase VI (CA6)	Saliva pH regulation	Caries[36,63,64]
	Matrix metalloproteinase 16 (MMP16)	Degradation of extracellular proteins	Caries[44,65]
	Mucin 5 (MUC5B)	Inhibits biofilm formation	Caries susceptibility[66]

quality and structure as well as lead to enamel defects and therefore predispose teeth to caries. Variants in ENAM gene (rs3796704 and rs7671281) have been shown to affect the microstructure of enamel in mammals.[18] Genetic variations in AMELX gene have been associated with amelogenesis imperfecta developmental conditions,[19] which affect the structure and clinical appearance of enamel of all or nearly all the teeth in about equal manner. Additionally, variations in AMELX gene, in particular rs17878486 located in the intron of the gene, have been associated with susceptibility to dental caries in adults[20–22] and children.[23] Furthermore, combined effect of the TUFT1 gene with a high level of *Streptococcus mutans* was observed to increase susceptibility to dental caries.[24]

Saliva composition, defense mechanisms genes, and oral microbiome

Saliva and salivary proteins play a role in caries formation by allowing the colonization of biofilms of cariogenic bacteria (actinomyces and *Streptococcus* species, such as *S mutans*) on teeth.[25–27] Salivary amylase (AMY1) is an enzyme that breaks down starches in the mouth. Variations in the gene encoding salivary amylase (AMY1) can impact an individual's ability to digest carbohydrates and may contribute to caries development. Variation in copy number of AMY1 gene has been associated with smooth-surface dental caries experience in adults.[28] Additionally, amylase enzyme activity was associated with dental caries in children: caries-free children had significantly higher alpha-amylase enzyme activity and children with inherently lower levels of alpha-amylase activity were more susceptible to dental caries.[29]

Additionally, salivary proteins including enzymes and antimicrobial peptides may affect individuals' susceptibility to dental caries. For example, lactotransferrin is a protein in saliva that has antibacterial properties and can limit the growth of cariogenic bacteria. Variations in the LTF gene may affect the levels and activity of lactotransferrin, impacting the ability to control oral bacteria.[30–32] Furthermore, cystatin S is an enzyme inhibitor that helps regulate the activity of proteases in saliva. Genetic variations in CST4 gene can alter its effectiveness in inhibiting proteases produced by cariogenic bacteria.[33]

Defensin beta 1 is an antimicrobial peptide found in the oral cavity, providing natural defense against oral pathogens. Genetic polymorphisms in DEFB1 gene encoding defensin beta have been shown to influence its antimicrobial activity, affecting the oral microbiome.[34,35]

Finally, genetic variations affecting the composition of an individual's oral microbiota and promoting the growth of cariogenic bacteria such as *S mutans*, a primary cariogenic bacterium responsible for initiating tooth decay, may contribute to an individual's susceptibility to dental caries and prognosis of restorative treatments.

Conclusions and clinical relevance

It is important to emphasize that dental caries is a complex condition and genetic susceptibility to dental caries is influenced by a combination of genes, along with environmental and behavioral factors. Genetic testing and counseling can help identify individuals who may be at higher risk for caries due to their genetic makeup. Personalized oral hygiene recommendations and preventive interventions can then be developed based on an individual's genetic profile, allowing for more effective caries prevention and management. Understanding genetic factors contributing to susceptibility to dental caries can help identify individuals who may benefit from more intensive preventive measures, tailored oral care recommendations, dietary guidelines, timely interventions, and therefore improved treatment outcomes.

Pharmacogenomics in Dentistry

There are wide interindividual differences in responses to medications and they depend on many factors including genetics. The study of the influence of genetic variations/polymorphisms on drug response is called pharmacogenomics (PGx).[67,68]

In a poll conducted among physicians from prestigious medical facilities, 99% of respondents agreed that PGx variations would affect a patient's response to medication therapy and that they ought to be taken into consideration when a drug-genome interaction was found to be a potentially significant clinical parameter (92%).[69]

Resources such as the Pharmacogenomics Knowledgebase (PharmGKB [https://www.pharmgkb.org/about]), Clinical Pharmacogenetics Implementation Consortium (https://cpicpgx.org/guidelines/), Dutch Pharmacogenetics Working Group,[70,71] Canadian Pharmacogenomics Network for Drug Safety (https://cpnds.ubc.ca/), and Food and Drug Administration provide clinically relevant, evidence-based, and peer-reviewed guidelines and information on how human genetic variation affects responses to medications. Resources such as PharmGKB provide knowledge about clinically actionable gene-drug associations and genotype-phenotype relationships that can aid in making well-informed decisions regarding the implementation of genetic testing and in utilizing drug-gene-disease associations to maximize therapeutic effects and minimize toxicity.[72,73] Research has also demonstrated that more than 80% of individuals may have a minimum of 1 functional gene variation influencing one of the top 100 prescribed drugs in the United States.[69]

Most existing pharmacogenomic information is related to gene variants encoding drug-metabolizing enzymes. Depending on the patient's status as a metabolizer, variations in these enzymes lead to variations in clinical efficacy and safety. Poor, intermediate, normal, extensive, rapid, ultrarapid, or indeterminate metabolizers are the common categories used to describe metabolizer phenotypes (**Table 2**)[72] https://cpicpgx.org/guidelines/

Given the danger of drug addiction and other side effects, personalized medicine employing PGx to safely and efficiently provide the right medication, at the right dose, to the right patient, is becoming increasingly vital.[72,83,84] Additionally, it would shorten hospital stays, lessen the likelihood of medication side effects, improve patient satisfaction, and eventually improve the prognosis for a number of diseases.[85] Nevertheless, there are a number of challenges in bringing the PGx recommendations into reality. Professionals who decide which medications to administer using PGx criteria lack professional training in PGx guidelines. It is imperative that PGx be included in clinical training programs and curricula.[72]

The sheer quantity of the people that would need to be tested, as well as the financial component and affordability, could make the implementation of a large, universal pharmacogenomic testing program difficult.[72]

External Apical Root Resorption/Orthodontically Induced Inflammatory Root Resorption

Tooth movement during orthodontic treatment can lead to external apical root resorption (EARR) in which the resorption specifically affects the apical one-third of the root. This change is permanent and can affect the longevity of the dentition.[86] Studies have indicated that approximately half of EARR is seen in orthodontically treated individuals and almost two-thirds of it affects the maxillary central incisor. Mechanical factors like the amount of force applied, direction of tooth movement, and type of appliance may influence the amount of EARR but several studies indicate that these factors only account for one-tenth to one-third of the overall root resorption (RR) cases,[87–89] and that

Table 2
A list of genes encoding metabolizing enzymes for different drugs and the therapeutic recommendations

Gene	Significant Information	Drug	Metabolizer Type (Therapeutic Recommendation by Clinical Pharmacogenetics Implementation Consortium/Dutch Pharmacogenetics Working Group/Food and Drug Administration)
CYP2D6	• It is essential for the metabolism of about 25% of drugs that are currently prescribed[74] • It exhibits unique genetic variations that change activity and impact drug metabolism.[72,75] • It affects how well patients respond to various analgesics, tricyclic antidepressants, antiarrhythmics, and other medications including antiemetics and antipsychotics.[74,76,77]	• Codeine • Tramadol • Venlafaxine • Amitriptyline • Nortriptyline	UM (Avoid/AD) PM (Avoid/AD) https://www.pharmgkb.org/chemical/PA449088/guidelineAnnotation/PA166104996 UM (Avoid/AD) PM (Avoid/AD) https://www.pharmgkb.org/chemical/PA451735/guidelineAnnotation/PA166228101 PM (AD) https://www.pharmgkb.org/chemical/PA451866/guidelineAnnotation/PA166288201 UM (DA/Avoid/AD) https://www.pharmgkb.org/chemical/PA448385/guidelineAnnotation/PA166104982 UM (Avoid/AD) IM (DA/CM) PM (Avoid/AD) https://www.pharmgkb.org/chemical/PA450657/guidelineAnnotation/PA166104998
CYP2C9	About 15% of drugs that undergo CYP450-catalyzed metabolism are metabolized by CYP2C9, and it also plays a key role in the metabolic clearance of a number of clinically used drugs with narrow therapeutic index.[72,78]	• Celecoxib • Flurbicoxib • Ibuprofen • Lornoxicam	IM (DA/CM) PM (DA/CM) https://www.pharmgkb.org/chemical/PA449957/guidelineAnnotation/PA166191841

Gene	Description	Drugs	Links
CYP2C19	The CYP2C19 gene exhibits considerable polymorphism, with significant variations in allele frequencies between populations.[79,80]	• Sertraline • Citalopram • Escitalopram • Amitriptyline CYP2C19 + CYP2D6 • Clopidogrel	PM (CM) https://www.pharmgkb.org/guidelineAnnotation/PA166104980 IM (DA),PM (DA) https://www.pharmgkb.org/guidelineAnnotation/PA166104977 UM (Avoid/AD), IM (DA), PM (DA) https://www.pharmgkb.org/guidelineAnnotation/PA166104975 UM, RM, PM (Avoid/AD) https://www.pharmgkb.org/chemical/PA448385/guidelineAnnotation/PA166105006 PM (Avoid/AD), IM (AD/ID) https://www.pharmgkb.org/guidelineAnnotation/PA166104948
CYP2B6	It plays a role in the metabolism of about 2%–10% of drugs used clinically.[72,81]	Sertraline (CYP2B6 + CYP2C19)	PM (DA/AD) https://www.pharmgkb.org/guidelineAnnotation/PA166127639
HLA-A	HLA-A*31:01 is more common in Caucasians (3%) and Hispanic/South Americans (6%).[72]	Carbamazepine	Positive (AD) https://www.pharmgkb.org/chemical/PA448785/guidelineAnnotation/PA166105008
HLA-B	HLA-B*15:02 is most pronounced in Asian populations. HLA-B*57:01-positive patients have an 80-fold elevated risk of flucloxacillin-induced liver injury.[72]	Carbamazepine, Flucloxacillin HLA-B*57:01	Positive (AD) https://www.pharmgkb.org/chemical/PA448785/guidelineAnnotation/PA166105008 Positive (AD) https://www.pharmgkb.org/chemical/PA16478/1042/guidelineAnnotation/PA166182810
G6PD	This housekeeping enzyme is essential for preventing reactive oxygen species from damaging cells. Deficiency causes hemolytic anemia.[82]	Acetaminophen Tramadol	Deficiency (AD) https://www.pharmgkb.org/labelAnnotation/PA166184224

Abbreviations: AD, alternative drug; CM, clinical monitoring; DA, dose adjustments according to Dutch Pharmacogenetics Working Group dosing guidelines; ID, increase dose, IM, intermediate metabolizer; PM, poor metabolizer; RM, rapid metabolizer; UM, ultrarapid metabolizer.

this type of RR can also be seen in individuals without orthodontic treatment like in patients with a history of trauma, and increased occlusal forces (bruxism). Therefore, it remains a major challenge to determine the reason why some individuals are more susceptible to EARR than others. It has been established that genetics accounts for about two-thirds of EARR seen in orthodontically treated patients.[86,90–92]

A number of effector cells, including odontoclasts, whose morphology and functions are strikingly similar to those of osteoclasts, are implicated in the process of RR.[93,94] Alveolar bone and RR is established when resident periodontal ligament and circulating mononuclear hematopoietic precursor cells, which have their origin from bone marrow, differentiate to form odontoclasts/osteoclasts.[93,95] Therefore, genes involved in bone and tooth root remodeling have been suggested to play a role in susceptibility to EARR (**Table 3**).[96]

Knowledge of the patient's genetic profile will allow for early identification of susceptible patients and might enable individualized treatment owing to the understanding of the molecular factors related to the etiology of EARR. The discovery of new biomarkers can hasten the formulation of medications that could prevent or minimize EARR in "high-risk" patients.

Chronic postsurgical pain

Chronic postsurgical pain (CPSP) or posttraumatic pain is defined as chronic pain that develops or increases in intensity after a surgical procedure or a tissue injury and persists beyond the healing process, that is, at least 3 months after the surgery or tissue trauma.[116] CPSP can occur as continuation of the acute postsurgical pain or after an asymptomatic phase.[117] Pain can be restricted to the surgical site, extend to the local areas innervated by nearby nerves, or refer to the entire dermatome. The level of pain is such that it lowers one's quality of life. Between 9% and 85% of patients undergoing surgical procedures can experience CPSP, implying that around 23 million people suffer from it annually.[118] The resulting medical costs and lost productivity are estimated to be in thousands of dollars.[119,120]

Based on family and twin research, the heritability of chronic pain susceptibility is estimated to be approximately 50%.[121] Comprehending the heritability of CPSP may prove beneficial in creating predictive algorithms that evaluate the preoperative risk of developing CPSP.[122] Genetic factors are responsible for 12% to 60% of susceptibility to chronic pain problems.[123]

The etiology of CPSP and chronic neuropathic pain is complex with multiple genetic and environmental factors and their interactions being implicated. Significant efforts have been made to identify a genetic susceptibility to CPSP and chronic neuropathic pain.[124–126] Combining the knowledge gained through genetic studies, such as genome-wide association studies and next-generation sequencing,[127,128] with biologic processes may allow for better understanding of the factors involved in the development of these conditions and to provide clinically applicable insights.[122,127–129] In the long term, this information will allow for the development of innovative diagnostic kits that could determine a person's risk of developing chronic pain allowing for more personalized approach to treatment (pharmacogenomic approach) focused on prevention rather than a reactive and symptomatic approach.[122,130,131] Numerous candidate genes for CPSP have already been found and confirmed, but there is still a great deal of genetic variants to be found (**Table 4**).[122]

Periodontal Disease

Periodontitis is a chronic inflammatory disease of the periodontal tissues associated with progressive destruction due to dysbiotic plaque formation.[151] The etiology of

Table 3
Genes and their polymorphisms that are implicated in external apical root resorption

Gene	Function/Role	Absence or Polymorphism
IL-1B: Interleukin 1 beta	A potent bone-resorptive cytokine[86,96]	A polymorphism in *IL-1B* gene, *(rs1143634),*[96] was implicated in approximately 15% of the variation in EARR of maxillary central incisors of orthodontic-treated individuals.[96–98]
IL-1RN: Interleukin 1 receptor antagonist	It inhibits the activities of interleukin 1-alpha (IL-1A) and interleukin 1-beta (IL1B).[99]	*IL-1RN* gene variants in allele 1 *(rs419598)* are linked to a higher likelihood of developing post-orthodontic EARR.[96,100–102]
P2RX7: Purinergic receptor P2X ligand-gated ion channel 7	This nonselective ion channel is expressed in the bone's clastic cells and appears to have a "protective" or "pro-osteogenic" effect on bone through stimulating osteoclast death/apoptosis and initiating bone growth.[91,96] It stimulates immune cells to secrete inflammatory cytokines including IL1B.[96,103]	It has been shown that P2X7R-mediated ATP signaling is required for the mechanically driven release of prostaglandins by bone cells and subsequent osteogenesis.[104] The lack/polymorphism of *P2X7R (rs1718119)* results in insufficient trabecular bone resorption and periosteal bone growth.[96,105] Increased EARR resulted from its absence.[106]
OPG: Osteoprotegerin (*TNFRSF11B:* tumor necrosis factor superfamily member 11B)	The RANK-RANKL interaction is negatively regulated by OPG, a soluble decoy receptor for RANKL that reduces RANK-RANKL interaction leading to the inhibition of osteoclastogenesis and bone remodeling.[96,107]	A polymorphism in the *OPG gene* (rs2073618) accounts for about 8% of EARR.[86,93,107]
RANK: Receptor activator of nuclear factor kappa B (*TNFRSF11A:* tumor necrosis factor superfamily member 11A)	The *TNFRSF11A* gene encodes the RANK, an essential signaling molecule in osteoclast formation and maturation.[97,108]	Polymorphism (SNP D18S64) has a potential mechanism in the pathogenesis of root resorption.[97,107,108]
RANKL: Receptor activator of nuclear factor kappa-B ligand (*TNFRSF11:* tumor necrosis factor superfamily member 11)	Osteoblasts, odontoblasts, fibroblasts from the pulp and PDL, and single odontoclasts express the membrane-bound cytokine RANKL, which plays an important role in promoting osteoclast/odontoclast development and activation.[96,107]	Lack of expression/polymorphism of the gene coding for Amelogenins, bone sialoprotein (BSP) induced a RANKL-mediated increase in the resorption process of the root cementum and bone surfaces.[93]

(continued on next page)

Table 3
(continued)

Gene	Function/Role	Absence or Polymorphism
OPN (osteopontin)/*SPP1* (secreted phosphoprotein 1)	It allows initiation of the intracellular signaling pathways in which osteoclasts develop the ruffled border that attaches clastic cells to the mineral component of bone/root surfaces that in turn leads to bone/root resorption. [91,93,109,110]	Polymorphism of *OPN* gene (*SPP1*) (rs9138 and rs11730582) and[111] suppressed proliferation of odontoclasts minimized the occurrence of external root resorption. [91,109,112]
TNFa (tumor necrosis factor alpha)	It is expressed in the PDL and alveolar bone during orthodontic tooth movement. In the presence of permissive levels of RANKL, it is involved in osteoclastogenesis and odontoclastogenesis. [113–115]	It exacerbates the process of orthodontically induced inflammatory bone resorption. [113]

Abbreviations: EARR, external apical root resorption; PDL, periodontal ligament.

Table 4

Genes significantly associated with chronic postsurgical pain

Gene Identifier	Gene Name	Associated Variants
COMT	Catechol-O-methyltransferase	rs4818, rs4633, rs6269, rs4680[132–134]
KCNS1	Potassium voltage-gated channel subfamily S	rs1072198, rs17641121, rs858003, rs2835925, rs2014712, and rs2545457[133,135–137]
DRD2	Dopamine receptor D2	rs4648317[129,138,139]
CHRNA6	Cholinergic receptor nicotinic alpha 6 subunit	rs7828365)[133,140]
P2X7R	Purinergic receptor P2X 7	rs208294[133,141–143]
IFNG1	Interferon gamma 1	rs2069727 and rs2069718[129,133,144]
GDF5	Growth differentiation factor 5	rs143384[124]
CACNG2	Gamma 2 subunit of the voltage dependent Ca2 + channel	rs4820242, rs2284015, rs2284017, rs2284018, and rs1883988[133,135,145]
BDNF	Brain derived neurotrophic factor	rs6265[120]
GCH1	GTP cyclohydrolase 1	rs411417 rs752688[135,138,139,146–148]
CACNA2D3	Calcium voltage-gated channel auxiliary subunit alpha2delta 3	rs6777055[135,149]
CTSG	cathepsin G	rs2070697 and rs2236742[135,150]

periodontal disease is complex with multiple genetic and environmental factors and their interactions playing a role in disease susceptibility and progression. It is highly prevalent leading to bleeding gums, clinical loss of attachment, periodontal pocketing, and radiographic visualization of alveolar bone loss.[151,152] Although the disease is rooted to plaque formation, a poor correlation between plaque accumulation and periodontal disease has been observed. These scenarios indicated the role of genetic factors in disease progression and host susceptibility.[153] Numerous genetic studies aiming at elucidating the genetic underpinnings of this multifactorial oral disease have been conducted. The genes found to be associated with periodontal disease are briefly summarized in the following sections and in **Table 5**.

Interleukins (IL): IL cytokines (pro-inflammatory) play key roles in the human immune response and are important for the maintenance of homeostasis in periodontium.[154] Polymorphisms of *IL-1, IL-1A* (rs1800587), and *IL-1B* (rs1143634) have been linked to severe risk of periodontitis and are considered as strong indicators of susceptibility to periodontal disease.[154] Additionally, polymorphisms in *IL-2* (rs2069762), *IL-6* (rs1800795 and rs2069827), and IL-6-1480 C/G have been associated with periodontitis. The *IL-6* polymorphism rs2069837 has been suggested to be protective against chronic periodontitis.[153] IL-10 (anti-inflammatory cytokine) is not commonly associated with periodontitis but certain polymorphisms such as *IL-10* (rs1800896) and *AGC* (rs1800872/rs1800896/rs1800871) have been associated with increased susceptibility to chronic periodontitis.[155] Two polymorphisms in IL-10 gene (rs61815643 and rs6667202) have been associated with aggressive periodontitis.[156,157]

Matrix metalloproteinases (MMPs): Polymorphism in *MMP* and *MMP-1* (rs1799750) was found to be associated with a severe form of chronic periodontitis.[158] The role of MMP-8 and MMP-9 in the pathogenesis of chronic periodontitis has been investigated extensively.[159,160] These enzymes are integral to the degradation of extracellular matrix components and have been implicated in the tissue destruction present in chronic periodontal disease, with numerous studies elucidating their role as key biomarkers of chronic periodontitis or contributors to disease progression and severity.[159–161] In addition to genetic factors, smoking[162] and diabetes mellitus[163,164] have been identified as significant risk factors for the development and progression of periodontal disease.

Bone morphogenetic protein (BMP): BMP-4 GAAA and GGGA haplotypes have been associated with periodontitis.[165] Aggressive periodontal disease has been linked to the *MP*/retinoic acid–inducible neural-specific 3 (*BRINP3*)protein. The increased expression of *BRINP3* leads to increased cell proliferation, migration, and programmed cell death in peri-implantitis.[166]

Antisense noncoding RNA in the INK4 locus (ANRIL): ANRIL polymorphisms rs1333042, rs1333048, rs2891168, and rs496892 have been associated with periodontitis.[167]

Serotonin transporter (5-HTT): Genetic variations in the 5-HTT gene have been suggested to play a role in susceptibility to or severity of periodontal disease.[168,169] Serotonin, regulated by 5-HTT, plays a pivotal role in modulating immune response, inflammation, and bone metabolism all of which are factors contributing to the pathogenesis of periodontitis. Interestingly, susceptibility to and development of periodontal disease have been associated with psychological conditions[169] and association between 5-HTT and depression, anxiety, and neuropsychiatric conditions have been well documented.[168,170] A list of genes and their polymorphisms that have been shown to be associated with periodontal disease is summarized in **Table 5**.

Implant failures

Endosseous dental implants are the standard treatment of choice due to their predictability and success rate.[165,186] Even with its high success rate and accurate clinical

Table 5
Genes associated with periodontal disease

Gene	Polymorphisms	Risk Association	Site of Action	Disease
IL-2	rs2069762	+ Risk	Transcription activity of these cytokines	Periodontitis[171]
IL-6	rs1800795 rs2069827 IL-6-1480 C/G	+ Risk	Suppression of osteoblast. Differentiation and promotion of osteoclasts. Bone resorption.[153,172]	Severe chronic periodontitis[173–175]
	rs2069837	++ Risk	Potential marker of protection against periodontitis.	Chronic periodontitis[153]
MMP-1	rs1799750	+ Risk	Degradation of basement membrane and extracellular matrix in tissues.[176]	Severe chronic periodontitis[177,178]
MMP-8	rs11225395	+ Risk	Facilitator of leukocytes and neutrophil granulocytes migration from the bloodstream to the periodontal sulcus. Expression induces inflammatory tissue damage.	Periodontitis and chronic periodontitis.[179,180]
TNF-α	rs1800629 rs1800469	+ Risk	Regulation of bone resorption.	Severe periodontitis[181–183]
TGF-β1	rs1800469	- Risk	Inflammatory and osteolytic process. Promote the MMP-mediated degradation of extracellular matrix components.	Severe periodontitis[184,185]

protocol, certain implants do fail.[186] This implies the association between host genetic factors and implant failure.[187] The chronic inflammatory process that affects the tissues around an implant and leads to loss of bone structure around the implant is peri-implantitis. An important factor in the development of peri-implantitis is genetic susceptibility (**Table 6**).[166]

IL: IL-1A and IL-1B were found in higher concentrations in the crevicular fluid and saliva of patients with active peri-implantitis and were correlated with severe peri-implant disease.[188–190] Peri-implantitis and early implant failure were significantly associated with *IL-1A* (rs1800587) and *IL-1B* (rs1143634),[190,191] osseointegration with *IL-1B* (rs1143634), and T allele of *IL-1B*-511 C/T 157 with an increased incidence of implant failure/loss. Investigations have revealed an increased association between smoking and polymorphisms in *IL-1A* (rs17561), and *IL-1B* (rs1143634) genes with peri-implant bone loss in dental implants (osseointegrated).[165,192,193] A recent meta-analysis points out that polymorphisms in *IL-1B*−511 (2/2) in Asian ethnicity were associated with an increased risk of early crestal bone loss and no significant association with *IL-1A* (rs1800587), *IL-1B* (rs1143634), and *IL-1* polymorphisms was reported*.[154] Another meta-analysis performed suggests an association between peri-implant disease and composite polymorphism genotype *IL-1A* (rs1800587) with *IL-1B* (+3953) and *IL-1B* (rs1143634).[194,195] Both studies suggest that due to limitations in the number of studies, the investigators could not draw a definitive conclusion and suggested more well-designed studies.[154,194] *IL-1B* (rs1143634) variant has an increased likelihood of implant loss with more intense inflammation, and is slowly being considered as a negative treatment factor during implant treatment.[194] *IL-4* polymorphisms IL-4+33 C/T have been positively associated with implant loss.[165,196,197] *IL-6* gene associations between the *IL6* (rs2069849 and rs2069843) with mini implant failure during orthodontic anchorage were found.[198] Rather, alleles and genotypes of *IL-2* (rs2069762) and *IL-6* (rs1800795) were not significantly associated with early implant failure.[199] IL-10, an anti-inflammatory cytokine, and *IL-10* polymorphisms were not significantly associated with peri-implant disease and dental implant failures.[184,200] IL-17 (pro-inflammatory) cytokine was found in higher concentrations in tissues adjacent to regions of bone degradation and chronic periodontitis. *IL-17* polymorphism rs10484879 is associated with both chronic periodontitis and peri-implant disease.[201]

Receptor activator of nuclear factor kappa-B ligand (RANKL): RANKL plays a vital role as a regulator of bone resorption, osteoclastogenesis, and osteoclast activation via the receptor activator of nuclear factor kappa-B ligand (RANK)-RANKL-osteoprotegerin pathway. *RANK* is a part of the tumor necrosis factor (*TNF*) superfamily and polymorphisms rs9533156 and rs9533156 were associated with peri-implantitis.[202,203]

MMPs: MMPs play a pathologic role in peri-implantitis–associated bone loss and are found in the peri-implant sulcular fluid. Polymorphism of *MMP-1* (rs1799750) was associated with an early implant loss in nonsmokers.[200] Also, the polymorphisms *MMP-1* (rs1144393 and rs1799750) and *MMP-8* (rs11225395) are strongly associated with dental implant loss.[197,204]

BMP: BMPs are growth factors facilitating bone osteogenesis. Polymorphism in *BRINP3* (rs1342913 and rs1935881) and low-level expression of *BRINP3* are linked to the development of peri-implantitis in the presence or absence of chronic periodontitis.[165,166] BMP-4 polymorphisms are associated with marginal implant bone loss prior to implant loading.[165]

Fibroblast growth factors (FGFs): FGF3 polymorphisms rs4631909 and *FGF10* CCTG haplotypes in C allele were associated with peri-implantitis whereas *FGF3* rs4631909 was found in healthy controls.[165]

Table 6
Genes implicated in implant failures

Gene	Polymorphisms	Risk Association	Site of Action	Disease
IL-1	IL-1B (rs1143634)	+ Risk Pro-inflammatory cytokine.	Inflammatory and bone loss induction via osteoclastogenesis[172] Promotes degradation of extracellular matrix components via MMP.[185]	Early implant loss, Peri-implant bone loss, Peri-implantitis – Bone loss.[172,202]
	IL-1B (C-511T)[208]	+ Risk		Early and delayed implant loss, Peri-implant marginal bone loss.[202]
	IL-1A (rs1800587) & IL-1B (rs1143634) mixed polymorphism	+ Risk Pro-inflammatory cytokine.	Increased bone loss	Early and delayed implant loss. Early peri-implant bone loss. Peri-implantitis.[202]
	IL-1RN	- Risk Anti-inflammatory cytokines	IL-1 receptor blocking, decrease in production of IL-6 in bone tissue.[172]	Early implant loss, peri-implantitis, implant loss.[202]
IL-4	rs2243250 rs2070874 rs79071878[196,209]	- Risk		No association
IL-6	rs2069843, rs2069849	+ Risk	Bone resorption and osteoclast activity[210,211]	Peri-implant mucositis Mini-implant loss[198]
IL-10	rs1800896, rs1800871, rs1800872[184]	- Risk Anti-inflammatory cytokines	Inhibition of production of IL-17 and RANKL Reduction of osteoclastogenesis[172]	Not associated with the risk of peri-implant disease
IL-17	rs10484879	+ Risk Pro-inflammatory cytokine	Promotion of osteoclastogenesis[172]	Early implant failure Peri-implantitis (chronic periodontitis)[165,172]
TNF-α	rs1800629[184]	- Risk		No association
TGF-β1	rs1800469[184]	- Risk Pro-inflammatory cytokine.	Inflammatory and osteolytic process. Promote the MMP-mediated degradation of extracellular matrix components[185]	Peri-implantitis

(continued on next page)

Table 6
(continued)

Gene	Polymorphisms	Risk Association	Site of Action	Disease
RANKL	rs35211496 (C/T)[202] rs9533156 (T/C)[203]	+ Risk Pro-inflammatory cytokine	Formation and activation of osteoclast.[172]	Early implant loss, peri-implant bone loss, peri-implantitis[202]
MMP1	rs1799750 rs1144393 and rs1799750	+ Risk Pro-inflammatory cytokine	Involved in extracellular matrix metabolism during implant osseointegration.[178]	Early implant loss in nonsmokers.[177] Implant loss.[197,204]
MMP-8	rs11225395[179]	+ Risk Pro-inflammatory cytokine	Influences other cytokines & enzymes.[212] Enhanced bone resorption by osteoclast and promotes bone defect formation.[172]	Early implant failure. Influence marginal bone loss around implants before implant loading.[172]
BMP4	GAAA and GGGA haplotypes[213] rs2761884[213]	+ Risk - Risk	Facilitator of osteogenesis[165]	Peri-implantitis Marginal bone loss prior to implant loading[214] Healthy peri-implant[213]
BRINP3	rs1935881 rs1342913	+ Risk	Cell proliferation, migration, and death[215]	Peri-implantitis[166]
FGF	FGF3 rs4631909, FGF10 CCTG	+ Risk	Regulator of cell proliferation, differentiation, and migration	Peri-implantitis[165]

Transforming growth factor (TGF): TNF-α (rs1800629), and TGF- β1(rs1800469) polymorphisms associated with severe periodontitis[181–183] were not found to be significantly associated with early implant failure.[184,205–207]

Oral lesions and management

The scope of practice of oral medicine may be defined as "care for oral health of patients with chronic recurrent and medically related disorders of the mouth and with their diagnosis and non-surgical management."[216] In this section, the authors will briefly discuss the role of genetics in better prognosis of oral lesions and oral oncology. The authors will also succinctly highlight the genetic disorders which affect oral health.

The oral lesions are classified based on their clinical presentation such as white or red lesions, ulcerated lesions, lumps and bumps, and pigmented lesions. They have various etiologies namely infective, idiopathic, inflammatory, reactive, and neoplastic changes.[217] Though genetics might not be primary cause of lesions development, certain inflammatory disorders contributing to lesion development may make use of immunogenetics and pharmacogenetics for the betterment of the prognosis.

One such inflammatory disorder most widely studied is Behçet's disease which is majorly characterized by oral ulcers apart from other symptoms.[218] The genetic studies so far have identified human leukocyte antigen susceptibility genes that may be used to prescribe personalized drugs.[219] Molar incisor hypomineralization (MIH) is an enamel condition present with rapid caries progression mainly affecting first molars and incisors and present with lesions ranging from white to brown in color. MIH has an etiology of gene-gene or gene-environment interaction and may be differentially diagnosed from other hypomineralized lesions especially amelogenesis imperfecta by characterizing the inherited genetic variants.[220,221] The rs5979395*G allele of the AMELX gene on X chromosome is found to be highly associated with MIH[46] while some variants in ENAM, AMELX, and MMP20 genes have been found to contribute to amelogenesis imperfecta.[45,222,223] The variants and their epigenetic effects have been established by various studies. It has been reported that the presentation of the systemic features of the disorder among patients vary depending on the genetic predisposition under the influence of environmental factors.[224] Recent studies on the oral microbiome suggest that microbiome dysgenesis allows the overgrowth of pathogenic bacteria which in turn establishes a mutualistic network with fungi thus creating an inflammatory environment that amplifies mucosal damage leading to development of lesions such as recurrent aphthous stomatitis and mucositis. There are studies which also show that identifying and appropriately treating this dysbiosis have good prognosis in lesion healing.[225] Similarly, microbiome analysis of samples from oral cancer lesions and normal oral sites of the same oral cancer patient revealed distinguished characteristics of the microbiota found in the lesion. Further studies are being carried out to understand whether dysbiosis has initiated the malignant transformation of oral mucosa.[226] Majority of the oral lesions include those that arise during the premalignant stage or during malignancy of head and neck cancers which is discussed in the following sections.

Oral cancer management

Head and neck cancer, which ranks as the sixth most prevalent cancer worldwide, is graded into oral and pharyngeal cancer and further into squamous cell carcinoma and adenocarcinoma.[227] Head and neck squamous cell carcinoma (HNSCC) contributes to 90% of the head and neck cancers and those that are human papillomavirus (HPV)-positive are known to have good prognosis.[228] Most of the recent research involves identifying the etiology and prognosis factors contributing to HPV-negative cancer especially oral squamous cell carcinomas (OSCCs) which have a poor prognosis with overall 50% 5-year survival rate[229] and are highly recurrent.

Most of the studies aiming to identify prognostic factors have included analyses of single-nucleotide polymorphisms, gene expression profiles, circulating microRNAs (miRNAs), DNA methylation status, or signature molecular profiling which is a combination of 1 or more screening methods. The good prognosis for an oral cancer treatment requires identifying the underlying genetic mutation and its appropriate targeted therapy also known as 'personalized treatment.' In the following section, the authors provide a summary of the common mutations and available therapies.

OSCC is known to follow a theory of "field cancerization" which involves several genetic and epigenetic factors in the initiation and multistep progression of cancer.[229] Though chromosome instability and loss of heterozygosity are commonly contributing to OSCC, they do not have any prognostic value and also similarly epigenetic alterations are not fully understood. Thus, it is well known that loss of function of TP53 gene contributes to more than 80% of OSCCs. Apart from TP53, the other genes whose point mutation contribute to cell cycle dysregulation and immortalization are CDKN2A, CCND1, PIK3CA, PTEN, and HRAS. Further point mutations with a prognostic value are summarized in **Table 7**.

Microribonucleic acids and oral cancer

miRNAs are short 22 bp nucleotide strands which are involved in almost all cellular functions and pathways, especially RNA silencing and post-transcriptional modulation in response to epigenetic changes. miRNAs also hold a promising significance as prognostic biomarkers in HNSCC and OSCC. Extensive reviews as reported by Mazumder and colleagues, 2019,[254] Ghafouri-Fard and colleagues, 2019,[255] Bhattacharjee and

Table 7 Genes associated with oral cancer prognosis		
Gene Identifier	**Chromosome Location**	**Prognostic Feature**
ATM	11q22–23	Poor prognosis[230,231]
CDKN2C	1p32.3	Large tumor recurrence, poor survival[232,233]
CYLD	16q	Invasion and inhibition of innate immunity, cisplatin resistance[234,235]
FBXW7	4q32	Contribute to radio resistance[236]
PTEN	10q23	Metastasis[232,237,238]
TP53	17p	Cisplatin resistance[239]
AKT-1	14q32	Increased aggressiveness, migration[237,240]
BCL-2	18q21	Poor prognosis, LNM, therapeutic resistance[241]
CCND1	11q13	Poor prognosis, aggressive tumor, LNM and invasive[242,243]
CTNNB1	3p22	LNM, poor prognosis, invasive[244,245]
DEK	6p22.3	LNM, poor survival[246]
FGFR4	5q35	Stage III, IV, and poor prognosis[247]
MDM2	12q15	Dysplastic lesions and poor prognosis[239,248]
MET	7q31	EMT, poor survival and poor prognosis[249]
PIK3CA	3q26	Stage II and invasive, resistance to cetuximab and palbociclib[250,251]
PTPN11	12q24	Poor prognosis, metastasis, and invasion[252,253]

Abbreviation: LNM, lymph node metastasis.

colleagues, 2023,[256] provide detailed insights into miRNAs which may be used as markers for prognosis and therapy. Some miRNAs which are potential prognostic markers are mir-371, mir-150, mir-21, and mir-7d. The markers mir-21 and mir-7d were also found to be significantly correlated with resistance to chemotherapy. The miRNAs which can be used to assess metastases are mir-134, mir-146a, mir-338, and mir-371. The miRNAs mir-375, mir-196, and mir-125b were significantly correlated with sensitivity to radiotherapy. miRNA sponges and miRNA masks are being created synthetically as potential treatment options to treat aggressive cancers. For example, miR-375 may be used as a successful tumor suppressor since when it was functionally restored it was found to suppress tumor aggressiveness.

Developmental disorders and defects

It is well established that the oral cavity development in a fetus begins even before 30 days and the tooth development begins at 30 days of the gestational process and continues into the teenage years when the wisdom tooth erupts at 19 years of age.[257] During this time, there are multiple opportunities for developmental disorders and disruptions. Though the pathoembryology is not well understood, it has been identified as complex since same genetic mutations can give rise to different phenotypes. Some of the genetic disorders affecting the oral mucosa include chondro-ectodermal dysplasia, dyskeratosis congenita, Ehlers-Danlos syndrome, keratosis follicularis, hereditary benign intraepithelial dyskeratosis, lipoid proteinosis, multiple hamartoma syndrome, pachyonychia congenita, Peutz-Jeghers syndrome, tuberous sclerosis, and white sponge nevus.[258] The developmental defects during embryonic development affecting the oral cavity include cleft lip and palate, craniosynostoses, hereditary anodontia, amelogenesis imperfecta and dentinogenesis imperfecta, and osteogenesis imperfecta. Developmental disorder affecting oral mucosa include cysts of the oral mucosa in newborns, Fordyce's granules, leukoedema; those affecting gingiva include retrocuspid papilla, and those affecting tongue include geographic tongue, fissured tongue, median rhomboid glossitis, hairy tongue, lingual varices, and lingual thyroid nodule. Though various genes contribute to the development of these disorders, the treatment or management does not depend on the genetic mutations.

SUMMARY

Precision dental practice can be developed upon understanding the genetic pathology behind dental development and its associated disorders and oral health. To enable this practice of precision medicine in dentistry and oral oncology, it is essential to understand individual's genetic predisposition, its influence by environmental interaction, epigenetic changes, and contribution to disease etiology. Understanding of the role of genetic variations in disease development and response to treatment would allow to formulate informed decisions on the treatment plans for better prognosis avoiding adverse drug reactions. The research pertaining to the role of genetics in prognosis of dental treatments is in a very nascent stage and more data including various ethnic groups and large sample size are required to frame guidelines to make precision medicine for dental and oral health a routine.

CLINICS CARE POINTS

- Integrating genetic information into personalized dental care may help optimize prevention, early detection, and management of dental conditions including but not limited to dental caries.

- Genetic information can tailor preventive strategies and early interventions, such as frequent check-ups and targeted treatments.
- PGx guidelines advocate the delivery of safe and effective medications through customized/individualized therapy by using genetic data to classify patients into distinct metabolizer profiles.
- Prior to receiving orthodontic therapy, a patient's genetic profile can be used to determine their vulnerability to EARR, which will require a more meticulous treatment strategy.
- It is possible to identify preoperative risks for CPSP to gain clinically useful insights into preventing the protracted suffering that follows surgery.
- The influence of genetics in assessing the prognosis of Implant surgeries will play a key role in Implant dentistry.
- This will help the clinicians in patient counseling and as well customize the treatment plan as per genetic predilections.
- This will help the clinicians in patient counseling and as well customize the treatment plan as per genetic predilections.
- A multidisciplinary team including dentists, geneticists, and counselors can be employed to ensure comprehensive care and ongoing monitoring for effective management of dental conditions and oral cancers.

DISCLOSURE

The authors have nothing to disclose.

REFERENCES

1. Gadbury-Amyot CC, Simmer-Beck ML, Lynch A, et al. Dental hygiene and direct access to care: past and present. J Dent Hyg 2023;97(5):24–34.
2. Lourenco MAG, Guimaraes TM, Miranda ABS, et al. Factors associated with total edentulism in the elderly and their impact on the self-perception of oral health and food. Int J Prosthodont (IJP) 2023;0(0). https://doi.org/10.11607/ijp.8534.
3. Moya-Lopez M, Gomez-De Diego R, Carrillo-Diaz M, et al. Eating Behaviours, Oral Hygiene, and Caries in a Population of Spanish Children with Divorced Parents: A Cross-Sectional Study. J Clin Med 2023;12(19).
4. Cogulu D, Saglam C. Genetic aspects of dental caries. Front Dent Med 2022. https://doi.org/10.3389/fdmed.2022.1060177.
5. Alotaibi RN, Howe BJ, Chernus JM, et al. Genome-Wide Association Study (GWAS) of dental caries in diverse populations. BMC Oral Health 2021;21(1):377.
6. Shaffer JR, Wang X, McNeil DW, et al. Genetic susceptibility to dental caries differs between the sexes: a family-based study. Caries Res 2015;49(2):133–40.
7. da Silva MK, de Carvalho ACG, Alves EHP, et al. Genetic Factors and the Risk of Periodontitis Development: Findings from a Systematic Review Composed of 13 Studies of Meta-Analysis with 71,531 Participants. Int J Dent 2017;2017: 1914073.
8. Loos BG, Van Dyke TE. The role of inflammation and genetics in periodontal disease. Periodontol 2020;83(1):26–39.
9. Coghill RC. Individual differences in the subjective experience of pain: new insights into mechanisms and models. Headache 2010;50(9):1531–5.
10. Fillingim RB. Individual differences in pain: understanding the mosaic that makes pain personal. Pain 2017;158(Suppl 1):S11–8.

11. Rabben T, Oye I. Interindividual differences in the analgesic response to ketamine in chronic orofacial pain. Eur J Pain 2001;5(3):233–40.
12. Nielsen CS, Stubhaug A, Price DD, et al. Individual differences in pain sensitivity: genetic and environmental contributions. Pain 2008;136(1–2):21–9.
13. WHO. Oral Health. Available at: https://www.who.int/news-room/fact-sheets/detail/oral-health. Accessed January 2024.
14. Teixeira R, Andrade NS, Queiroz LCC, et al. Exploring the association between genetic and environmental factors and molar incisor hypomineralization: evidence from a twin study. Int J Paediatr Dent 2018;28(2):198–206.
15. Vieira AR. Genetics and caries: prospects. Braz Oral Res 2012;26(Suppl 1):7–9.
16. Opal S, Garg S, Jain J, et al. Genetic factors affecting dental caries risk. Aust Dent J 2015;60(1):2–11.
17. Wang X, Willing MC, Marazita ML, et al. Genetic and environmental factors associated with dental caries in children: the Iowa Fluoride Study. Caries Res 2012;46(3):177–84.
18. Lucas P, Constantino P, Wood B, et al. Dental enamel as a dietary indicator in mammals. Bioessays 2008;30(4):374–85.
19. Crawford PJ, Aldred M, Bloch-Zupan A. Amelogenesis imperfecta. Orphanet J Rare Dis 2007;2:17.
20. Gachova D, Lipovy B, Deissova T, et al. Polymorphisms in genes expressed during amelogenesis and their association with dental caries: a case-control study. Clin Oral Invest 2023;27(4):1681–95.
21. Li X, Liu D, Sun Y, et al. Association of genetic variants in enamel-formation genes with dental caries: A meta- and gene-cluster analysis. Saudi J Biol Sci 2021;28(3):1645–53.
22. Reza Khami M, Asgari S, Valizadeh S, et al. AMELX and ENAM Polymorphisms and Dental Caries. Int J Dent 2022;2022:8501179.
23. Devang Divakar D, Alanazi SAS, Assiri MYA, et al. Association between ENAM polymorphisms and dental caries in children. Saudi J Biol Sci 2019;26(4):730–5.
24. Slayton RL, Cooper ME, Marazita ML. Tuftelin, mutans streptococci, and dental caries susceptibility. J Dent Res 2005;84(8):711–4.
25. Stromberg N, Esberg A, Sheng N, et al. Genetic- and lifestyle-dependent dental caries defined by the acidic proline-rich protein genes PRH1 and PRH2. EBioMedicine 2017;26:38–46.
26. Dawes C. Salivary flow patterns and the health of hard and soft oral tissues. J Am Dent Assoc 2008;139(Suppl):18S–24S.
27. Esberg A, Sheng N, Marell L, et al. Streptococcus mutans adhesin biotypes that match and predict individual caries development. EBioMedicine 2017;24:205–15.
28. Stangvaltaite-Mouhat L, Puriene A, Aleksejuniene J, et al. Amylase Alpha 1 Gene (AMY1) Copy Number Variation and Dental Caries Experience: A Pilot Study among Adults in Lithuania. Caries Res 2021;55(3):174–82.
29. Parsaie Z, Rezaie P, Azimi N, et al. Relationship between salivary alpha-amylase enzyme activity, anthropometric indices, dietary habits, and early childhood dental caries. Int J Dent 2022;2022:2617197.
30. Azevedo LF, Pecharki GD, Brancher JA, et al. Analysis of the association between lactotransferrin (LTF) gene polymorphism and dental caries. J Appl Oral Sci 2010;18(2):166–70.
31. Li X, Su Y, Liu D, et al. The association between genetic variants in lactotransferrin and dental caries: a meta- and gene-based analysis. BMC Med Genet 2020;21(1):114.

32. Singh PK, Parsek MR, Greenberg EP, et al. A component of innate immunity prevents bacterial biofilm development. Nature 2002;417(6888):552–5.

33. Pappa E, Vougas K, Zoidakis J, et al. Downregulation of salivary proteins, protective against dental caries, in type 1 diabetes. Proteomes 2021;9(3).

34. Ozturk A, Famili P, Vieira AR. The antimicrobial peptide DEFB1 is associated with caries. J Dent Res 2010;89(6):631–6.

35. Wu L, Li Z, Zhou J, et al. An association analysis for genetic factors for dental caries susceptibility in a cohort of Chinese children. Oral Dis 2022;28(2):480–94.

36. Sharifi R, Shayan A, Jamshidy L, et al. A systematic review and meta-analysis of CA VI, AMBN, and TUFT1 polymorphisms and dental caries risk. Meta Gene 2021.

37. Chisini LA, Cademartori MG, Conde MCM, et al. Genes in the pathway of tooth mineral tissues and dental caries risk: a systematic review and meta-analysis. Clin Oral Invest 2020;24(11):3723–38.

38. Kuchler EC, Pecharki GD, Castro ML, et al. Genes involved in the enamel development are associated with calcium and phosphorus level in saliva. Caries Res 2017;51(3):225–30.

39. Sharma A, Patil SS, Muthu MS, et al. Single nucleotide polymorphisms of enamel formation genes and early childhood caries - systematic review, gene-based, gene cluster and meta-analysis. J Indian Soc Pedod Prev Dent 2023;41(1):3–15.

40. Cabay RJ. An overview of molecular and genetic alterations in selected benign odontogenic disorders. Arch Pathol Lab Med 2014;138(6):754–8.

41. Americano GC, Jacobsen PE, Soviero VM, et al. A systematic review on the association between molar incisor hypomineralization and dental caries. Int J Paediatr Dent 2017;27(1):11–21.

42. Sharifi R, Jahedi S, Mozaffari HR, et al. Association of LTF, ENAM, and AMELX polymorphisms with dental caries susceptibility: a meta-analysis. BMC Oral Health 2020;20(1):132.

43. Werneck RI, Mira MT, Trevilatto PC. A critical review: an overview of genetic influence on dental caries. Oral Dis 2010;16(7):613–23.

44. Zaorska K, Szczapa T, Borysewicz-Lewicka M, et al. Prediction of early childhood caries based on single nucleotide polymorphisms using neural networks. Genes 2021;12(4).

45. Jeremias F, Koruyucu M, Kuchler EC, et al. Genes expressed in dental enamel development are associated with molar-incisor hypomineralization. Arch Oral Biol 2013;58(10):1434–42.

46. Jeremias F, Pierri RA, Souza JF, et al. Family-based genetic association for molar-incisor hypomineralization. Caries Res 2016;50(3):310–8.

47. Chaussain C, Bouazza N, Gasse B, et al. Dental caries and enamelin haplotype. J Dent Res 2014;93(4):360–5.

48. Gerreth K, Zaorska K, Zabel M, et al. Association of ENAM gene single nucleotide polymorphisms with dental caries in Polish children. Clin Oral Invest 2016; 20(3):631–6.

49. Zanolli C, Hourset M, Esclassan R, et al. Neanderthal and Denisova tooth protein variants in present-day humans. PLoS One 2017;12(9):e0183802.

50. Daubert DM, Kelley JL, Udod YG, et al. Human enamel thickness and ENAM polymorphism. Int J Oral Sci 2016;8(2):93–7.

51. Nibali L, Di Iorio A, Tu YK, et al. Host genetics role in the pathogenesis of periodontal disease and caries. J Clin Periodontol 2017;44(Suppl 18):S52–78.

52. Piekoszewska-Zietek P, Turska-Szybka A, Olczak-Kowalczyk D. Single nucleotide polymorphism in the aetiology of caries: systematic literature review. Caries Res 2017;51(4):425–35.

53. Weber ML, Hsin HY, Kalay E, et al. Role of estrogen related receptor beta (ESRRB) in DFN35B hearing impairment and dental decay. BMC Med Genet 2014;15:81.

54. Shaffer JR, Carlson JC, Stanley BO, et al. Effects of enamel matrix genes on dental caries are moderated by fluoride exposures. Hum Genet 2015;134(2): 159–67.

55. Chisini LA, Santos FDC, de Carvalho RV, et al. Impact of tooth mineral tissues genes on dental caries: A birth-cohort study. J Dent 2023;133:104505.

56. Bartlett JD. Dental enamel development: proteinases and their enamel matrix substrates. ISRN Dent 2013;2013:684607.

57. Smith CEL, Kirkham J, Day PF, et al. A Fourth KLK4 Mutation Is Associated with Enamel Hypomineralisation and Structural Abnormalities. Front Physiol 2017; 8:333.

58. Antunes LA, Antunes LS, Kuchler EC, et al. Analysis of the association between polymorphisms in MMP2, MMP3, MMP9, MMP20, TIMP1, and TIMP2 genes with white spot lesions and early childhood caries. Int J Paediatr Dent 2016;26(4): 310–9.

59. Tannure PN, Kuchler EC, Lips A, et al. Genetic variation in MMP20 contributes to higher caries experience. J Dent 2012;40(5):381–6.

60. Filho AV, Calixto MS, Deeley K, et al. MMP20 rs1784418 Protects Certain Populations against Caries. Caries Res 2017;51(1):46–51.

61. Kor M, Pouramir M, Khafri S, et al. Association between dental caries, obesity and salivary alpha amylase in adolescent girls of babol city, Iran-2017. J Dent 2021;22(1):27–32.

62. Mejia-Benitez MA, Bonnefond A, Yengo L, et al. Beneficial effect of a high number of copies of salivary amylase AMY1 gene on obesity risk in Mexican children. Diabetologia 2015;58(2):290–4.

63. Yildiz G, Ermis RB, Calapoglu NS, et al. Gene-environment interactions in the etiology of dental caries. J Dent Res 2016;95(1):74–9.

64. Esberg A, Haworth S, Brunius C, et al. Carbonic Anhydrase 6 Gene Variation influences Oral Microbiota Composition and Caries Risk in Swedish adolescents. Sci Rep 2019;9(1):452.

65. Lewis DD, Shaffer JR, Feingold E, et al. Genetic Association of MMP10, MMP14, and MMP16 with Dental Caries. Int J Dent 2017;2017:8465125.

66. Cavallari T, Salomao H, Moyses ST, et al. The impact of MUC5B gene on dental caries. Oral Dis 2018;24(3):372–6.

67. Evans WE, McLeod HL. Pharmacogenomics–drug disposition, drug targets, and side effects. N Engl J Med 2003;348(6):538–49.

68. Rollinson V, Turner R, Pirmohamed M. Pharmacogenomics for primary care: an overview. Genes 2020;11(11).

69. Tagwerker C, Carias-Marines MJ, Smith DJ. Effects of pharmacogenomic testing in clinical pain management: retrospective study. JMIRx Med 2022; 3(2):e32902.

70. Beunk L, Nijenhuis M, Soree B, et al. Dutch Pharmacogenetics Working Group (DPWG) guideline for the gene-drug interaction between CYP2D6, CYP3A4 and CYP1A2 and antipsychotics. Eur J Hum Genet 2024;32(3):278–85.

71. Yoon DY, Lee S, Ban MS, et al. Pharmacogenomic information from CPIC and DPWG guidelines and its application on drug labels. Transl Clin Pharmacol 2020;28(4):189–98.

72. Brandl E, Halford Z, Clark MD, et al. Pharmacogenomics in pain management: a review of relevant gene-drug associations and clinical considerations. Ann Pharmacother 2021;55(12):1486–501.

73. Haidar CE, Petry N, Oxencis C, et al. ASHP statement on the pharmacist's role in clinical pharmacogenomics. Am J Health Syst Pharm 2022;79(8):704–7.

74. Muralidharan A, Smith MT. Pain, analgesia and genetics. J Pharm Pharmacol 2011;63(11):1387–400.

75. Ingelman-Sundberg M. Genetic polymorphisms of cytochrome P450 2D6 (CYP2D6): clinical consequences, evolutionary aspects and functional diversity. Pharmacogenomics J 2005;5(1):6–13.

76. Lotsch J, Geisslinger G, Tegeder I. Genetic modulation of the pharmacological treatment of pain. Pharmacol Ther 2009;124(2):168–84.

77. Zhou SF. Polymorphism of human cytochrome P450 2D6 and its clinical significance: part II. Clin Pharmacokinet 2009;48(12):761–804.

78. Daly AK, Rettie AE, Fowler DM, et al. Pharmacogenomics of CYP2C9: Functional and Clinical Considerations. J Pers Med 2017;8(1).

79. Hicks JK, Bishop JR, Sangkuhl K, et al. Clinical pharmacogenetics implementation consortium (CPIC) Guideline for CYP2D6 and CYP2C19 genotypes and dosing of selective serotonin reuptake inhibitors. Clin Pharmacol Ther 2015; 98(2):127–34.

80. Sim SC, Risinger C, Dahl ML, et al. A common novel CYP2C19 gene variant causes ultrarapid drug metabolism relevant for the drug response to proton pump inhibitors and antidepressants. Clin Pharmacol Ther 2006;79(1):103–13.

81. Hedrich WD, Hassan HE, Wang H. Insights into CYP2B6-mediated drug-drug interactions. Acta Pharm Sin B 2016;6(5):413–25.

82. Richardson SR, O'Malley GF. Glucose-6-phosphate dehydrogenase deficiency. StatPearls 2024.

83. Cornett EM, Carroll Turpin MA, Pinner A, et al. Pharmacogenomics of pain management: the impact of specific biological polymorphisms on drugs and metabolism. Curr Oncol Rep 2020;22(2):18.

84. Dowell D, Haegerich TM, Chou R. CDC guideline for prescribing opioids for chronic pain–United States, 2016. JAMA 2016;315(15):1624–45.

85. Kaye AD, Koress CM, Novitch MB, et al. Pharmacogenomics, concepts for the future of perioperative medicine and pain management: A review. Best Pract Res Clin Anaesthesiol 2020;34(3):651–62.

86. Hartsfield JK Jr, Everett ET, Al-Qawasmi RA. Genetic Factors in External Apical Root Resorption and Orthodontic Treatment. Crit Rev Oral Biol Med 2004;15(2): 115–22.

87. Baumrind S, Korn EL, Boyd RL. Apical root resorption in orthodontically treated adults. Am J Orthod Dentofacial Orthop 1996;110(3):311–20.

88. Horiuchi A, Hotokezaka H, Kobayashi K. Correlation between cortical plate proximity and apical root resorption. Am J Orthod Dentofacial Orthop 1998; 114(3):311–8.

89. Linge L, Linge BO. Patient characteristics and treatment variables associated with apical root resorption during orthodontic treatment. Am J Orthod Dentofacial Orthop 1991;99(1):35–43.

90. Harris EF, Kineret SE, Tolley EA. A heritable component for external apical root resorption in patients treated orthodontically. Am J Orthod Dentofacial Orthop 1997;111(3):301–9.

91. Nieto-Nieto N, Solano JE, Yanez-Vico R. External apical root resorption concurrent with orthodontic forces: the genetic influence. Acta Odontol Scand 2017; 75(4):280–7.

92. Sharab LY, Morford LA, Dempsey J, et al. Genetic and treatment-related risk factors associated with external apical root resorption (EARR) concurrent with orthodontia. Orthod Craniofac Res 2015;18(Suppl 1):71–82.

93. Iglesias-Linares A, Hartsfield JK Jr. Cellular and Molecular Pathways Leading to External Root Resorption. J Dent Res 2017;96(2):145–52.

94. Wang Z, McCauley LK. Osteoclasts and odontoclasts: signaling pathways to development and disease. Oral Dis 2011;17(2):129–42.

95. Hienz SA, Paliwal S, Ivanovski S. Mechanisms of Bone Resorption in Periodontitis. J Immunol Res 2015;2015:615486.

96. Pereira S, Lavado N, Nogueira L, et al. Polymorphisms of genes encoding P2X7R, IL-1B, OPG and RANK in orthodontic-induced apical root resorption. Oral Dis 2014;20(7):659–67.

97. Al-Qawasmi RA, Hartsfield JK Jr, Everett ET, et al. Genetic predisposition to external apical root resorption. Am J Orthod Dentofacial Orthop 2003;123(3): 242–52.

98. Bastos Lages EM, Drummond AF, Pretti H, et al. Association of functional gene polymorphism IL-1beta in patients with external apical root resorption. Am J Orthod Dentofacial Orthop 2009;136(4):542–6.

99. Medicine NLo. IL1RN interleukin 1 receptor antagonist [Homo sapiens (human)], Available at: https://www.ncbi.nlm.nih.gov/gene/3557, Accessed January 2024. 2024.

100. Iglesias-Linares A, Yanez-Vico R, Ballesta-Mudarra S, et al. Postorthodontic external root resorption is associated with IL1 receptor antagonist gene variations. Oral Dis 2012;18(2):198–205.

101. Iglesias-Linares A, Yanez-Vico RM, Ballesta-Mudarra S, et al. Interleukin 1 receptor antagonist (IL1RN) genetic variations condition post-orthodontic external root resorption in endodontically-treated teeth. Histol Histopathol 2013;28(6): 767–73.

102. Linhartova P, Cernochova P, Izakovicova Holla L. IL1 gene polymorphisms in relation to external apical root resorption concurrent with orthodontia. Oral Dis 2013;19(3):262–70.

103. Ferrari D, Pizzirani C, Adinolfi E, et al. The P2X7 receptor: a key player in IL-1 processing and release. J Immunol 2006;176(7):3877–83.

104. Li J, Liu D, Ke HZ, et al. The P2X7 nucleotide receptor mediates skeletal mechanotransduction. J Biol Chem 2005;280(52):42952–9.

105. Ke HZ, Qi H, Weidema AF, et al. Deletion of the P2X7 nucleotide receptor reveals its regulatory roles in bone formation and resorption. Mol Endocrinol 2003;17(7):1356–67.

106. Viecilli RF, Katona TR, Chen J, et al. Orthodontic mechanotransduction and the role of the P2X7 receptor. Am J Orthod Dentofacial Orthop 2009;135(6):694 e1–e16 [discussion 694-5].

107. Kalra S, Gupta P, Tripathi T, et al. External apical root resorption in orthodontic patients: molecular and genetic basis. J Fam Med Prim Care 2020;9(8): 3872–82.

108. Neela PK, Atteeri A, Mamillapalli PK, et al. Genetics of dentofacial and orthodontic abnormalities. Glob Med Genet 2020;7(4):95–100.

109. Sodek J, Ganss B, McKee MD. Osteopontin. Crit Rev Oral Biol Med 2000;11(3): 279–303.

110. Denhardt DT, Noda M, O'Regan AW, et al. Osteopontin as a means to cope with environmental insults: regulation of inflammation, tissue remodeling, and cell survival. J Clin Invest 2001;107(9):1055–61.

111. Iglesias-Linares A, Yanez-Vico RM, Moreno-Fernandez AM, et al. Osteopontin gene SNPs (rs9138, rs11730582) mediate susceptibility to external root resorption in orthodontic patients. Oral Dis 2014;20(3):307–12.

112. Chung CJ, Soma K, Rittling SR, et al. OPN deficiency suppresses appearance of odontoclastic cells and resorption of the tooth root induced by experimental force application. J Cell Physiol 2008;214(3):614–20.

113. Yamaguchi M, Fukasawa S. Is inflammation a friend or foe for orthodontic treatment?: inflammation in orthodontically induced inflammatory root resorption and accelerating tooth movement. Int J Mol Sci 2021;22(5).

114. Bletsa A, Berggreen E, Brudvik P. Interleukin-1alpha and tumor necrosis factor-alpha expression during the early phases of orthodontic tooth movement in rats. Eur J Oral Sci 2006;114(5):423–9.

115. Garlet TP, Coelho U, Silva JS, et al. Cytokine expression pattern in compression and tension sides of the periodontal ligament during orthodontic tooth movement in humans. Eur J Oral Sci 2007;115(5):355–62.

116. Schug SA, Lavand'homme P, Barke A, et al. The IASP classification of chronic pain for ICD-11: chronic postsurgical or posttraumatic pain. Pain 2019;160(1): 45–52.

117. Fregoso G, Wang A, Tseng K, et al. Transition from acute to chronic pain: evaluating risk for chronic postsurgical pain. Pain Physician 2019;22(5):479–88.

118. Correll D. Chronic postoperative pain: recent findings in understanding and management. F1000Res 2017;6:1054.

119. Chidambaran V, Gang Y, Pilipenko V, et al. Systematic Review and Meta-Analysis of Genetic Risk of Developing Chronic Postsurgical Pain. J Pain 2020;21(1–2):2–24.

120. Tian Y, Liu X, Jia M, et al. Targeted Genotyping Identifies Susceptibility Locus in Brain-derived Neurotrophic Factor Gene for Chronic Postsurgical Pain. Anesthesiology 2018;128(3):587–97.

121. Young EE, Lariviere WR, Belfer I. Genetic basis of pain variability: recent advances. J Med Genet 2012;49(1):1–9.

122. Clarke H, Katz J, Flor H, et al. Genetics of chronic post-surgical pain: a crucial step toward personal pain medicine. Can J Anaesth 2015;62(3):294–303.

123. Dourson AJ, Willits A, Raut NGR, et al. Genetic and epigenetic mechanisms influencing acute to chronic postsurgical pain transitions in pediatrics: Preclinical to clinical evidence. Can J Pain 2022;6(2):85–107.

124. Yan S, Nie H, Bu G, et al. The effect of common variants in GDF5 gene on the susceptibility to chronic postsurgical pain. J Orthop Surg Res 2021;16(1):420.

125. Duan G, Xiang G, Zhang X, et al. A single-nucleotide polymorphism in SCN9A may decrease postoperative pain sensitivity in the general population. Anesthesiology 2013;118(2):436–42.

126. Sessle BJ. Chronic Orofacial Pain: Models, Mechanisms, and Genetic and Related Environmental Influences. Int J Mol Sci 2021;22(13).

127. Koboldt DC, Steinberg KM, Larson DE, et al. The next-generation sequencing revolution and its impact on genomics. Cell 2013;155(1):27–38.

128. Rizzo JM, Buck MJ. Key principles and clinical applications of "next-generation" DNA sequencing. Cancer Prev Res 2012;5(7):887–900.

129. Chidambaran V, Ashton M, Martin LJ, et al. Systems biology-based approaches to summarize and identify novel genes and pathways associated with acute and chronic postsurgical pain. J Clin Anesth 2020;62:109738.

130. Katz J, Seltzer Z. Transition from acute to chronic postsurgical pain: risk factors and protective factors. Expert Rev Neurother 2009;9(5):723–44.

131. Seltzer Z, Dorfman R. Identifying genetic and environmental risk factors for chronic orofacial pain syndromes: human models. J Orofac Pain. Fall 2004; 18(4):311–7.

132. George SZ, Wallace MR, Wright TW, et al. Evidence for a biopsychosocial influence on shoulder pain: pain catastrophizing and catechol-O-methyltransferase (COMT) diplotype predict clinical pain ratings. Pain 2008;136(1–2):53–61.

133. Hoofwijk DM, van Reij RR, Rutten BP, et al. Genetic polymorphisms and their association with the prevalence and severity of chronic postsurgical pain: a systematic review. Br J Anaesth 2016;117(6):708–19.

134. Rut M, Machoy-Mokrzynska A, Reclawowicz D, et al. Influence of variation in the catechol-O-methyltransferase gene on the clinical outcome after lumbar spine surgery for one-level symptomatic disc disease: a report on 176 cases. Acta Neurochir 2014;156(2):245–52.

135. James SK. Chronic postsurgical pain: is there a possible genetic link? Br J Pain 2017;11(4):178–85.

136. Costigan M, Belfer I, Griffin RS, et al. Multiple chronic pain states are associated with a common amino acid-changing allele in KCNS1. Brain 2010;133(9): 2519–27.

137. Tsantoulas C. Emerging potassium channel targets for the treatment of pain. Curr Opin Support Palliat Care 2015;9(2):147–54.

138. Montes A, Roca G, Sabate S, et al. Genetic and Clinical Factors Associated with Chronic Postsurgical Pain after Hernia Repair, Hysterectomy, and Thoracotomy: A Two-year Multicenter Cohort Study. Anesthesiology 2015;122(5):1123–41.

139. van Reij RRI, Joosten EAJ, van den Hoogen NJ. Dopaminergic neurotransmission and genetic variation in chronification of post-surgical pain. Br J Anaesth 2019;123(6):853–64.

140. Wieskopf JS, Mathur J, Limapichat W, et al. The nicotinic alpha6 subunit gene determines variability in chronic pain sensitivity via cross-inhibition of P2X2/3 receptors. Sci Transl Med 2015;7(287):287ra72.

141. Song J, Ying Y, Wang W, et al. The role of P2X7R/ERK signaling in dorsal root ganglia satellite glial cells in the development of chronic postsurgical pain induced by skin/muscle incision and retraction (SMIR). Brain Behav Immun 2018;69:180–9.

142. Sorge RE, Trang T, Dorfman R, et al. Genetically determined P2X7 receptor pore formation regulates variability in chronic pain sensitivity. Nat Med 2012;18(4): 595–9.

143. Wang W, Zhong X, Li Y, et al. Rostral ventromedial medulla-mediated descending facilitation following P2X7 receptor activation is involved in the development of chronic post-operative pain. J Neurochem 2019;149(6):760–80.

144. Stephens K, Cooper BA, West C, et al. Associations between cytokine gene variations and severe persistent breast pain in women following breast cancer surgery. J Pain 2014;15(2):169–80.

145. Nissenbaum J, Devor M, Seltzer Z, et al. Susceptibility to chronic pain following nerve injury is genetically affected by CACNG2. Genome Res 2010;20(9): 1180–90.

146. Hokama Y, Asahina AY, Hong TW, et al. Causitive toxin(s) in the death of two Atlantic dolphins. J Clin Lab Anal 1990;4(6):474–8.

147. Latremoliere A, Costigan M. GCH1, BH4 and pain. Curr Pharmaceut Biotechnol 2011;12(10):1728–41.

148. Smith SB, Reenila I, Mannisto PT, et al. Epistasis between polymorphisms in COMT, ESR1, and GCH1 influences COMT enzyme activity and pain. Pain 2014;155(11):2390–9.

149. Naureen Z, Lorusso L, Manganotti P, et al. Genetics of pain: From rare Mendelian disorders to genetic predisposition to pain. Acta Biomed 2020;91(13-S): e2020010.

150. Liu X, Tian Y, Meng Z, et al. Up-regulation of Cathepsin G in the Development of Chronic Postsurgical Pain: An Experimental and Clinical Genetic Study. Anesthesiology 2015;123(4):838–50.

151. Papapanou PN, Sanz M, Buduneli N, et al. Periodontitis: Consensus report of workgroup 2 of the 2017 World Workshop on the Classification of Periodontal and Peri-Implant Diseases and Conditions. J Periodontol 2018;89(Suppl 1): S173–82.

152. Armitage GC. Development of a classification system for periodontal diseases and conditions. Ann Periodontol 1999;4(1):1–6.

153. Farhat SB, de Souza CM, Braosi AP, et al. Complete physical mapping of IL6 reveals a new marker associated with chronic periodontitis. J Periodontal Res 2017;52(2):255–61.

154. Agrawal KK, Anwar M, Gupta C, et al. Association of interleukin-1 gene polymorphism and early crestal bone loss around submerged dental implants: A systematic review and meta-analysis. J Indian Prosthodont Soc 2021;21(2):116–24.

155. Emampanahi M, Masoudi Rad S, Saghaeian Jazi M, et al. Association between interleukin-10 gene polymorphisms and severe chronic periodontitis. Oral Dis 2019;25(6):1619–26.

156. Schaefer AS, Bochenek G, Manke T, et al. Validation of reported genetic risk factors for periodontitis in a large-scale replication study. J Clin Periodontol 2013; 40(6):563–72.

157. Taiete T, Casati MZ, Stolf CS, et al. Validation of reported GLT6D1 (rs1537415), IL10 (rs6667202), and ANRIL (rs1333048) single nucleotide polymorphisms for aggressive periodontitis in a Brazilian population. J Periodontol 2019;90(1): 44–51.

158. Luchian I, Goriuc A, Sandu D, et al. The Role of Matrix Metalloproteinases (MMP-8, MMP-9, MMP-13) in Periodontal and Peri-Implant Pathological Processes. Int J Mol Sci 2022;23(3).

159. Sorsa T, Alassiri S, Grigoriadis A, et al. Active MMP-8 (aMMP-8) as a Grading and Staging Biomarker in the Periodontitis Classification. Diagnostics 2020;10(2).

160. Verstappen J, Von den Hoff JW. Tissue inhibitors of metalloproteinases (TIMPs): their biological functions and involvement in oral disease. J Dent Res 2006; 85(12):1074–84.

161. Li G, Yue Y, Tian Y, et al. Association of matrix metalloproteinase (MMP)-1, 3, 9, interleukin (IL)-2, 8 and cyclooxygenase (COX)-2 gene polymorphisms with chronic periodontitis in a Chinese population. Cytokine 2012;60(2):552–60.

162. Heikkinen AM, Sorsa T, Pitkaniemi J, et al. Smoking affects diagnostic salivary periodontal disease biomarker levels in adolescents. J Periodontol 2010;81(9): 1299–307.

163. Atanasova T, Stankova T, Bivolarska A, et al. Matrix Metalloproteinases in Oral Health-Special Attention on MMP-8. Biomedicines 2023;11(6).

164. Sapna G, Gokul S, Bagri-Manjrekar K. Matrix metalloproteinases and periodontal diseases. Oral Dis 2014;20(6):538–50.

165. Chen X, Zhao Y. Genetic Involvement in Dental Implant Failure: Association With Polymorphisms of Genes Modulating Inflammatory Responses and Bone Metabolism. J Oral Implantol 2019;45(4):318–26.

166. Casado PL, Aguiar DP, Costa LC, et al. Different contribution of BRINP3 gene in chronic periodontitis and peri-implantitis: a cross-sectional study. BMC Oral Health 2015;15:33.

167. Ozturk A, Ada AO. The roles of ANRIL polymorphisms in periodontitis: a systematic review and meta-analysis. Clin Oral Invest 2022;26(2):1121–35.

168. Wu L, Deng T, Wang CY, et al. Serotonin Transporter (5-HTT) Gene Polymorphisms and Susceptibility to Chronic Periodontitis: A Case-Control Study. Front Genet 2019;10:706.

169. Costa JE, Gomes CC, Cota LO, et al. Polymorphism in the promoter region of the gene for 5-HTT in individuals with aggressive periodontitis. J Oral Sci 2008;50(2):193–8.

170. Borkowska A, Bielinski M, Szczesny W, et al. Effect of the 5-HTTLPR polymorphism on affective temperament, depression and body mass index in obesity. J Affect Disord 2015;184:193–7.

171. Scarel-Caminaga RM, Trevilatto PC, Souza AP, et al. Investigation of an IL-2 polymorphism in patients with different levels of chronic periodontitis. J Clin Periodontol 2002;29(7):587–91.

172. Chmielewski M, Pilloni A. Current Molecular, Cellular and Genetic Aspects of Peri-Implantitis Disease: A Narrative Review. Dent J 2023;11(5).

173. Franch-Chillida F, Nibali L, Madden I, et al. Association between interleukin-6 polymorphisms and periodontitis in Indian non-smokers. J Clin Periodontol 2010;37(2):137–44.

174. Nibali L, D'Aiuto F, Donos N, et al. Association between periodontitis and common variants in the promoter of the interleukin-6 gene. Cytokine 2009; 45(1):50–4.

175. Trevilatto PC, Scarel-Caminaga RM, de Brito RB Jr, et al. Polymorphism at position -174 of IL-6 gene is associated with susceptibility to chronic periodontitis in a Caucasian Brazilian population. J Clin Periodontol 2003;30(5):438–42.

176. Li D, Cai Q, Ma L, et al. Association between MMP-1 g.-1607dupG polymorphism and periodontitis susceptibility: a meta-analysis. PLoS One 2013;8(3): e59513.

177. Santos MC, Campos MI, Souza AP, et al. Line SR. Analysis of MMP-1 and MMP-9 promoter polymorphisms in early osseointegrated implant failure. Int J Oral Maxillofac Implants 2004;19(1):38–43.

178. Leite MF, Santos MC, de Souza AP, et al. Osseointegrated implant failure associated with MMP-1 promotor polymorphisms (-1607 and -519). Int J Oral Maxillofac Implants 2008;23(4):653–8.

179. Costa-Junior FR, Alvim-Pereira CC, Alvim-Pereira F, et al. Influence of MMP-8 promoter polymorphism in early osseointegrated implant failure. Clin Oral Invest 2013;17(1):311–6.

180. Zhang L, Li X, Yan H, et al. Salivary matrix metalloproteinase (MMP)-8 as a biomarker for periodontitis: A PRISMA-compliant systematic review and meta-analysis. Medicine (Baltim) 2018;97(3):e9642.

181. de Souza AP, Trevilatto PC, Scarel-Caminaga RM, et al. Analysis of the TGF-beta1 promoter polymorphism (C-509T) in patients with chronic periodontitis. J Clin Periodontol 2003;30(6):519–23.

182. Shi LX, Zhang L, Zhang DL, et al. Association between TNF-alpha G-308A (rs1800629) polymorphism and susceptibility to chronic periodontitis and type 2 diabetes mellitus: A meta-analysis. J Periodontal Res 2021;56(2):226–35.

183. Zhang X, Zhu X, Sun W. Association Between Tumor Necrosis Factor-alpha (G-308A) Polymorphism and Chronic Periodontitis, Aggressive Periodontitis, and Peri-implantitis: A Meta-analysis. J Evid Based Dent Pract 2021;21(3):101528.

184. Jamshidy L, Tadakamadla SK, Choubsaz P, et al. Association of IL-10 and TNF-alpha Polymorphisms with Dental Peri-Implant Disease Risk: A Meta-Analysis, Meta-Regression, and Trial Sequential Analysis. Int J Environ Res Publ Health 2021;18(14).

185. Suzuki A, Horie T, Numabe Y. Investigation of molecular biomarker candidates for diagnosis and prognosis of chronic periodontitis by bioinformatics analysis of pooled microarray gene expression datasets in Gene Expression Omnibus (GEO). BMC Oral Health 2019;19(1):52.

186. Deas DE, Mikotowicz JJ, Mackey SA, et al. Implant failure with spontaneous rapid exfoliation: case reports. Implant Dent 2002;11(3):235–42.

187. Alvim-Pereira F, Montes CC, Mira MT, et al. Genetic susceptibility to dental implant failure: a critical review. Int J Oral Maxillofac Implants 2008;23(3):409–16.

188. Huynh-Ba G, Lang NP, Tonetti MS, et al. Association of the composite IL-1 genotype with peri-implantitis: a systematic review. Clin Oral Implants Res 2008;19(11):1154–62.

189. Cardoso JM, Ribeiro AC, Palos C, et al. Association between IL-1A and IL-1B gene polymorphisms with peri-implantitis in a Portuguese population-a pilot study. PeerJ 2022;10:e13729.

190. Eguia Del Valle A, Lopez-Vicente J, Martinez-Conde R, et al. Current understanding of genetic polymorphisms as biomarkers for risk of biological complications in implantology. J Clin Exp Dent 2018;10(10):e1029–39.

191. Liao J, Li C, Wang Y, et al. Meta-analysis of the association between common interleukin-1 polymorphisms and dental implant failure. Mol Biol Rep 2014;41(5):2789–98.

192. Feloutzis A, Lang NP, Tonetti MS, et al. IL-1 gene polymorphism and smoking as risk factors for peri-implant bone loss in a well-maintained population. Clin Oral Implants Res 2003;14(1):10–7.

193. Lin YH, Huang P, Lu X, et al. The relationship between IL-1 gene polymorphism and marginal bone loss around dental implants. J Oral Maxillofac Surg 2007;65(11):2340–4.

194. Mohammadi H, Roochi MM, Sadeghi M, et al. Association between Interleukin-1 Polymorphisms and Susceptibility to Dental Peri-Implant Disease: A Meta-Analysis. Pathogens 2021;10(12).

195. Jin Q, Teng F, Cheng Z. Association between common polymorphisms in IL-1 and TNFalpha and risk of peri-implant disease: A meta-analysis. PLoS One 2021;16(10):e0258138.

196. Pigossi SC, Alvim-Pereira F, Alvim-Pereira CC, et al. Association of interleukin 4 gene polymorphisms with dental implant loss. Implant Dent 2014;23(6):723–31.

197. Zhang F, Finkelstein J. The relationship between single nucleotide polymorphisms and dental implant loss: a scoping review. Clin Cosmet Invest Dent 2019;11:131–41.

198. Reichow AM, Melo AC, de Souza CM, et al. Outcome of orthodontic mini-implant loss in relation to interleukin 6 polymorphisms. Int J Oral Maxillofac Surg 2016; 45(5):649–57.

199. Campos MI, Godoy dos Santos MC, Trevilatto PC, et al. Interleukin-2 and interleukin-6 gene promoter polymorphisms, and early failure of dental implants. Implant Dent 2005;14(4):391–6.

200. Pigossi SC, Alvim-Pereira F, Montes CC, et al. Genetic association study between Interleukin 10 gene and dental implant loss. Arch Oral Biol 2012;57(9): 1256–63.

201. Kadkhodazadeh M, Baghani Z, Ebadian AR, et al. IL-17 gene polymorphism is associated with chronic periodontitis and peri-implantitis in Iranian patients: a cross-sectional study. Immunol Invest 2013;42(2):156–63.

202. Kadkhodazadeh M, Baghani Z, Ebadian AR, et al. Receptor activator of nuclear factor kappa-B gene polymorphisms in Iranian periodontitis and peri-implantitis patients. J Periodontal Implant Sci 2014;44(3):141–6.

203. Kadkhodazadeh M, Ebadian AR, Gholami GA, et al. Analysis of RANKL gene polymorphism (rs9533156 and rs2277438) in Iranian patients with chronic periodontitis and periimplantitis. Arch Oral Biol 2013;58(5):530–6.

204. Ferrer N, Aceituno-Antezana O, Astudillo-Rozas W, et al. Genetic Polymorphisms Associated with Early Implant Failure: A Systematic Review. Int J Oral Maxillofac Implants 2021;36(2):219–33.

205. Dos Santos MC, Campos MI, Souza AP, et al. Analysis of the transforming growth factor-beta 1 gene promoter polymorphisms in early osseointegrated implant failure. Implant Dent 2004;13(3):262–9.

206. Mo YY, Zeng XT, Weng H, et al. Association between tumor necrosis factor-alpha G-308A polymorphism and dental peri-implant disease risk: A meta-analysis. Medicine (Baltim) 2016;95(35):e4425.

207. Santiago Junior JF, Biguetti CC, Matsumoto MA, et al. Can Genetic Factors Compromise the Success of Dental Implants? A Systematic Review and Meta-Analysis. Genes 2018;9(9).

208. Dirschnabel AJ, Alvim-Pereira F, Alvim-Pereira CC, et al. Analysis of the association of IL1B(C-511T) polymorphism with dental implant loss and the clusterization phenomenon. Clin Oral Implants Res 2011;22(11):1235–41.

209. Scarel-Caminaga RM, Trevilatto PC, Souza AP, et al. Investigation of IL4 gene polymorphism in individuals with different levels of chronic periodontitis in a Brazilian population. J Clin Periodontol 2003;30(4):341–5.

210. Ishimi Y, Miyaura C, Jin CH, et al. IL-6 is produced by osteoblasts and induces bone resorption. J Immunol 1990;145(10):3297–303.

211. Takeuchi T, Yoshida H, Tanaka S. Role of interleukin-6 in bone destruction and bone repair in rheumatoid arthritis. Autoimmun Rev 2021;20(9):102884.

212. Schminke B, Vom Orde F, Gruber R, et al. The pathology of bone tissue during peri-implantitis. J Dent Res 2015;94(2):354–61.

213. Coelho RB, Goncalves RJ, Villas-Boas Rde M, et al. Haplotypes in BMP4 and FGF Genes Increase the Risk of Peri-Implantitis. Braz Dent J 2016;27(4):367–74.

214. Shimpuku H, Nosaka Y, Kawamura T, et al. Bone morphogenetic protein-4 gene polymorphism and early marginal bone loss around endosseous implants. Int J Oral Maxillofac Implants 2003;18(4):500–4.

215. Connelly JJ, Shah SH, Doss JF, et al. Genetic and functional association of FAM5C with myocardial infarction. BMC Med Genet 2008;9:33.
216. Lin YM, Simms ML, Atkin PA. Oral medicine in regional oral and maxillofacial surgery units: a five-year review. Br Dent J 2023.
217. Zahid E, Bhatti O, Zahid MA, et al. Overview of common oral lesions. Malays Fam Physician 2022;17(3):9–21.
218. Mahmoudi M, Aslani S, Meguro A, et al. A comprehensive overview on the genetics of Behcet's disease. Int Rev Immunol 2022;41(2):84–106.
219. Salmaninejad A, Zamani MR, Shabgah AG, et al. Behcet's disease: An immunogenetic perspective. J Cell Physiol 2019;234(6):8055–74.
220. Almuallem Z, Busuttil-Naudi A. Molar incisor hypomineralisation (MIH) - an overview. Br Dent J 2018.
221. Jeremias F, Bussaneli DG, Restrepo M, et al. Inheritance pattern of molar-incisor hypomineralization. Braz Oral Res 2021;35:e035.
222. Hocevar L, Kovac J, Podkrajsek KT, et al. The possible influence of genetic aetiological factors on molar-incisor hypomineralisation. Arch Oral Biol 2020;118: 104848.
223. Pang L, Li X, Wang K, et al. Interactions with the aquaporin 5 gene increase the susceptibility to molar-incisor hypomineralization. Arch Oral Biol 2020;111: 104637.
224. Lygidakis NA, Garot E, Somani C, et al. Best clinical practice guidance for clinicians dealing with children presenting with molar-incisor-hypomineralisation (MIH): an updated European Academy of Paediatric Dentistry policy document. Eur Arch Paediatr Dent 2022;23(1):3–21.
225. Min Z, Yang L, Hu Y, et al. Oral microbiota dysbiosis accelerates the development and onset of mucositis and oral ulcers. Front Microbiol 2023;14:1061032.
226. Shitozawa Y, Haro K, Ogawa M, et al. Differences in the microbiota of oral rinse, lesion, and normal site samples from patients with mucosal abnormalities on the tongue. Sci Rep 2022;12(1):16839.
227. Alfouzan AF. Head and neck cancer pathology: Old world versus new world disease. Niger J Clin Pract 2019;22(1):1–8.
228. Nan Z, Dou Y, Chen A, et al. Identification and validation of a prognostic signature of autophagy, apoptosis and pyroptosis-related genes for head and neck squamous cell carcinoma: to imply therapeutic choices of HPV negative patients. Front Immunol 2022;13:1100417.
229. Li CC, Shen Z, Bavarian R, et al. Oral Cancer: Genetics and the Role of Precision Medicine. Dent Clin North Am 2018;62(1):29–46.
230. Bau DT, Chang CH, Tsai MH, et al. Association between DNA repair gene ATM polymorphisms and oral cancer susceptibility. Laryngoscope 2010;120(12): 2417–22.
231. Lindemann A, Takahashi H, Patel AA, et al. Targeting the DNA Damage Response in OSCC with TP53 Mutations. J Dent Res 2018;97(6):635–44.
232. Batta N, Pandey M. Mutational spectrum of tobacco associated oral squamous carcinoma and its therapeutic significance. World J Surg Oncol 2019;17(1):198.
233. Rao SK, Pavicevic Z, Du Z, et al. Pro-inflammatory genes as biomarkers and therapeutic targets in oral squamous cell carcinoma. J Biol Chem 2010; 285(42):32512–21.
234. Gillison ML, Akagi K, Xiao W, et al. Human papillomavirus and the landscape of secondary genetic alterations in oral cancers. Genome Res 2019;29(1):1–17.

235. Suenaga N, Kuramitsu M, Komure K, et al. Loss of Tumor Suppressor CYLD Expression Triggers Cisplatin Resistance in Oral Squamous Cell Carcinoma. Int J Mol Sci 2019;20(20).

236. Arita H, Nagata M, Yoshida R, et al. FBXW7 expression affects the response to chemoradiotherapy and overall survival among patients with oral squamous cell carcinoma: A single-center retrospective study. Tumour Biol 2017;39(10). 1010428317731771.

237. Cohen Y, Goldenberg-Cohen N, Shalmon B, et al. Mutational analysis of PTEN/ PIK3CA/AKT pathway in oral squamous cell carcinoma. Oral Oncol 2011;47(10): 946–50.

238. Liu M, Song H, Xing Z, et al. Correlation between PTEN gene polymorphism and oral squamous cell carcinoma. Oncol Lett 2019;18(2):1755–60.

239. Patel KR, Vajaria BN, Singh RD, et al. Clinical implications of p53 alterations in oral cancer progression: a review from India. Exp Oncol 2018;40(1):10–8.

240. Nakashiro K, Tanaka H, Goda H, et al. Identification of Akt1 as a potent therapeutic target for oral squamous cell carcinoma. Int J Oncol 2015;47(4):1273–81.

241. Pavithra V, Kumari K, Haragannavar VC, et al. Possible Role of Bcl-2 Expression in Metastatic and Non Metastatic Oral Squamous Cell Carcinoma. J Clin Diagn Res 2017;11(9):ZC51–4.

242. Deepak Roshan VG, Sinto MS, Thomas S, et al. Cyclin D1 overexpression associated with activation of STAT3 in oral carcinoma patients from South India. J Cancer Res Therapeut 2018;14(2):403–8.

243. Sabir M, Baig RM, Mahjabeen I, et al. Significance of cyclin D1 polymorphisms in patients with head and neck cancer. Int J Biol Markers 2013;28(1):49–55.

244. Cai ZG, Shi XJ, Gao Y, et al. beta-catenin expression pattern in primary oral squamous cell carcinoma. Chin Med J (Engl) 2008;121(19):1866–70.

245. Kumar R, Samal SK, Routray S, et al. Identification of oral cancer related candidate genes by integrating protein-protein interactions, gene ontology, pathway analysis and immunohistochemistry. Sci Rep 2017;7(1):2472.

246. Nakashima T, Tomita H, Hirata A, et al. Promotion of cell proliferation by the proto-oncogene DEK enhances oral squamous cell carcinogenesis through field cancerization. Cancer Med 2017;6(10):2424–39.

247. Chou CH, Hsieh MJ, Chuang CY, et al. Functional FGFR4 Gly388Arg polymorphism contributes to oral squamous cell carcinoma susceptibility. Oncotarget 2017;8(56):96225–38.

248. Ralhan R, Sandhya A, Meera M, et al. Induction of MDM2-P2 transcripts correlates with stabilized wild-type p53 in betel- and tobacco-related human oral cancer. Am J Pathol 2000;157(2):587–96.

249. Sun Z, Liu Q, Ye D, et al. Role of c-Met in the progression of human oral squamous cell carcinoma and its potential as a therapeutic target. Oncol Rep 2018; 39(1):209–16.

250. Murugan AK, Munirajan AK, Tsuchida N. Genetic deregulation of the PIK3CA oncogene in oral cancer. Cancer Lett 2013;338(2):193–203.

251. Wan X, Li X, Yang J, et al. Genetic association between PIK3CA gene and oral squamous cell carcinoma: a case control study conducted in Chongqing, China. Int J Clin Exp Pathol 2015;8(10):13360–6.

252. Wang HC, Chiang WF, Huang HH, et al. Src-homology 2 domain-containing tyrosine phosphatase 2 promotes oral cancer invasion and metastasis. BMC Cancer 2014;14:442.

253. Zhang J, Zhang F, Niu R. Functions of Shp2 in cancer. J Cell Mol Med 2015; 19(9):2075–83.

254. Mazumder S, Datta S, Ray JG, et al. Liquid biopsy: miRNA as a potential biomarker in oral cancer. Cancer Epidemiol 2019;58:137–45.
255. Ghafouri-Fard S, Gholipour M, Taheri M, et al. MicroRNA profile in the squamous cell carcinoma: prognostic and diagnostic roles. Heliyon 2020;6(11):e05436.
256. Bhattacharjee B, Syeda AF, Rynjah D, et al. Pharmacological impact of micro-RNAs in head and neck squamous cell carcinoma: Prevailing insights on molecular pathways, diagnosis, and nanomedicine treatment. Front Pharmacol 2023; 14:1174330.
257. Carachi R, Doss SHE. Clinical embryology: an atlas of congenital malformations. New York, NY: Springer International Publishing; 2019. https://doi.org/10.1007/978-3-319-26158-4.
258. Pinna R, Cocco F, Campus G, et al. Genetic and developmental disorders of the oral mucosa: Epidemiology; molecular mechanisms; diagnostic criteria; management. Periodontol 2000 2019;80(1):12–27.

Systemic Factors Affecting Orthodontic Treatment Outcomes and Prognosis – Part 1

Sumit Gupta, BDS, MDS[a],*, Anil Ardeshna, DMD, MDS[b],
Paul Emile Rossouw, BSc, BCHD(Dent), BCHD-Hons(Child Dent), MCHD (Ortho),
PhD, Cert (Ortho), PhD (Dental Science), FRCD(C)[c],
Manish Valiathan, BDS, MDS, DDS, MSD[d]

KEYWORDS

- Renal diseases • Liver diseases • Orthodontic treatment • Periodontal issues
- Tooth eruption • Osteoporosis

KEY POINTS

- Renal diseases impact dental health, causing delayed tooth eruption and gingival overgrowth, necessitating orthodontic caution and collaboration with physicians.
- Liver diseases correlate with periodontal issues; hepatitis transmission risk requires stringent infection control measures during orthodontic procedures.
- Osteoporosis affects orthodontic treatment due to bisphosphonate use, potentially inhibiting tooth movement, while orofacial muscle dysfunctions like open bite require specialized care.
- Ehlers-Danlos syndrome demands careful orthodontic management due to collagen-related fragility, rapid tooth movement, and heightened risk of periodontal problems and orthodontic relapse.
- Autoimmune diseases such as diabetes mellitus and juvenile idiopathic arthritis require tailored orthodontic approaches considering oral complications and joint involvement, emphasizing collaboration and cautious treatment planning.

INTRODUCTION

The objective of orthodontic treatment is to set an appropriate treatment plan to attain the best balance and harmony of facial lines (esthetic), a healthy oral environment,

[a] Diplomate, American Board of Orofacial Pain, Private Practice, Rak Dental Care & Implant Centre, Ras Al Khaimah, United Arab Emirates; [b] Diplomate American Board of Orthodontics, Department of Orthodontics, Rutgers School of Dental medicine, 110 Bergen Street, Newark, NJ 07101, USA; [c] Division of Orthodontics and Dentofacial Orthopedics, University of Rochester Eastman Institute of Oral Health, 625 Elmwood Avenue, Box 683, Rochester, NY 14620, USA; [d] Department of Orthodontics, Case Western Reserve University, 9601 Chester Avenue, Cleveland, OH 44106, USA
* Corresponding author. 304 NS Tower, Al Qassimi Street, Corniche, PO Box 11939, Ras Al Khaimah, UAE.
E-mail address: drsumitg29@gmail.com

Dent Clin N Am 68 (2024) 693–706
https://doi.org/10.1016/j.cden.2024.05.004
0011-8532/24/© 2024 Elsevier Inc. All rights are reserved, including those for text and data mining, AI training, and similar technologies.

dental.theclinics.com

functional dentition, and stable result.[1] However, few studies have shown that it is necessary to adjust or change a treatment plan, especially when associated with a systemic disorder.[2–5]

There is also an increased demand for contemporary orthodontic treatment regardless of hidden medical disorders. Thus, early diagnosis may lead to adequate management of an underlying disease that may prove difficult to overcome because of hidden difficulties during and after orthodontic treatment. Moreover, it is important to recognize and incorporate orthodontic treatment goals to accommodate systemic disease problems to warrant attaining the noted treatment goals. The following 2 articles, part 1 and 2, will address some of these problems to equip the clinician with an understanding and knowledge to manage examples of systemic disease during orthodontic treatment.[2–5]

MALIGNANCIES

Modern methods of cancer treatment have significantly increased survival rates, leading to an increasing number of children requiring orthodontic treatment after their cancer treatment.[6] Cancer and its treatments, particularly in childhood, can significantly impact orthodontic treatment. Radiotherapy can lead to cranio-facial growth interference, mandibular retrognathia, and other complications, making orthodontic treatment more challenging. Disturbances in tooth development, root resorption, and bone density are common in long-term survivors of childhood cancer, but orthodontic treatment does not produce harmful side effects in these patients.[7,8] Similarly, chemotherapy and radiotherapy may have lasting effects on systemic health, influencing factors like bone density, healing capabilities, and susceptibility to infections. Side effects such as mucosa inflammation and recurrence, necessities an optimized treatment plan for oncological patients.[9] Moreover, the use of ionizing radiation affects the shear strength and failure mode of ceramic orthodontic brackets bonded with different composites.[10]

Survivors of childhood cancer are particularly at risk for late dental effects, emphasizing the long-term implications of cancer treatments on dental health.[11] Furthermore, the use of bisphosphonates in cancer treatment has been increasingly recognized for its significant impact on dental treatments.[12] Malignancies, especially those involving the head and neck region, may necessitate alterations in the standard diagnostic imaging protocols. Radiographic assessments, such as cone-beam computed tomography scans, play a pivotal role in orthodontic records. However, alterations in anatomy due to tumor growth or changes induced by cancer treatments may obscure critical structures, influencing the accuracy of cephalometric analyses and 3-dimensional reconstructions.

The impact of cancer treatments on dental and skeletal structures is a critical consideration in orthodontic treatment planning.[13] Cancer therapies can compromise the mechanical properties of oral tissues, leading to increased susceptibility to trauma and delayed healing, as orthodontic forces may need to be modified to accommodate compromised tissue integrity.[14] The study by Cuoghi and colleagues (2016) delves into the correlation between pain and tissue damage in response to orthodontic tooth movement, shedding light on the complexities of tissue response to mechanical forces.[15] Furthermore, the prevalence, intensity, and extent of impacts on daily performances related to wearing orthodontic appliances among cancer survivors need to be assessed to understand the full scope of the impact.[16] Cancer survivors undergoing orthodontic treatment experience lower long-term stability of treatment compared to generally healthy individuals.[17] Additionally, cancer survivors, especially male patients, report a significantly lower quality of life during orthodontic treatment.[18] The impact of orthodontic treatment on the oral health quality of life is significantly higher in male cancer survivor patients compared to the control group.[9] This emphasizes the importance of considering the positive impact of orthodontic treatment on the quality of life of cancer survivor patients.

NEUROLOGIC DISORDERS

Neurologic disorders affect a diverse demographic, including children, adolescents, and adults. The challenges in providing orthodontic treatment to these individuals stem from the need for individualized care plans, considering the dynamic nature of neurodevelopmental disorders and their influence on craniofacial growth patterns, patient compliance, effect on tooth movement, and oral hygiene.

Multiple sclerosis (MS) is a condition characterized by the demyelination, neurodegeneration, and autoimmune response within the central nervous system, typically impacting younger individuals.[19] The prevalence of MS estimated to be 2.2 million worldwide indicating a 10.4% increase in age-standardized prevalence since 1990. The prevalence of MS is influenced by a complex interplay of genetic, environmental, and demographic factors, leading to varying prevalence rates across different regions globally.[20,21] Patients with MS are almost universally infected with Epstein-Barr virus (EBV), and the risk of developing the disease increases with the level of EBV-specific antibody titers.[22] The symptoms of MS relevant to orthodontic care include fatigue, weakness, decreased balance, spasticity, gait problems, depression, cognitive issues, bladder, visual and sensory loss, neuropathic pain, and muscle weakness.[23] These symptoms may impact a patient's ability to maintain oral hygiene, attend dental appointments, or undergo orthodontic procedures. For instance, muscle weakness and decreased balance may affect a patient's ability to perform oral care tasks effectively, such as brushing with a regular brush, elastics, removable appliances, or aligner wear.[24] Additionally, bladder and bowel deficits may necessitate accommodations during dental visits. Furthermore, depression and cognitive issues can impact a patient's overall experience and may require special attention and support during dental and orthodontic care.

Epilepsy is a neurologic disorder characterized by recurrent unprovoked seizures, often resulting from brain damage due to injury, infection, birth trauma, or cerebrovascular accidents. It can also be associated with genetic syndromes such as Down's syndrome or Sturge-Weber syndrome.[25] The estimates of prevalence of epilepsy in the United States (US) from 1% to 5 to 9 per 1000 individuals affecting an estimated 3 million Americans. When considering orthodontic treatment for patients with epilepsy, several factors should be taken into account. Patients should continue their antiepileptic medication as prescribed and should not be overly fatigued during appointments. Additionally, the orthodontist should ensure that the patient has eaten normally before each appointment. It is important for the orthodontic team to be well-trained in seizure management, and patients should be informed about the risk of soft tissue and dental injuries during a seizure.[26,27] Furthermore, the potential side effects of antiepileptic medications, such as gingival overgrowth associated with phenytoin, should be monitored, and removable appliances should be used with caution due to the risk of dislodgement during a seizure.[28] Given the potential for metal in fixed orthodontic appliances to distort MRI images, the use of ceramic brackets maybe more appropriate.[29]

Children with attention-deficit/hyperactivity disorder (ADHD) present unique challenges in orthodontic treatment, encompassing behavioral, attentional, cooperative, hygiene, and dental trauma aspects.[30] These challenges are further compounded by the potential adverse effects of orthodontic interventions, such as root resorption, pain, and periodontal disease. Interventions aimed at enhancing adherence, including the use of rewards, provision of written information, and plaque demonstration, have been identified as effective strategies. Moreover, patient anxiety and paternal attitudes have been recognized as influential factors affecting compliance during treatment. Children with ADHD are prone to distraction, have limited sustained attention span, and may exhibit motor overactivity, emphasizing the need for specialized approaches. Additionally, children with ADHD have been found to experience dental injuries more frequently than previously described. Furthermore, the use of methylphenidate in the treatment of ADHD has been associated with a high risk of dental trauma, necessitating careful consideration in orthodontic treatment planning.[31] Moreover, children with ADHD have exhibited a higher prevalence of caries and periodontal problems compared to their peers without ADHD, underscoring the importance of addressing oral health concerns in this population.[32] The impact of ADHD on sleep-disordered breathing and malocclusion has also been recognized, highlighting the need for comprehensive assessment and management of orthodontic concerns in children with ADHD.[33]

Cerebral palsy (CP) is a non-progressive neurologic disorder that affects movement and posture, resulting from injury to the developing brain. The most common form of CP is spastic, accounting for nearly 80% of all cases. Individuals with CP are more susceptible to malocclusions, particularly class II malocclusion, increased open bite, and overjet.[34,35] Additionally, they are prone to dental caries, oral hygiene challenges, and dental erosion, often associated with gastroesophageal reflux.[36] Furthermore, delayed or advanced dental maturity may be expected in patients with CP compared with healthy individuals. The use of botulinum toxin for spasticity, a prevalent symptom in children with CP, has been extensively evaluated. Moreover, children with CP often require general anesthesia for dental management due to impaired reflexes, involuntary movements, muscle spasms, and cognitive impairment.

Functional and fixed orthodontic treatment, including rapid maxillary expansion and vertical control, can lead to improvements in occlusion, facial esthetics, speech, and oral function.[37]

RESPIRATORY DISEASES

Respiratory diseases encompass a broad spectrum of disorders affecting the respiratory system, including the lungs, airways, and other breathing structures.[38] Patients with respiratory diseases may face challenges during orthodontic treatment due to several factors. One major factor is the impact of respiratory diseases on patients' compliance with oral hygiene advice. Patients with respiratory diseases may have difficulty maintaining proper oral hygiene, which can lead to an increased risk of dental caries and periodontal disease during orthodontic treatment. Mouth breathing and altered breathing patterns and also create malocclusions (X). Orthodontic treatment planning must integrate preventive measures to address these implications for long-term oral health. Furthermore, respiratory diseases can also affect the duration of orthodontic treatment. Patients with respiratory diseases may experience prolonged orthodontic treatment time due to factors such as increased treatment sensitivity, reduced immune function, and potential disruptions in treatment due to respiratory symptoms or flare-ups. Dental procedures, including orthodontic treatments, can produce aerosols, which increase the risk of transmission of acute viral respiratory tract infections. After the coronavirus disease 2019 pandemic, the concerns regarding aerosols and respiratory diseases have become more significant. Orthodontic procedures that involve the use of instruments like high-speed handpieces and ultrasonic scalers can generate aerosols that may contain viral particles.

Asthma is a chronic respiratory disease that affects millions globally.[39] It has been associated with various oral conditions such as periodontal disease.[40] It has also been implicated with an increased risk of root resorption. However, others did not find a significant association.[41-43] Asthma medications can affect orthodontic treatment in several ways. Montelukast, a medication used to manage asthma, may cause a slight delay in orthodontic tooth movement and decreased osteoclast activity, but the differences are not statistically significant.[44] Steroid inhalers can lead to oral candidiasis.[45]

Furthermore, genetic analyses have revealed associations between obstructive sleep apnea (OSA)–a condition often comorbid with asthma–and cardiometabolic health. Children diagnosed with asthma may experience more severe malocclusions than their non-asthmatic counterparts. These malocclusions can lead to mouth breathing patterns, which might exacerbate dental problems such as tooth decay due to reduced saliva flow caused by mouth breathing.

Cystic fibrosis (CF) represents the most prevalent life-limiting autosomal recessive disorder among individuals of European descent, typically manifesting in childhood. It primarily affects the exocrine glands of the lungs, liver, pancreas, and intestines, leading to progressive multisystem failure and disability. Oral manifestations of CF include hypoplastic enamel and delayed tooth eruption. While tetracycline staining of teeth was reported in the past, alternative medications are now utilized, and antibiotic treatment has been associated with a lower prevalence of dental disease. Given the systemic nature of CF and its impact on respiratory health, it is essential to consider potential implications for orthodontic treatment. Although direct evidence on the specific effects of CF on orthodontic interventions is limited, the underlying pathophysiology and associated complications warrant attention. Notably, individuals with CF are prone to respiratory infections and compromised lung function due to mucus accumulation in the airways.[46]

Numerous studies have underscored the link between abnormal breathing patterns, such as mouth breathing, and alterations in craniofacial development and malocclusions.[47,48] The work of Guilleminault highlights how mouth breathing, often associated with OSA, can lead to maxillary constriction and mandibular retrognathia, necessitating specialized orthodontic interventions.[49] Patients with respiratory disorders, particularly those with nasal airway resistance, may encounter challenges in adapting and tolerating to orthodontic appliances bulky headgear might be contraindicated for sleep apnea patients, while lip bumpers can benefit mouth breathers. Beyond mouth breathing, tongue posture significantly influences airway patency and craniofacial development.[50,51] Myofunctional therapy can be effective in improving upper airway dimensions, potentially complementing orthodontic interventions.[52] Mouth breathing and altered breathing patterns have been linked to periodontal issues.[51]

ALLERGIES

The biocompatibility of orthodontic materials and their potential to elicit allergic reactions have been subjects of investigation.[53-55] The literature suggests a bidirectional interaction, wherein orthodontic appliances may exacerbate allergic responses, while allergic conditions may compromise the efficacy of orthodontic interventions.

Allergic reactions to various components of orthodontic appliances, such as nickel, latex, or auto-polymerized acrylic resin, have been extensively documented.[56,57] These reactions can lead to heightened discomfort, inflammation, and delayed healing and compromised treatment timelines.[58] The inflammatory response associated with allergies may also contribute to delayed tissue healing, influencing the overall success of orthodontic interventions.[59]

Nickel allergy is a common concern in orthodontics, with studies suggesting a low but existing prevalence of nickel allergy in orthodontic patients.[56,60,61] The prevalence of nickel allergy is estimated to be 11% in women and 2% in men, with sensitization to nickel increasing due to the widespread use of jewelry containing the metal. However, there is evidence suggesting that orthodontic treatment with nickel-containing metallic appliances before ear piercing may reduce the likelihood of nickel allergy.[61] The release of nickel ions from metallic orthodontic appliances during treatment has been demonstrated in both in vitro and in vivo studies, emphasizing the importance of considering the biocompatibility of these materials.[62] The immune response to nickel often manifests as a type IV cell-mediated delayed hypersensitivity reaction.[63] This reaction is commonly associated with the leaching of nickel from orthodontic appliances, leading to contact dermatitis or mucositis upon re-exposure to the metal.[64] Oral clinical signs and symptoms of nickel allergy include a range of manifestations such as a burning sensation, gingival hyperplasia, and stomatitis with mild-to-severe erythema. Furthermore, individuals with a history of atopic dermatitis to nickel-containing metals should be treated with caution during orthodontic treatment.[54]

Orthodontists should replace Ni-Ti archwires with alternative materials such as stainless steel archwires with low nickel content, titanium molybdenum alloy, and fiber-reinforced composite wires. Additionally, alternative nickel-free bracket materials including ceramic and polycarbonate can be used, or fixed appliances may be substituted with plastic aligners.

The use of auto-polymerized acrylic resin in orthodontic appliances has been associated with hypersensitivity reactions in patients.[65] These reactions have been linked to the release of toxic components, known as haptens, from the resin, including formaldehyde, benzyl peroxide, plasticizers such as dibutyl phthalate, and residual methyl methacrylate monomer. The leaching of residual monomer into the oral environment has been identified as a primary cause of these reactions, with concentrations of 1.5% to 4.5% in self-curing acrylic resins and 0.3% in heat-curing resins. International standards limit residual monomer levels to 4.5% for self-curing and 2.2% for heat-curing acrylic resins.[66] Residual monomer leaching from the resin into the oral environment can cause local and systemic reactions. Studies have shown that acrylic resins, especially chemically activated ones, can be cytotoxic due to high residual monomer levels. The cytotoxic effects of acrylic resins have been assessed through various in vitro tests, such as the MTT test, which measures cell viability. Different polymerization methods and the composition of acrylic resins have been found to influence their cytotoxicity.[67] Additionally, the leached products from acrylic resins have been shown to affect lipid metabolism, induce membrane alterations, and inhibit cellular growth.

The prevalence of potential type I hypersensitivity to latex is lower than 1% in the general population, but it ranges between 6% and 12% among dental professionals.[68] The increase in allergic reactions to natural rubber latex (NRL) over the past 2 decades has been attributed to the expanded use of latex-based gloves, particularly powdered gloves, which serve as the primary reservoir of latex allergens.[69,70] Specific guidelines in Europe and the US have successfully reduced its incidence in high-risk populations within the medical field.[71] Additionally, orthodontic elastics used for intermaxillary forces application are identified as another potential source of latex protein, leading to both type I and type IV hypersensitivity reactions.[72] Latex allergy is an immunoglobin (Ig) E-mediated immediate hypersensitivity response to NRL protein, presenting with various clinical signs such as contact urticaria, angioedema, asthma, and anaphylaxis.

The clinical effects of latex allergy are attributable to either type I or type IV hypersensitivity reactions.[73]

Allergies have been suggested as a potential factor associated with root resorption in orthodontic treatment.[41] Those with higher levels of IL-17, demonstrated increased orthodontic root resorption (Shimizu and colleagues, 2013). However, statistical significance of this association was not consistent across studies.[54,74–76]

RENAL DISEASES

As per the Centers for Disease Control and Prevention, about 10000 children and adolescents in the US are currently dealing with kidney failure and are undergoing treatment through dialysis or kidney transplantation.[77]

Dentally, chronic kidney disease (CKD) may cause delayed tooth eruption. The etiology of this is unclear but maybe due to overall impaired somatic growth. Panoramic radiographs reveal atypical features such as a bone with a ground glass appearance due to poor calcification, absence of lamina dura, hypercementosis, and constriction of the dental pulp chamber.

Radiographic dental findings in CKD patients are associated with hyperparathyroidism that is associated with CKD and renal osteodystrophy. Increased activity of osteoclasts influences all bones, encompassing the jaws and the alveolar bone.[77]

Orthodontists commonly encounter cases of chronic renal failure. Orthodontic treatment is considered appropriate for patients with well-controlled disease. However, if the renal failure is in an advanced stage and dialysis is imminent, it is advisable to postpone the treatment.[77]

In individuals with chronic renal failure who are not dependent on dialysis, it is advisable for the orthodontist to confer with the patient's physician. If the renal failure has progressed significantly, and dialysis is on the horizon, orthodontic treatment should be postponed.[78]

Renal transplant patients utilize combinations of immunosuppressant drugs, including Azathioprine, Prednisolone, Cyclosporin, Tacrolimus, and Mycophenolate Mofetil, to prevent graft rejection. Additionally, patients may receive calcium channel antagonists such as Amlodipine or Nifedipine. Children who have undergone renal transplants frequently experience drug-induced gingival overgrowth due to the prolonged use of these medications.[78]

The extent of gingival hyperplasia varies widely among individuals. Orthodontic appliances, particularly fixed ones, can elicit a significant response in the gingival tissues, even if there is no pre-existing gingival overgrowth before orthodontic treatment. Regular visits to a hygienist are essential for these patients throughout their orthodontic treatment.[78] In some cases, there might be a recurrence of gingival overgrowth, requiring surgical intervention during orthodontic treatment. Patients and parents should be informed about this possibility in advance.[78]

LIVER DISEASES

Patients with liver diseases have high prevalence of periodontal disease. In liver cirrhosis it ranges between 25% and 69%. Xerostomia is also another common finding in these patients.[79]

Hepatitis B, C, and D are transmitted through blood and can be contracted via contaminated sharps and droplet infection. It is crucial to treat all patients as potentially infected, and universal cross-infection control measures should be implemented. Orthodontic procedures that generate aerosols include interproximal stripping for enamel removal, clearing residual cement after debonding, and prophylaxis.[80]

MUSCULOSKELETAL PROBLEMS

Osteoporosis: It is a prevalent metabolic bone disease characterized by the progressive reduction of bone density and deterioration of bone structure. While it is more frequently observed in women post-menopause, it can also affect men. In cases of confirmed osteoporosis in women, bisphosphonate drugs are the primary choice of treatment.[81] The administration of bisphosphonates appears to be linked with adverse clinical outcomes, extended treatment duration, and alterations in the roots and adjacent tissues of orthodontic patients.[80]

The success of orthodontic treatment relies on osteoclastic activity, which facilitates tooth movement. The extent of tooth inhibition is expected to be influenced by the potency of the osteoclastic inhibition specific to bisphosphonate and the dosage administered at the particular site. It is presumed that inhibition of tooth movement occurs to a greater extent and more rapidly with high intravenous doses compared to lower oral doses.[82]

Orofacial muscles dysfunction: In individuals with orofacial dysfunction and syndromes, open bite is commonly observed. Patients with open bites typically exhibit weak orofacial muscles, anterior positioning of the tongue, mouth breathing, and an open mouth posture. Progressive myopathies like Myotonic Dystrophy Type 1 and Duchenne Muscular Dystrophy frequently present with malocclusions, particularly lateral and anterior open bites.[81]

Ehlers-Danlos syndrome (EDS): It encompasses a group of inherited conditions impacting the structure and function of collagen proteins, resulting in functionally weaker or decreased production of collagen. Common features include elastic skin, hypermobile joints, and fragile bony tissues. Dental characteristics relevant to EDS include joint hypermobility, dystrophic scars, poor wound healing, and a tendency to bleed excessively. In cases where the temporomandibular joint (TMJ) is notably affected, shorter appointment durations with frequent rests and regular TMJ assessments may be necessary. Certain forms of EDS can make patients more susceptible to periodontal problems and caries due to tooth morphology. During orthodontic treatment, teeth are likely to move rapidly due to collagenous laxity. There is also an elevated risk of damaging the fragile periodontal ligament, emphasizing the need for the use of light forces whenever possible. Additionally, there is a high potential for orthodontic relapse, making the consideration of both bonded and removable retainers important.[83]

AUTOIMMUNE DISEASES

Diabetes Mellitus: Being aware of the oral complications associated with diabetes mellitus, dental practitioners should take them into consideration when treating patients with DM.[84] It is advisable not to proceed with orthodontic treatment for patients with uncontrolled diabetes. In cases where the patient's metabolic control is not optimal (HbA1c $\geq$ 9%), diligent efforts should be made to enhance blood glucose control. For DM patients with well-managed medical conditions and no complications, routine dental procedures can be carried out without specific precautions.[84] Yet, there is still an increased likelihood of gingival inflammation, likely attributed to impaired neutrophil function. Throughout the course of treatment, orthodontists should closely monitor the periodontal health of patients with diabetes. Additionally, scheduling extended orthodontic appointments in the morning, following the patient's insulin injection and a regular breakfast, is recommended.[78]

Juvenile Idiopathic Arthritis (JIA): It is an inflammatory disease with destructive effects, primarily affecting children and leading to joint pain, swelling, and limitations in range-of-motion.[81] More prevalent in females, JIA typically begins before the age of 16 and involves progressive destruction of articular surfaces in various joints, including hands, wrists, fingers, toes, knees, shoulders, and elbows.[81] The TMJ is affected in 45% of JIA case. Nine orthodontic issues associated with JIA include mandibular retrognathia, condylar hypoplasia, a steep mandibular plane angle, open bite, antegonial notching, increased lower face height, and skeletal class II. Many of these problems are linked to condylar bone resorption. Facial asymmetry can result from unilateral TMJ involvement.[85] Approximately 70% of patients experience remission during adolescence.[81]

In the initial stages of managing the condition, non-steroidal anti-inflammatory drugs are employed.[83] While some individuals may remain asymptomatic and can be treated with intracapsular steroid injections, others may experience condylar hypoplasia, leading to a growth rotation that is both downward and backward.[83]

Upon achieving control over inflammation, the objective of orthodontic treatment is to restore optimal occlusion and mandibular function. Daily mandibular physical therapy, emphasizing a gradual increase in mandibular movement and the prevention of further joint stiffness, can complement this goal. It is advised to avoid the use of heavy class II elastics as they can exert excessive stress on the joints. The utilization of functional appliances remains a topic of debate, with questions surrounding whether these appliances amplify stress on the TMJ or act as joint protectors by relieving pressure on the condyles. Orthognathic surgery is typically deferred until growth is complete, except in instances of TMJ ankylosis, which necessitate earlier surgical intervention.[85]

SUMMARY

The number of medically compromised patients seeking orthodontic care is increasing and this trend is likely to continue. While orthodontic therapy is typically viewed as being of low risk compared to more invasive dental procedures, specific orthodontic treatments could be potentially harmful to certain patient populations. Continuous education and appropriate intervention studies are needed to reduce the complication of these hazards. Orthodontists must maintain up-to-date measures in respect to dealing with newer modes of orthodontic practice, developments in orthodontic materials, as well as be aware of personal health and management for special medical care for this professional group. It is imperative to exercise prevention as a most important aspect of risk management.

Orthodontists must understand these hazards and their outcome, to ensure that we can be successful practitioners.

CLINICS CARE POINTS

Malignancies

- Cancer therapies can compromise the mechanical properties of oral tissues, leading to increased susceptibility to trauma and delayed healing.
- Orthodontic forces may need to be modified to accommodate compromised tissue integrity.

Neurological disorders

Multiple sclerosis (MS)
- Patients with MS are almost universally infected with Epstein-Barr virus (EBV).
- Symptoms of MS may impact a patient ability to maintain oral hygiene, attend dental appointments, or undergo orthodontic procedures.

Epilepsy
- Patients should continue their antiepileptic medication as prescribed and should not be overly fatigued during appointments.
- The potential side effects of antiepileptic medications, such as gingival overgrowth associated with phenytoin, should be monitored.
- Removable appliances should be used with caution due to the risk of dislodgement during a seizure.

Attention-deficit/hyperactivity disorder (ADHD)
- Children with ADHD exhibit a higher prevalence of caries and periodontal problems thereby requiring strict oral hygiene maintenance.

Respiratory Diseases

Asthma
- Montelukast, a medication used to manage asthma, may cause a slight delay in orthodontic tooth movement.
- Steroid inhalers can lead to oral candidiasis.

Cystic Fibrosis (CF)
- Oral manifestations of CF include hypoplastic enamel and delayed tooth eruption.

Allergies

- In patients with Nickel allergies, replace Ni-Ti arch wires with alternative materials such as stainless steel with low nickel content, titanium molybdenum alloy, fiber-reinforced composite wires.

Renal diseases

- Chronic kidney disease may cause delayed tooth eruption.

- If the renal failure is in an advanced stage and dialysis is imminent, it is advisable to postpone orthodontic treatment.

Liver diseases

- Patients with liver diseases have high prevalence of periodontal disease and also xerostomia.

Musculoskeletal problems

- In patients with Ehler Danlos syndrome, where the temporomandibular joint (TMJ) is notably affected, shorter appointment durations with frequent rests and regular TMJ assessments may be necessary.

REFERENCES

1. Tweed CH. Evolutionary Trends in Orthodontics, Past, Present, and Future. Am J Orthod 1953.
2. Hall J, Payne AGT, Purton DG, et al. Immediately Restored, Single-Tapered Implants in the Anterior Maxilla: Prosthodontic and Aesthetic Outcomes After 1 Year. Clin Implant Dent Relat Res 2007;9(1):34–45.
3. Kinzer GA, Kokich VO. Managing Congenitally Missing Lateral Incisors. Part II: Tooth-Supported Restorations. J Esthetic Restor Dent 2005;17(2):76–84.
4. Polder BJ, Van't Hof MA, van der Linden FPGM, et al. A Meta-analysis of the Prevalence of Dental Agenesis of Permanent Teeth. Community Dent Oral Epidemiol 2004;32(3):217–26.
5. Zachrisson BU, Rosa M, Toreskog S. Congenitally Missing Maxillary Lateral Incisors: Canine Substitution. Am J Orthod Dentofacial Orthop 2011;139(4). 434, 436, 438 passim.

6. Michalak I, Kusmierczyk D, Bluj-Komarnitka K, et al. Radiological imaging and orthodontic treatment in the case of growing patients after oncological treatment: Case reports. Dent Med Probl 2019;56(2):209–15.

7. Kaste SC, Goodman P, Leisenring W, et al. Impact of radiation and chemotherapy on risk of dental abnormalities: a report from the Childhood Cancer Survivor Study. Cancer 2009;115(24):5817–27.

8. Venkataraghavan K, Patil S, Guvva S, et al. Abnormal odontogenesis following management of childhood cancer (retinoblastoma): review and a new variant. J Contemp Dent Pract 2013;14(2):360–4.

9. Mitus-Kenig M, Derwich M, Czochrowska E, et al. Quality of Life in Orthodontic Cancer Survivor Patients-A Prospective Case-Control Study. Int J Environ Res Public Health 2020;17(16):5824.

10. Tomasin Neto A, Amaral F, Romano F. Effects of ionizing radiation and different resin composites on shear strength of ceramic brackets: an in vitro study. Dental Press J Orthod 2022;27(2):e2219330.

11. Gawade PL, Hudson MM, Kaste SC, et al. A systematic review of dental late effects in survivors of childhood cancer. Pediatr Blood Cancer 2014;61(3):407–16.

12. Rayman S, Almas K, Dincer E. Bisphosphonate-related jaw necrosis: a team approach management and prevention. Int J Dent Hyg 2009;7(2):90–5.

13. Carrillo CM, Correa FN, Lopes NN, et al. Dental anomalies in children submitted to antineoplastic therapy. Clinics (Sao Paulo) 2014;69(6):433–7.

14. Meeran NA. Biological response at the cellular level within the periodontal ligament on application of orthodontic force - An update. J Orthod Sci 2012;1(1):2–10.

15. Cuoghi OA, Topolski F, de Faria LP, et al. Pain and Tissue Damage in Response to Orthodontic Tooth Movement: Are They Correlated? J Contemp Dent Pract 2016; 17(9):713–20.

16. Bernabe E, Sheiham A, de Oliveira CM. Impacts on daily performances related to wearing orthodontic appliances. Angle Orthod 2008;78(3):482–6.

17. Mitus-Kenig M, Derwich M, Czochrowska E, et al. Cancer survivors present significantly lower long-term stability of orthodontic treatment: a prospective case-control study. Eur J Orthod 2021;43(6):631–8.

18. Proc P, Szczepanska J, Herud A, et al. Comparative Study of Malocclusions between Cancer Patients and Healthy Peers. Int J Environ Res Public Health 2022; 19(7):4045.

19. Dobson R, Giovannoni G. Multiple sclerosis - a review. Eur J Neurol 2019;26(1): 27–40.

20. Baranzini SE, Oksenberg JR. The Genetics of Multiple Sclerosis: From 0 to 200 in 50 Years. Trends Genet 2017;33(12):960–70.

21. Giovannoni G, Ebers G. Multiple sclerosis: the environment and causation. Curr Opin Neurol 2007;20(3):261–8.

22. Serafini B, Rosicarelli B, Franciotta D, et al. Dysregulated Epstein-Barr virus infection in the multiple sclerosis brain. J Exp Med 2007;204(12):2899–912.

23. Ntranos A, Lublin F. Diagnostic Criteria, Classification and Treatment Goals in Multiple Sclerosis: The Chronicles of Time and Space. Curr Neurol Neurosci Rep 2016;16(10):90.

24. Bakathir MA. Orthodontic treatment for a patient with multiple sclerosis. J Orthod Sci 2017;6(3):110–3.

25. Kurtzke JF. Epilepsy: Frequency, Causes and Consequences. Arch Neurol 1992.

26. Sanders BJ, Weddell JA, Dodge NN. Managing patients who have seizure disorders: dental and medical issues. J Am Dent Assoc 1995;126(12):1641–7.

27. Sheller B. Orthodontic Management of Patients With Seizure Disorders. Semin Orthod 2004.
28. Cornacchio AL, Burneo JG, Aragon CE. The effects of antiepileptic drugs on oral health. J Can Dent Assoc 2011;77:b140.
29. Goswami M, Johar S, Khokhar A. Oral Health Considerations and Dental Management for Epileptic Children in Pediatric Dental Care. Int J Clin Pediatr Dent 2023;16(1):170–6.
30. Chau YC, Lai KY, McGrath CP, et al. Oral health of children with attention deficit hyperactivity disorder. Eur J Oral Sci 2017;125(1):49–54.
31. Katz-Sagi H, Redlich M, Brinsky-Rapoport T, et al. Increased dental trauma in children with attention deficit hyperactivity disorder treated with methylphenidate–a pilot study. J Clin Pediatr Dent 2010;34(4):287–9.
32. Ehlers V, Callaway A, Wantzen S, et al. Oral Health of Children and Adolescents With or Without Attention Deficit Hyperactivity Disorder (ADHD) Living in Residential Care in Rural Rhineland-Palatinate, Germany. BMC Oral Health 2019;19(1):258.
33. Hansen C, Markstrom A, Sonnesen L. Sleep-disordered breathing and malocclusion in children and adolescents-a systematic review. J Oral Rehabil 2022;49(3): 353–61.
34. Almotareb FL, Al-Shamahy HA. Comparison of the prevalence of malocclusion and oral habits between children with cerebral palsy and healthy children. BMC Oral Health 2024;24(1):72.
35. Miamoto CB, Ramos-Jorge ML, Pereira LJ, et al. Severity of malocclusion in patients with cerebral palsy: determinant factors. Am J Orthod Dentofacial Orthop 2010;138(4):394 e1–e94 e5.
36. Abanto J, Ortega AO, Raggio DP, et al. Impact of oral diseases and disorders on oral-health-related quality of life of children with cerebral palsy. Spec Care Dent 2014;34(2):56–63.
37. Iscan HN, Metin-Gursoy G, Kale-Varlik S. Functional and fixed orthodontic treatment in a child with cerebral palsy. Am J Orthod Dentofacial Orthop 2014;145(4): 523–33.
38. GBDCRD Collaborators. Global burden of chronic respiratory diseases and risk factors, 1990-2019: an update from the Global Burden of Disease Study 2019. EClinicalMedicine 2023;59:101936.
39. Curto A, Mihit F, Curto D, et al. Assessment of Orthodontic Treatment Need and Oral Health-Related Quality of Life in Asthmatic Children Aged 11 to 14 Years Old: A Cross-Sectional Study. Children (Basel) 2023;10(2):176.
40. Moraschini V, Calasans-Maia JA, Calasans-Maia MD. Association between asthma and periodontal disease: A systematic review and meta-analysis. J Periodontol 2018;89(4):440–55.
41. Dos Santos CCO, Bellini-Pereira SA, Medina MCG, et al. Allergies/asthma and root resorption: a systematic review. Prog Orthod 2021;22(1):8.
42. McNab S, Battistutta D, Taverne A, et al. External apical root resorption of posterior teeth in asthmatics after orthodontic treatment. Am J Orthod Dentofacial Orthop 1999;116(5):545–51.
43. Sameshima GT, Sinclair PM. Characteristics of patients with severe root resorption. Orthod Craniofac Res 2004;7(2):108–14.
44. Asaad H, Al-Sabbagh R, Al-Tabba D, et al. Effect of the leukotriene receptor antagonist montelukast on orthodontic tooth movement. J Oral Sci 2017;59(2): 297–302.
45. Ellepola ANB, Samaranayake LP. Inhalational and Topical Steroids, and Oral Candidosis: A Mini Review. Oral Dis 2001;7(4):211–6.

46. Coffey N, F OL, Burke F, et al. Oral care considerations for people with cystic fibrosis: a cross-sectional qualitative study. BDJ Open 2023;9(1):11.

47. Behrents RG, Shelgikar AV, Conley RS, et al. Obstructive sleep apnea and orthodontics: An American Association of Orthodontists White Paper. Am J Orthod Dentofacial Orthop 2019;156(1):13–28 e1.

48. Cistulli PA. Craniofacial abnormalities in obstructive sleep apnoea: implications for treatment. Respirology 1996;1(3):167–74.

49. Guilleminault C, Sullivan SS, Huang YS. Sleep-disordered breathing, orofacial growth, and prevention of obstructive sleep apnea. Sleep Med Clin 2019;14(1):13–20.

50. Lin L, Zhao T, Qin D, et al. The impact of mouth breathing on dentofacial development: A concise review. Front Public Health 2022;10:929165.

51. Tamkin J. Impact of airway dysfunction on dental health. Bioinformation 2020;16(1):26–9.

52. Camacho M, Certal V, Abdullatif J, et al. Myofunctional therapy to treat obstructive sleep apnea: a systematic review and meta-analysis. Sleep 2015;38(5):669–75.

53. Alencar LBBd, Sousa SCAd, Silva IL, et al. Allergic reactions in orthodontic patients: a review. Int J Odontostomatol 2021;15(1):132–6.

54. Salve RS and Khatri JM. Allergies and Its Management in Orthodontics. Int J Appl Dent Sci, 8 (1): 15–19.

55. Syed M, Chopra R, Sachdev V. Allergic reactions to dental materials-a systematic review. J Clin Diagn Res 2015;9(10):ZE04–9.

56. Golz L, Papageorgiou SN, Jager A. Nickel hypersensitivity and orthodontic treatment: a systematic review and meta-analysis. Contact Dermatitis 2015;73(1):1–14.

57. Sifakakis I, Eliades T. Adverse reactions to orthodontic materials. Aust Dent J 2017;62(Suppl 1):20–8.

58. Fletcher R, Harrison W, Crighton A. Dental material allergies and oral soft tissue reactions. Br Dent J 2022;232(9):620–5.

59. Salve RS, Khatri JM. Allergies and its management in orthodontics. Int J Appl Decis Sci 2022.

60. Zigante M, Rincic Mlinaric M, Kastelan M, et al. Symptoms of titanium and nickel allergic sensitization in orthodontic treatment. Prog Orthod 2020;21(1):17.

61. Fors R, Stenberg B, Stenlund H, et al. Nickel allergy in relation to piercing and orthodontic appliances–a population study. Contact Dermatitis 2012;67(6):342–50.

62. Sallam RA. Metal ions release in saliva from Fixed Orthodontic appliances: A Systematic Review. Arab J Nucl Sci Appl 2020;53(2):201–7.

63. Kim JY, Huh K, Lee KY, et al. Nickel induces secretion of IFN-gamma by splenic natural killer cells. Exp Mol Med 2009;41(4):288–95.

64. Noble J, Ahing SI, Karaiskos NE, et al. Nickel allergy and orthodontics, a review and report of two cases. Br Dent J 2008;204(6):297–300.

65. Gonçalves TS, Morganti MA, Campos LC, et al. Allergy to auto-polymerized acrylic resin in an orthodontic patient. Am J Orthod Dentofacial Orthop 2006;129(3):431–5.

66. Kedjarune U, Charoenworaluk N, Koontongkaew S. Release of methyl methacrylate from heat-cured and autopolymerized resins: cytotoxicity testing related to residual monomer. Aust Dent J 1999;44(1):25–30.

67. Ata SO, Yavuzyılmaz H. *In Vitro* comparison of the cytotoxicity of acetal resin, heat-polymerized resin, and auto-polymerized resin as denture base materials. J Biomed Mater Res B Appl Biomater 2009;91(2):905–9.

68. Hain MA, Longman LP, Field EA, et al. Natural rubber latex allergy: implications for the orthodontist. J Orthod 2007;34(1):6–11.
69. Palosuo T, Makinen-Kiljunen S, Alenius H, et al. Measurement of natural rubber latex allergen levels in medical gloves by allergen-specific IgE-ELISA inhibition, RAST inhibition, and skin prick test. Allergy 1998;53(1):59–67.
70. Toraason M, Sussman G, Biagini R, et al. Latex allergy in the workplace. Toxicol Sci 2000;58(1):5–14.
71. Wagner S, Breiteneder H. Hevea brasiliensis latex allergens: current panel and clinical relevance. Int Arch Allergy Immunol 2005;136(1):90–7.
72. Nettis E, Assennato G, Ferrannini A, et al. Type I allergy to natural rubber latex and type IV allergy to rubber chemicals in health care workers with glove-related skin symptoms. Clin Exp Allergy 2002;32(3):441–7.
73. Taylor JS, Erkek E. Latex allergy: diagnosis and management. Dermatol Ther 2004;17(4):289–301.
74. Murata N, Ioi H, Ouchi M, et al. Effect of allergen sensitization on external root resorption. J Dent Res 2013;92(7):641–7.
75. Owman-Moll P, Kurol J. Root resorption after orthodontic treatment in high- and low-risk patients: analysis of allergy as a possible predisposing factor. Eur J Orthod 2000;22(6):657–63.
76. Pastro JDV, Nogueira ACA, Salvatore de Freitas KM, et al. Factors associated to apical root resorption after orthodontic treatment. Open Dent J 2018;12:331–9.
77. Velan E, Sheller B. Oral health in children with chronic kidney disease. Pediatr Nephrol 2021;36(10):3067–75.
78. Burden D, Mullally B, Sandler J. Orthodontic treatment of patients with medical disorders. Eur J Orthod 2001;23(4):363–72.
79. Aberg F, Helenius-Hietala J. Oral health and liver disease: bidirectional associations-a narrative review. Dent J (Basel) 2022;10(2):16.
80. Zymperdikas VF, Yavropoulou MP, Kaklamanos EG, et al. Effects of systematic bisphosphonate use in patients under orthodontic treatment: a systematic review. Eur J Orthod 2020;42(1):60–71.
81. Patel A, Burden DJ, Sandler J. Medical disorders and orthodontics. J Orthod 2009;36(Suppl):1–21.
82. Zahrowski JJ. Bisphosphonate treatment: an orthodontic concern calling for a proactive approach. Am J Orthod Dentofacial Orthop 2007;131(3):311–20.
83. Alawsi F, Sawbridge D, Fitzgerald R. Orthodontics in patients with significant medical co-morbidities. J Orthod 2020;47(1_suppl):4–24.
84. Bensch L, Braem M, Van Acker K, et al. Orthodontic treatment considerations in patients with diabetes mellitus. Am J Orthod Dentofacial Orthop 2003;123(1):74–8.
85. Alqahtani H. Medically compromised patients in orthodontic practice: Review of evidence and recommendations. Int Orthod 2019;17(4):776–88.

Systemic Factors Affecting Orthodontic Treatment Outcomes and Prognosis–Part 2

Anil Ardeshna, DMD, MDS[a],*, Sumit Gupta, BDS, MDS[b],
Paul Emile Rossouw, BSc, BCHD(Dent), BCHD-Hons (Child Dent), MCHD (Ortho),
Cert (Ortho), PhD (Dental Science), FRCD(C)[c],
Manish Valiathan, BDS, MDS, DDS, MSD[d]

KEYWORDS

- Orthodontic treatment • Medical conditions • Dental health • Patient management

KEY POINTS

- Congenital heart disease patients with prosthetic devices, increase the risk of infective endocarditis (IE) with associated antibiotic prophylaxis considerations.
- In patients with IE, presence of orthodontic appliances may accumulate more plaque thereby increasing the risk of bacteremia.
- Orthodontic treatment is not contraindicated in patients with bleeding disorders but should be undertaken only after thorough history taking and consultation with the patient's hematologist.
- Nutritional deficiencies like vitamin, iron, and protein can pose various challenges to the orthodontist and should be managed before orthodontic treatment is started leading to better results.
- Various drugs significantly impact orthodontic treatment and related bone remodeling activity and a thorough knowledge of this is key to a successful orthodontic treatment result.

INTRODUCTION

Systemic disorders change the treatment approach and objective of patients compromised with the various disorders reviewed in Part 1 and now provide a continuation of the management in Part 2. However, it depends upon the comprehensive knowledge of an orthodontist regarding systemic disorders and possible orthodontic treatment

[a] Department of Orthodontics, Rutgers School of Dental Medicine, Newark, NJ, USA; [b] Private Practice, Rak Dental Care & Implant Centre, Ras Al Khaimah, United Arab Emirates; [c] Division of Orthodontics and Dentofacial Orthopedics, University of Rochester, Eastman Institute for Oral Health; [d] Department of Orthodontics, Case Western Reserve University, 9601 Chester Avenue, Cleveland, OH 44106, USA
* Corresponding author.
E-mail address: ardeshap@sdm.rutgers.edu

Dent Clin N Am 68 (2024) 707–724
https://doi.org/10.1016/j.cden.2024.05.005
0011-8532/24/© 2024 Elsevier Inc. All rights are reserved, including those for text and data mining, AI training, and similar technologies.

dental.theclinics.com

approach to gain successful results. Part 2 of this 2-part series on systemic problems serves as a continuation of the pursuit of knowledge to enhance the clinician's treatment planning acumen. Hence, it is of immense significance to recognize the systemic disease processes and concomitant clinical management. Orthodontic treatment is an elective procedure, and clinicians should consider all treatment options to ensure a satisfactory risk-benefit ratio for each patient. When appropriate, orthodontic treatment options should be clearly defined. Treatment options must also be effective and evidence-based, hence, providing the information for consideration in the 2 consecutive parts. If required, treatment delay until the medical problem is in remission is recommended.

Cardiovascular Disorders

Children and adults with cardiovascular disorders are often encountered in orthodontic practice. In spite of orthodontics being perceived as the least invasive form of all dental disciplines, the potential risks for cardiac compromised patients cannot be overlooked and requires special considerations and precautions to keep complications to the minimal.

The most common cardiovascular conditions seen in younger patients who form the majority of an orthodontic practice include congenital heart disease (CHD), infective endocarditis (IE), cardiomyopathies, and dysrhythmias whereas in adult patients, hypertension is the most common.

Congenital heart disease

With an overall live birth prevalence of 700 to 1200/100,000 in western populations majority of the CHDs are unlikely to be of a direct significance to the orthodontist as most of the significant cardiac defects are corrected surgically early in infancy or childhood.[1] The exception to this is a potential delay in tooth eruption and enamel defects if ameloblasts are affected during tooth formation that can lead to the formation of thinner and/or softer enamel. Consequently, these teeth are more prone to caries and difficult to restore,[2] posing a challenge to orthodontists. These patients are also likely to be more susceptible to gingival tissue problems with orthodontic appliances.[3]

CHD patients who have prosthetic devices, or which cause cyanosis, increase the risk of IE with associated antibiotic prophylaxis considerations.[4]

Infective endocarditis

IE is a rare but potentially fatal condition characterized by inflammation of the endocardium, particularly affecting the heart valves. It has high mortality and morbidity, serious complications being stroke and even death.[5] A necessary prerequisite for the development of IE is bacteraemia. Studies have shown that the organism found in periodontal pockets were commonly associated with IE and most commonly encountered organisms are Alpha–hemolytic Streptococci (Streptococcus viridans) causing atleast 50% of native valve IE and Staphylococcus aureus.[6–8]

IE has an incidence rate of less than 10 per 100,000.[9,10] Primary prevention of IE is very important because of the potential complications associated with it.

A direct link between IE and orthodontic treatment has never been established.[3] However, orthodontic patients should be made aware of the potential risk of IE, the need to avoid bacteremia and the importance of maintaining good oral hygiene. Presence of orthodontic appliances may accumulate more plaque thereby increasing the risk of bacteremia. Any invasive procedures which have the potential risk of transient bacteremia should be accompanied by appropriate antibiotic prophylaxis.[11]

Antibiotic prophylaxis is not recommended for routine follow ups and adjustments of fixed and removable orthodontic appliances.[12] However, any orthodontic procedure assaulting gingival and periodontal health requires antibiotic prophylaxis to minimize chances of bacteremia. The current American Heart Association Guidelines recommends antibiotic prophylaxis during placement of orthodontic bands and for high risk patients during debanding.[6] Placement of bands may push bacterial deposits from the tooth surface into the gingival sulcus by hydraulic effect of the bonding cement leading to bacteremia.[13]

Also antibiotic prophylaxis is required during placement of separators.[14,15] Elastomeric rings retain plaque more and occlusal forces on separators may traumatize the gingival margin enough allowing bacteria to enter the blood stream.[16,17] Antibiotic prophylaxis is also recommended for procedures like impression taking, removal of palatal expander, removal of Haas type palatal expander, surgical exposure of impacted teeth, orthodontic traction of teeth using gold chains, interproximal reduction, placement of temporary anchorage devices, before any tooth extractions as part of orthodontic treatment plan, when orthognathic surgery is planned and for soft tissue trauma caused by loose detached orthodontic appliances.[6,12,18]

Other orthodontic considerations for infective endocarditis patients
1. Orthodontists should determine the patient's level of risk for IE before starting therapy by consulting the patient's primary physician.
2. Patient's pretreatment and intra treatment oral hygiene status should be impeccable and the same should be instructed clearly to the patient verbally as well as in the written.
3. Regular supportive therapy from the oral hygienist.
4. Recommend the use of Chlorhexidine Gluconate (0.12% or 0.2%) mouthwash to reduce plaque and gingival inflammation.[19–21]
5. Bonding should be preferred over banding.
6. Use of smooth finished appliances which cause less mucosal and gingival irritation.
7. Securing arch wires with elastomeric modules rather than wire ligatures and preference of self-ligating brackets over conventional brackets as they may help reduce mucosal injury[22] (Maheshwari and colleagues, 2012).
8. Avoidance of fixed palatal acrylic appliances, such as Nance button and rapid palatal expanders which can cause mucosal inflammation.
9. Removal of excessive adhesives and thorough cleaning to minimize plaque accumulation.
10. Placing and removal of brackets, archwires, and ligature ties carefully to avoid mucosal injury.[22]
11. Use of clear aligner therapy as it is a minimally invasive removable orthodontic treatment modality.[23]

Hypertension
High blood pressure is the major risk factor for cardiovascular disease and a major cause of renal failure and stroke. Hypertension affects over 1 billion people worldwide with a prevalence of around 30% to 45% of the general population, increasing steeply with age. Elective orthodontic treatment should be deferred for uncontrolled hypertensive patients until blood pressure is controlled. However, there are no contraindications for orthodontic treatment of well controlled hypertensive patients.

Orthodontic considerations for hypertensive patients

1. Minimize stress by minimal or no waiting time before appointments and shorter duration of each appointment.

2. In cases where calcium channel blockers are prescribed which can cause gingival hyperplasia, patient's primary physician should be consulted to suggest an alternative drug.

Hematological Disorders

Blood disorders, either acquired or inherited, can affect the management of patients in a daily orthodontic practice. Hemophilia and sickle cell anemia are common hematological disorders where orthodontic considerations are important.

Hemophilia

Hemophilia, a disorder due to deficiency of some coagulation factors, is considered as one of the most common congenital bleeding disorder.[24] Hemophilia A is an X linked recessive hereditary disorder caused by deficiency of Factor VIII whereas Hemophilia B (Christmas Disease) is due to deficiency of Factor IX.

Orthodontic treatment is not contraindicated in patients with bleeding disorders but should be undertaken only after thorough history taking and consultation with the patient's hematologist.[25] Gingival bleeding and post extraction hemorrhage is frequently seen in hemophilic patients. Patients with hemophilia require special considerations in regards to viral infection risk and bleeding risk.[26]

Orthodontic Consideration for Hemophilic Patients

1. Hemophilic patients usually receive multiple blood transfusions increasing the risk of hepatitis and thereby requiring special precautions to prevent the possible spread of hepatitis virus.
2. Maintenance of excellent atraumatic oral hygiene to avoid inflamed and oedematous gingiva.[27]
3. Shorter treatment duration to reduce complications.[28]
4. Fixed appliances especially self-ligating brackets preferred over removable appliances to reduce gingival trauma.[22]
5. Elastomeric modules over wire ligatures.
6. Bonding over Banding and preformed bands over custom made bands.
7. Avoid extractions and surgery. If required, to be done after transfusion in a hospital set up.
8. Nerve block anesthetic injections are contraindicated and prevent the risk of hematoma formation.[29]
9. Extra oral anchorage instead of temporary anchorage devices to prevent bleeding risk.
10. Avoid high orthodontic forces to lessen periodontal complications.
11. Aspirin and non-steroidal anti-inflammatory drugs (NSAIDs) are not recommended for pain management as they can increase bleeding tendency. Safest alternative is acetaminophen.[30]

Sickle cell anemia

Sickle cell anemia is a genetic disorder characterized by an HbS hemoglobin gene mutation. Deoxygenation induces the red blood cells to deform into a sickle shape restricting their movement through blood capillaries thereby causing hypoxia and severe pain.[31]

Sickle cell anemia patients present to orthodontists with problems like enamel hypoplasia, delayed tooth eruption, Class II Malocclusion, prognathic midface, retrognathic mandible, increased overjet and overbite, increased vertical dimension.[32,33]

Orthodontic considerations for sickle cell anemia patients

1. Non-extraction approach to reduce risk of osteomyelitis.[33,34] If extractions are necessary, should be done in hospital setting under local anesthetic as general anesthetics can cause hypoxia.[34]
2. Avoidance of orthognathic surgery.
3. Early morning appointments, minimizing stress.
4. Light orthodontic forces are desirable to reduce risk of pulpal necrosis.
5. Rest periods between activation should be increased to allow local microcirculation.[34]
6. In case of clear aligners, reduce tooth movements by increasing duration of wear of each aligner.
7. Avoid bleeding during orthodontic procedures.

Eating Disorders

The most common eating disorders are anorexia nervosa (AN) and bulimia nervosa (BN), most commonly seen in females and having their onset during the early teens, often continuing as a chronic disorder. AN is characterized by excessive fear of body image distortion by gaining excess weight and hence opt for restricted eating.[35] BN is characterized by binge eating along with voluntary purging, use of enemas and laxatives, and excessive exercise. Dental manifestations of both these disorders include dental caries, erosion, hypersensitivity, xerostomia, raised occlusal restorations, and salivary gland hypertrophy posing challenges to orthodontists.[31]

Orthodontists play an important role in early identification of signs and symptoms of eating disorders. They should deal with these patients sensitively, have confidential discussions, and make appropriate referrals.

Endocrine Disorders

Thyroid disorders

Thyroid dysfunction, either hypothyroidism or hyperthyroidism, is the second most common endocrine disorder, occurring most frequently in females, especially those over 50 year old and affects bone turnover.

In hypothyroidism, problems include slower metabolism, low bone turnover, delayed eruption of teeth, poor periodontal health, delayed wound healing, impaction of second M and macroglossia, increased risk of root resorption, and somewhat decreased rate of tooth movement under orthodontic forces.[36,37] Thyroid hormone supplements taken by many hypothyroidism patients often increase the rate of orthodontic tooth movement, increased bone remodeling, increased bone resorptive activity, and reduced bone density. Hypothyroidism patients are susceptible to central nervous system depressants such as sedatives, hypnotics, and antianxiety agents.

In hyperthyroidism, orthodontic problems include high bone turnover, accelerated tooth eruption (Paumpros and colleagues, 1994), increased rate of tooth movement, increased susceptibility to caries, periodontal disease, maxillary or mandibular osteoporosis, and burning mouth syndrome.[38] These patients have increased levels of stress and anxiety and a surgical procedure can trigger a thyrotoxic crisis. It is difficult to sedate a hyperthyroidism patient because of high metabolic and heart rate. Atropine and Scopolamine should therefore be avoided in these patients.

Orthodontic considerations in patients with thyroid disorder

1. Stress free procedures with shorter duration.
2. Avoid use of adrenaline due to spread of infections foci.

3. Avoid excessive radiation exposure and use of thyroid collar during radiation exposure.
4. NSAIDs and aspirin are not recommended.[38]

Addison's disease

Addison's disease, with a prevalence of 9.3 to 14/10,000 (Vaidya and colleagues, 2009), is characterized by adrenal suppression and is associated with peripheral vascular collapse and even cardiac arrest. Orthodontists should identify the clinical manifestations like perioperative hypotension and ways for preventing acute adrenal insufficiency in patients seeking orthodontic treatment. Orthodontic procedures for patients on long term steroids do not warrant supplementation with additional steroids (Gibbon and Ferguson, 2004).

Orthodontic considerations in patients with adrenal insufficiency

1. Working in close liaison with the patient's endocrinologist to determine whether patients require supplemental steroids.
2. Minor oral surgical procedures should be performed under steroid coverage.
3. Postpone orthodontic treatment in patients on high steroid doses.
4. Reduced orthodontic forces (Kalia and colleagues, 2004).

Pregnancy

The role of hormonal changes during pregnancy is well known, however most pregnant patients are generally healthy and need not be denied orthodontic treatment. But orthodontists should keep in mind the following important factors before initiating orthodontic treatment in pregnant patients.

1. Pregnancy associated gingivitis which is usually seen in the first trimester due to an increased level of progesterone and estrogen causing an exaggerated inflammatory reaction.
2. Pregnancy diabetes because of hormonal changes.
3. Root, bone resorption and tooth movements affected by hormonal changes.

Orthodontic considerations in pregnant patients

1. Meticulous oral hygiene regimen to reduce risk of gingival problems.
2. Shorter, stress free morning appointments and allowing patients to change positions frequently.
3. Avoiding unpleasant taste and odors which can trigger nausea, gagging, and vomiting.
4. Avoid x-rays, drug therapy, and extractions in the first trimester.
5. Avoiding supine position during late pregnancy.
6. Rate of tooth movements may be decreased during pregnancy, accordingly treatment time to be extended.
7. Minimize exaggerated inflammatory reaction response to pregnancy induced hormonal alterations, therefore use of light orthodontic forces.
8. Steel ligatures over elastomeric modules as latter are considered less hygienic.[39]

CONGENITAL DISORDERS
Missing or Peg Shaped Maxillary Lateral Incisors

A congenitally absent maxillary lateral incisor occurs twice as often on the left side and is the second most common tooth agenesis, excluding third molars. This absence occurs approximately between 1.55% to 1.78% of the population [Polder and colleagues 2004]. A peg-shaped maxillary permanent lateral incisor might have a 55% chance of having a similar small lateral incisor on the contralateral side [Hua and colleagues 2013].[40]

Orthodontic Management

Missing or malformed maxillary lateral incisors can be successfully treated by either replacing or restoring the lateral incisor, or by canine substitution and reshaping the canine to simulate the lateral incisor.[41]

The treatment options may also include dental implants and tooth-supported restorations such as a resin-bonded bridge, a cantilever bridge, and a conventional full-coverage bridge.[42–45] These patients are usually managed by an interdisciplinary treatment approach.[43] The patient's age, dentofacial morphology, profile, crowding, and preferences determine the treatment decisions, which have lifelong consequences.[46–48] Autotransplantation of developing teeth is also documented as a predictable treatment modality for missing teeth.[49–51] [Czochrowska and colleagues 2000; Czochrowska and colleagues 2002; Plakwicz and colleagues 2016].

CRANIOFACIAL ANOMALIES

Craniofacial anomalies and dysmorphologies present in various formats and the etiology include chromosomal disorders (purely genetic), multifactorial disorders (genetic and environmental), disorders caused by teratogens (non-genetic, environmental influences such as viral infections, drugs, and irradiation, to which the mother was exposed to during pregnancy), as well as disorders of unknown etiology.[52]

Herewith, an overview of 2 common disorders representing examples of Class II and Class III malocclusions.

Treacher Collins Syndrome

An autosomal dominant genetic disorder with an incidence of 1:50,000 births. Most cases (90%) are a result of a mutation in the TCOF1 gene on chromosome 5. New mutations amount to 60% and 40% are passed down to siblings.[52,53] Characteristics include a narrow face with down-slanting palpebral fissures, lower eyelid colobomas, external ear malformations and sometimes ears can be entirely absent with conductive hearing loss, and addition, the nose appears large due to malar and mandibular hypoplasia. Obstructive sleep apnea may be present and cleft palate occurs in approximately one-third of cases. Individuals usually have a normal intelligence and life span is not affected.[52,53] The receding and vertical mandibular pattern creates an image of an extreme Class II malocclusion. Failure of neural crest cells to migrate into the first and second branchial arches leads to dysplasia, hypoplasia, or aplasia of the musculoskeletal derivatives of these arches. Therefore, the abnormalities are bilateral and symmetric.

Treatment usually entails the following.[52,53]

1. Various plastic and oral, maxilla-facial surgical procedures to improve craniofacial features such as malar augmentation, mandibular, and maxillary hypoplasia.
2. Cleft-lip and palate, if present, follows the conventional time sensitive procedures.
3. Hearing aids are often variable.
4. Rhinoplasty to compensate for the deficient upper and lower jaws. In the early years, it may require the placement of a tracheostomy tube to assist them with breathing.

CROUZON SYNDROME

An autosomal dominant genetic disorder characterized by premature fusion of certain skull bones (craniosynostosis). The early sutural fusion affects the craniofacial shape. Individuals generally have normal intelligence, but some reduced intellectual capacity has been reported. Appropriate treatment ensures productive and active involvement in mainstream society. It is a disorder of the 1st branchial arch with an incidence of 1:60,000. The syndrome has the typical triad of characteristics: (1) Craniosynostosis; (2) midface hypoplasia (Class III appearance) including relative prognathism, anterior open bite, high vaulted palate, posterior crossbite, and severe dental crowding. Obstructive sleep apnea is common, and a tracheotomy is often seen early in life. A cleft palate can be associated with this syndrome (but is not as common as it is in Aperts syndrome); (3) Exophthalmos with hypertelorism and often seen strabismus of the eyes (squint or crossed eyes).[52,54]

Treatment in Crouzon Syndrome is focused on relieving synostosis of the sutures, reshaping calvaria, distraction osteogenesis, fronto-orbital advancement with LeFort III or monobloc osteotomy, orthodontic treatment and LeFort II/III, Rhinoplasty/genioplasty.[52,54,55]

Genetic Counseling

Genetic counseling plays an important role as a preventive tool to establish correct genetic diagnosis and to determine if the anomaly is isolated or associated with a syndrome. If syndromic, is it inherited or de novo and an assessment of a recurrence in the future can be made. A prenatal diagnosis can assist a genetic counselor to educate and guide parents to an appropriate course of action based on the risk, family goals, ethical and religious standards or help the parents adjust for the future.[52]

NUTRITIONAL DEFICIENCIES

The World Health Organization use catchphrases: "Nutrition is the science of food and its relationship to health" and "Malnutrition is the cellular imbalance between the supply of the nutrients and the energy which the body's demand for them to ensure growth, maintenance, and specific functions".[56–59] Malnutrition thus develops when the body does not get the right number of vitamins, minerals, and other nutrients, which is essential to maintain healthy tissues and organ functions. Moreover, such nutritional deficiencies can affect the oral structures.[57] To illustrate this impact on the healthy body a few common deficiencies will be reviewed.

1. Protein/calorie malnutrition: Delayed tooth eruption, reduced tooth size, decreased enamel solubility, salivary gland dysfunction.[59]
2. Vitamin A deficiency: Decreased epithelial tissue development that could lead to gingivitis, periodontitis and hyperplasia of the gingiva, impaired tooth formation, enamel hypoplasia. There are 2 main sources of vitamin A: animal sources (liver, including fish liver, egg yolk [not the white] and dairy products such as milk [including human breast milk], cheese and butter, meat) and plant sources (mangos, papaya, many of the squashes, carrots, sweet potatoes, and maize [but not the white varieties]), dark green leafy vegetables such as spinach or amaranth as well as red palm oil and biruti palm oil (Note: if these oils are boiled to remove their color the vitamin A is destroyed). All the sources of vitamin A need some fat in the diet to aid absorption.[56,59,60]

3. Vitamin C deficiency (Scurvy): Irregular dentin formation, dental pulpal changes, bleeding gums, delayed wound healing, defective collagen formation. Fruit and vegetables are the best sources of this vitamin.[59,61]

4. Vitamin D/Calcium phosphorus deficiency: Vitamin D is both a nutrient we eat and a hormone our bodies make. It is a fat-soluble vitamin that helps the body absorb and retain calcium and phosphorus; moreover, both are critical for building bone. Lowered plasma calcium, hypomineralization, compromised tooth integrity, delayed eruption pattern, absence of lamina dura, abnormal alveolar bone patterns. Few foods naturally contain vitamin D, though some foods are fortified with the vitamin. The best way to get enough vitamin D is taking a supplement because it is hard to eat enough through food.[56,59,62]

5. Vitamin B1 (Thiamine/Thiamin) deficiency leads to: Cracked lips and angular cheilosis. In general, its presence keeps the nervous system healthy. Thiamin is found in many types of food. Good sources include: peas, some fresh fruits (such as bananas and oranges), nuts, whole grain breads, some fortified breakfast cereals, and liver.[56,59]

6. Vitamin B2 (Riboflavin) and Vitamin B3 (Niacin) deficiency lead to: Inflammation of the tongue, angular cheilosis and ulcerative gingivitis. In general, symptoms of a deficiency include confusion. Vitamin B1 and B2 deficiencies are rare in the United States. Vitamin B1 and B2 help convert food into energy. Vitamin B1 has neurologic benefits, and vitamin B2 helps maintain proper eyesight.[56,59] Sources of vitamin B1 include: whole grains, fortified bread, cereal, pasta, and rice, pork, fish, legumes, including black beans and soybeans, nuts and seeds. Good sources of vitamin B2 include eggs, organ meats such as kidney and liver, lean meats, low-fat milk and plain yoghurt, green vegetables, including broccoli and spinach, fortified breakfast cereals, whole grains, and mushrooms. Ultraviolet (UV) light can destroy riboflavin, so ideally these foods should be kept out of direct sunlight.

7. Vitamin B3 (Niacin): Vitamin B3 deficiencies are very rare in the United States. In severe cases, low B3 can lead to a serious condition called pellagra. Cardinal signs of pellagra are in health care referred to as the "3 Ds": diarrhea, dermatitis, and dementia. Vitamin B3 deficiency also leads to: rough skin that turns red or brown in the sun, a bright red tongue, vomiting, constipation or diarrhea, fatigue, aggressive, paranoid, or suicidal behavior, and hallucinations. Vitamin B3, helps: the body release energy from food, keep the nervous system and skin healthy. There are 2 forms of niacin: nicotinic acid and nicotinamide. Both are found in food. Good sources of niacin include: meat, fish, wheat flour, and eggs.[59]

8. Vitamin B6 (Pyridoxine) deficiency leads to: Periodontal disease, anemia, skin problems, such as itchy skin rashes, cracks around the mouth, painful tongue, burning sensation in the oral cavity. Vitamin B6 deficiency is uncommon. Vitamin B6 is found in a wide variety of foods. Sources include: pork, poultry, such as chicken or turkey, organ meats, some fish, peanuts, soya beans, wheatgerm, oats, potatoes and other starchy vegetables, fruits such as bananas, except for citrus fruits, milk, and some fortified breakfast cereals.[56,59]

9. Vitamin B9 (Folate) deficiency leads to: Megaloblastic anemia, which causes weakness, fatigue, trouble concentrating, irritability, headache, heart palpitations, shortness of breath, open sores in the mouth, tongue swelling, changes in skin, hair, or fingernail color. Pregnant women with a folate deficiency could result in their babies being born with neural tube defects, such as spina bifida. In addition, folic acid is recommended before pregnancy and during early pregnancy, to help protect the fetus from cleft lip and palate. Vitamin B9 deficiency is rare in the United States, but a deficiency can result from a low ingestion of fresh fruit and

vegetables. Celiac disease and certain medications (example Dilantin) may also result in vitamin B9 deficiency. Folate is found in many foods. Good sources include: broccoli, brussels sprouts, leafy green vegetables, such as cabbage, kale, spring greens and spinach, peas, chickpeas and kidney beans, liver, breakfast cereals fortified with folic acid.

10. Vitamin B12 deficiency leads to: Angular cheilosis, halitosis, bone loss, hemorrhagic gingivitis, detachment of periodontal fibers, and painful ulcers in the mouth. Good sources include: meat, fish, milk, cheese, eggs, and some fortified breakfast cereals. Vitamin B deficiency can cause diseases such as beriberi, pellagra or anemia. People who are vitamin B deficient may feel tired, numbness or weakness, among other symptoms.[56,59]

11. Iron deficiency lead to: Salivary gland dysfunction, very red, painful tongue with a burning sensation, dysphagia, and angular cheilosis.[56,59]

Caries and periodontal disease evolve more quickly in undernourished populations; demineralization is followed by cavitation and the pathology of periodontitis starts in the gingiva and invades the periodontal ligament up to the alveolar bone. The most important risk factor in the development of periodontal disease and caries is represented by inadequate oral hygiene. Malnutrition and bad oral hygiene represent the 2 important factors that predispose to necrotizing gingivitis.[63]

DRUG RELATED SYSTEMIC FACTORS AND ORTHODONTIC TREATMENT
Pain Medication

Orthodontic patients often take analgesics for pain during treatment. But various analgesics have different capacities to inhibit prostaglandins, and these differences might affect tooth movement. Nonsteroidal anti-inflammatory analgesics such as aspirin (acetylsalicylic acid) and ibuprofen diminish the number of osteoclasts, probably by inhibiting the secretion of prostaglandins, thereby reducing orthodontic tooth movement. Acetaminophen (Tylenol or Paracetamol) do not affect orthodontic tooth movement, and it might be the analgesic of choice for treating pain associated with orthodontic treatment.[64]

Speed of Tooth Movement

Systemic factors such as the use of drugs significantly impact orthodontic tooth movement and thus related bone remodeling activity.[65] Various medications such as estrogen, androgen, and calcitonin (systemic hormones) play a role in an increase in bone mineral content, bone mass, and a decrease in the rate of bone resorption which delays orthodontic treatment. However, an increase in tooth movement can occur as a result of thyroid hormones and corticosteroids (used for many inflammatory and autoimmune diseases) but this effect could have an unfavorable effect on the stability of the orthodontic result. It might be advisable to postpone orthodontic treatment for patients taking acute doses. Bisphosphonates, vitamin D metabolites, and fluorides may cause a reduction of orthodontic tooth movement and nonsteroidal anti-inflammatory analgesics cause a reduction in bone resorption that also impacts the speed of tooth movement. Clinical prescription of the noted medications should be well researched before use to ensure limited detrimental treatment effects.[65]

Bisphosphonates

Bisphosphonates are used to manage osteopenia and osteoporosis or to treat hypercalcemia caused by bone metastasis in cancer patients. Excess bisphosphonates (approximately 50%) is excreted unchanged by the kidneys; the remainder that is absorbed, has a high affinity for bony tissues that prevents the resorption of trabecular bone by osteoclasts and hence preserve bone density. The medical benefits of bisphosphonates are well known as also noted previously; however, a number of side effects exist including delayed tooth eruption, inhibited tooth movement, impaired bone healing, and bisphosphonate-induced osteonecrosis of the jaws (Maxilla and Mandible).[66] This can be exacerbated by the following factors: corticosteroid treatment, chemotherapy, medical comorbidities such as diabetes mellitus, the presence of dental disease, dental extractions, oral bone surgery, trauma from poorly fitted dental appliances, smoking, and alcohol abuse. Bisphosphonates have a long half-life of 10 years, thus an extended period of the effects can have a severe impact on general health, but also in particular, limit orthodontic treatment. Orthodontic treatment can only be considered after medical consultations and if possible, treatment should be carried out prior to bisphosphonate treatment. In patients at high risk of osteonecrosis of the jaws, it may be better to accept the malocclusion and consider the benefits of cosmetic dentistry.[65,66]

Drug-Induced Gingival Hyperplasia

The clinical signs of drug-induced gingival hyperplasia can vary in severity from minor overgrowth to complete coverage of standing teeth. These effects are compounded by poor oral hygiene, but can occur in the absence of plaque. Displacement of teeth can also occur resulting in further esthetic and functional problems. The main drugs that cause drug-induced gingival hyperplasia are phenytoin, cyclosporine, and calcium channel blockers including nifedipine, diltiazem, and amlodipine.[67] There are a few alternatives for reducing gingival overgrowth. One possibility is to use a different drug. There is usually spontaneous regression of the gingival hyperplasia, provided the oral hygiene is excellent. In some patients, however, the drug is critical to control either their epilepsy, transplant, and cardiac condition. In these cases, intensive periodontal treatment with excision of the hyperplastic tissue is necessary. The risk of drug-induced gingival overgrowth demands a team approach with the patient, patient's physician, dentist, periodontist, hygienist, and the orthodontist. Treatment should follow a preventative approach to ensure excellent oral hygiene. Avoid impingement of the gingiva by orthodontic appliances for example, use small, low profile brackets, and avoid excess composite around the margins of the attachments. Restrict the use of bands if possible as they appear to be associated with more gingival inflammation compared to smaller bonded attachments.[68]

Occupational Hazards in Orthodontics

Occupational hazards develop because of risks in the working conditions during execution of tasks as part of your occupation. In Orthodontics, these hazards can be broadly categorized as health hazards imposing threat to a person's biological balance from exposure to physical factors (example: light, noise, vibrations, heat, trauma), chemical factors (example: etching material, composite-resin, disinfectants and fluids used in radiology) and biological factors (example: cross infections) and other hazards causing risk to professional's well-being like musculoskeletal problems and psychological factors.[69] Ramazzini, the father of occupational medicine, was the first one to recognize the role of occupation in dynamics of health and disease.[70]

Orthodontists are exposed to several occupational hazards which include exposure to infections (including human immunodeficiency virus, viral hepatitis, coronavirus disease 2019 [COVID-19], and respiratory syncytial virus [RSV]).[71,72] Hepatitis C virus transmission risk is 1.8% and is the most serious viral hepatitis infection because of its ability to produce chronic infection in as many as 85% of those infected.[71,73–77]

Protection from x-ray radiation is essential when obtaining radiographs and non-ionizing radiation from the use of blue and UV light to cure various dental and orthodontic materials can damage the eyes.[68,71,78] Protective eyewear is essential to use in reducing the risk from blood-borne pathogens during procedures in which splatter or the use of aerosols might occur. Protective eyewear not only shields during splatter, but it is important to protect eyes from debris during procedures as well as from harming curing lights to reduce the risk of ocular injuries.[71,79–82]

Noise is always present during the work of dental staff divided into distracting noise and destructive noise. Orthodontists and dentists, in particular, are at risk for noise-induced hearing loss. Although hearing loss may not be symptomatic, the first complication and the reason for seeking a hearing evaluation may be tinnitus.[71,83] The sources of dental sounds inducing hearing loss that can be diminished are high-speed turbine handpieces, low-speed handpieces, high-velocity suction, ultrasonic instruments and cleaners, vibrators and other mixing devices, and model trimmers. At last, it should be worth mentioning that air conditioners and office music played too loud.[69,71,83]

Contact dermatitis can occur in the orthodontic office because of contact with resin-composite materials or latex allergies.[84,85] Respiratory disorders can also occur as a result of bad airflow or air exchange in the office.[86,87] Percutaneous exposure incidents remain a main concern, as exposure to serious infectious agents is a virtual risk. Minimizing percutaneous exposure incidents and their consequences should continue to be considered, including sound infection control practices, continuing education, and vaccination against hepatitis B, COVID-19, and RSV.[69,88] Basically, for any infection control strategies, dentists should be aware of individual protective measures and appropriate sterilization or other high-level disinfection utilities.[69,71] Strained posture at work disturbs the musculoskeletal alignment and leads to a stooped spine and muscle and joint pains.[71,89,90] Orthodontic practice is stressful. Not only physical impairments, but job-related psychological disorders may also affect a dentist's health. Risk factors include job-related stress, tension, depression, emotional exhaustion, and depersonalization.[69,71,91]

SUMMARY

A complete medical history, as well as excellent communication must exist amongst the orthodontist, patient, and the patient's physician. In addition, clinical alertness is critical in the successful care of the medically compromised patient population. Occupational hazards in dental medicine are numerous; however, unfortunately education on occupational health is not always a standard part of the curriculum of dental schools. A change in this respect should be encouraged if the adverse effects of systemic disorders need to be avoided or diminished in the practice of orthodontics. It is imperative for the clinician to be aware of how systemic disorders impact an orthodontic treatment plan and, thus, alter a treatment modality when required with the medically compromised patients in mind. Moreover, a comprehensive knowledge and understanding of the relationship of systemic disorders with the craniofacial and dental environment enables a successful clinical outcome of orthodontic treatment.

CLINICS CARE POINTS: KEY CONSIDERATIONS AND PITFALLS

Cardiovascular Disorders
- Congenital Heart Disease (CHD):
  - Expect delays in tooth eruption and enamel defects.
  - Check with physician if antibiotic prophylaxis is required.

- Infective Endocarditis (IE):
  - Maintain rigorous oral hygiene practices.
  - Administer antibiotics during procedures that could cause bacteremia.
- Hypertension:
  - Schedule stress-free and shorter dental appointments.
  - Monitor for gingival hyperplasia, a side effect of some antihypertensive medications.

Hematological Disorders
- Hemophilia:
  - Utilize brackets such as self-ligating to minimize bleeding risks.
  - Ensure patients have adequate transfusion support for any surgical procedures such as canine exposure.
- Sickle Cell Anemia:
  - Non-extraction treatments maybe preferable with light orthodontic forces.
  - Avoid stressful and prolonged appointments to prevent sickle cell crises.

Endocrine Disorders
- Thyroid Disorders:
  - In hypothyroidism, monitor for delays in tooth eruption and root resorption.
  - In hyperthyroidism, be aware of the potential for accelerated tooth movement and manage accordingly.
- Addison's Disease:
  - Coordinate with the endocrinologist for steroid supplementation before procedures.
  - Carefully manage orthodontic treatment during periods of high steroid doses to avoid complications.

Pregnancy
- Maintain good oral hygiene to manage pregnancy gingivitis.
- Avoid radiographs, drug therapy, and extractions, especially during the first trimester.

Congenital Disorders
- Missing/Peg-Shaped Maxillary Lateral Incisors:
  - Consider options like canine substitution or interdisciplinary approaches.
  - Tailor treatment plans based on the patient's age and individual preferences.

Craniofacial Anomalies
- Treacher Collins Syndrome:
  - Implement a combination of surgical and orthodontic interventions.
  - Address potential issues such as obstructive sleep apnea.
- Crouzon Syndrome:
  - Plan for early intervention for craniosynostosis and Class III malocclusions.
  - Employ a multidisciplinary approach to treatment for best outcomes.

DISCLOSURE

No Disclosures or conflicts of interests.

REFERENCES

1. Geva T, Martins JD, Wald RM. Atrial septal defects. Lancet 2014;383(9932): 1921–32.
2. Nosrati E, Eckert GJ, Kowolik MJ, et al. Gingival evaluation of the pediatric cardiac patient. Pediatr Dent 2013;35(5):456–62.
3. Gaidry D, Kudlick EM, Hutton JG Jr, et al. A survey to evaluate the management of orthodontic patients with a history of rheumatic fever or congenital heart disease. Am J Orthod 1985;87(4):338–44.
4. Garrocho-Rangel A, Echavarria-Garcia AC, Rosales-Berber MA, et al. Dental management of pediatric patients affected by pulmonary atresia with ventricular

septal defect: a scoping review. Med Oral Patol Oral Cir Bucal 2017;22(4): e458–66.

5. Taubert KA, Dajani AS. Preventing bacterial endocarditis: American Heart Association guidelines. Am Fam Physician 1998;57(3):457–68.

6. Wilson WR, Taubert KA, Gewitz MH, et al. Prevention of infective endocarditis: guidelines from the American Heart Association. J Am Dent Assoc 2007; 138(6):739–60.

7. Moreillon P, Que YA. Infective endocarditis. Lancet 2004;363(9403):139–49.

8. Selton-Suty C, Celard M, Le Moing V, et al. Preeminence of Staphylococcus aureus in infective endocarditis: a 1-year population-based survey. Clin Infect Dis 2012;54(9):1230–9.

9. DeSimone DC, Tleyjeh IM, Correa de Sa DD, et al. Temporal trends in infective endocarditis epidemiology from 2007 to 2013 in Olmsted County, MN. Am Heart J 2015;170(4):830–6.

10. Thornhill MH, Jones S, Prendergast B, et al. Quantifying infective endocarditis risk in patients with predisposing cardiac conditions. Eur Heart J 2018;39(7): 586–95.

11. Dajani AS, Bisno AL, Chung KJ, et al. Prevention of bacterial endocarditis. Recommendations by the American Heart Association. JAMA 1990;264(22):2919–22.

12. Gürel HG, Basciftci FA, Arslan U. Transient bacteremia after removal of a bonded maxillary expansion appliance. Am J Orthod Dentofacial Orthop 2009;135(2): 190–3.

13. Erverdi N, Kadir T, Ozkan H, et al. Investigation of bacteremia after orthodontic banding. Am J Orthod Dentofacial Orthop 1999;116(6):687–90.

14. Leong JW, Kunzel C, Cangialosi TJ. Management of the American Heart Association's guidelines for orthodontic treatment of patients at risk for infective endocarditis. Am J Orthod Dentofacial Orthop 2012;142(3):348–54.

15. Umeh OD, Sanu OO, Utomi IL, et al. Factors associated with odontogenic bacteraemia in orthodontic patients. J West Afr Coll Surg 2016;6(2):52–77.

16. Forsberg CM, Brattström V, Malmberg E, et al. Ligature wires and elastomeric rings: two methods of ligation, and their association with microbial colonization of Streptococcus mutans and lactobacilli. Eur J Orthod 1991;13(5):416–20.

17. McLaughlin JO, Coulter WA, Coffey A, et al. The incidence of bacteremia after orthodontic banding. Am J Orthod Dentofacial Orthop 1996;109(6):639–44.

18. Rosa EA, Rached RN, Tanaka O, et al. Preliminary investigation of bacteremia incidence after removal of the Haas palatal expander. Am J Orthod Dentofacial Orthop 2005;127(1):64–6.

19. Stirrups DR, Laws EA, Honigman JL. The effect of a chlorhexidine gluconate mouthrinse on oral health during fixed appliance orthodontic treatment. Br Dent J 1981;151(3):84–6.

20. Brightman LJ, Terezhalmy GT, Greenwell H, et al. The effects of a 0.12% chlorhexidine gluconate mouthrinse on orthodontic patients aged 11 through 17 with established gingivitis. Am J Orthod Dentofacial Orthop 1991;100(4):324–9.

21. Lang NP, Hotz P, Graf H, et al. Effects of supervised chlorhexidine mouthrinses in children. A longitudinal clinical trial. J Periodontal Res 1982;17(1):101–11.

22. Burden D, Mullally B, Sandler J. Orthodontic treatment of patients with medical disorders. Eur J Orthod 2001;23(4):363–72.

23. Chhibber A, Agarwal S, Yadav S, et al. Which orthodontic appliance is best for oral hygiene? A randomized clinical trial. Am J Orthod Dentofacial Orthop 2018;153(2):175–83.

24. Jover-Cervero A, Poveda Roda R, Bagan JV, et al. Dental treatment of patients with coagulation factor alterations: an update. Med Oral Patol Oral Cir Bucal 2007;12(5):E380–7.
25. Grossman RC. Orthodontics and dentistry for the hemophilic patient. Am J Orthod 1975;68(4):391–403.
26. Harrington B. Primary dental care of patients with haemophilia. Haemophilia 2000;6(Suppl 1):7–12.
27. Gupta A, Epstein JB, Cabay RJ. Bleeding disorders of importance in dental care and related patient management. J Can Dent Assoc 2007;73(1):77–83.
28. van Venrooy JR, Proffit WR. Orthodontic care for medically compromised patients: possibilities and limitations. J Am Dent Assoc 1985;111(2):262–6.
29. Piot B, Sigaud-Fiks M, Huet P, et al. Management of dental extractions in patients with bleeding disorders. Oral Surg Oral Med Oral Pathol Oral Radiol Endod 2002; 93(3):247–50.
30. Kumar JN, Kumar RA, Varadarajan R, et al. Specialty dentistry for the hemophiliac: is there a protocol in place? Indian J Dent Res 2007;18(2):48–54.
31. Patel A, Burden DJ, Sandler J. Medical disorders and orthodontics. J Orthod 2009;36(Suppl):1–21.
32. Oredugba FA, Savage KO. Anthropometric finding in Nigerian children with sickle cell disease. Pediatr Dent 2002;24(4):321–5.
33. Amoah KG, Newman-Nartey M, Ekem I. The orthodontic management of an adult with sickle cell disease. Ghana Med J 2015;49(3):214–8.
34. Alves PV, Alves DK, de Souza MM, et al. Orthodontic treatment of patients with sickle-cell anemia. Angle Orthod 2006;76(2):269–73.
35. Ashcroft A, Milosevic A. The eating disorders: 1. Current scientific understanding and dental implications. Dent Update 2007;34(9):544–6, 49-50, 53-546.
36. Young ER. The thyroid gland and the dental practitioner. J Can Dent Assoc 1989; 55(11):903–7.
37. Chandna S, Bathla M. Oral manifestations of thyroid disorders and its management. Indian J Endocrinol Metab 2011;15(Suppl 2):S113–6.
38. Pinto A, Glick M. Management of patients with thyroid disease: oral health considerations. J Am Dent Assoc 2002;133(7):849–58.
39. Michalowicz BS, DiAngelis AJ, Novak MJ, et al. Examining the safety of dental treatment in pregnant women. J Am Dent Assoc 2008;139(6):685–95.
40. Hua F, He H, Ngan P, et al. Prevalence of peg-shaped maxillary permanent lateral incisors: a meta-analysis. Am J Orthod Dentofacial Orthop 2013;144(1):97–109.
41. Miller WB, McLendon WJ, Hines FB 3rd. Two treatment approaches for missing or peg-shaped maxillary lateral incisors: a case study on identical twins. Am J Orthod Dentofacial Orthop 1987;92(3):249–56.
42. Kinzer GA, Kokich VO Jr. Managing congenitally missing lateral incisors. Part II: tooth-supported restorations. J Esthet Restor Dent 2005;17(2):76–84.
43. Kokich VO Jr, Kinzer GA, Janakievski J. Congenitally missing maxillary lateral incisors: restorative replacement. Counterpoint. Am J Orthod Dentofacial Orthop 2011;139(4):435–7, 39 passim.
44. Polder BJ, Van't Hof MA, Van der Linden FP, et al. A meta-analysis of the prevalence of dental agenesis of permanent teeth. Community Dent Oral Epidemiol 2004;32(3):217–26.
45. Zachrisson BU, Rosa M, Toreskog S. Congenitally missing maxillary lateral incisors: canine substitution. Point. Am J Orthod Dentofacial Orthop 2011;139(4). https://doi.org/10.1016/j.ajodo.2011.02.003.

46. Hall JA, Payne AG, Purton DG, et al. Immediately restored, single-tapered implants in the anterior maxilla: prosthodontic and aesthetic outcomes after 1 year. Clin Implant Dent Relat Res 2007;9(1):34–45.

47. Oyama K, Kan JY, Rungcharassaeng K, et al. Immediate provisionalization of 3.0-mm-diameter implants replacing single missing maxillary and mandibular incisors: 1-year prospective study. Int J Oral Maxillofac Implants 2012;27(1):173–80.

48. Vanlıoglu BA, Özkan Y, Evren B, et al. Experimental custom-made zirconia abutments for narrow implants in esthetically demanding regions: a 5-year follow-up. Int J Oral Maxillofac Implants 2012;27(5):1239–42.

49. Czochrowska EM, Stenvik A, Album B, et al. Autotransplantation of premolars to replace maxillary incisors: a comparison with natural incisors. Am J Orthod Dentofacial Orthop 2000;118(6):592–600.

50. Czochrowska EM, Stenvik A, Bjercke B, et al. Outcome of tooth transplantation: survival and success rates 17-41 years posttreatment. Am J Orthod Dentofacial Orthop 2002;121(2):110–9 [quiz: 93].

51. Plakwicz P, Fudalej P, Czochrowska EM. Transplant vs implant in a patient with agenesis of both maxillary lateral incisors: a 9-year follow-up. Am J Orthod Dentofacial Orthop 2016;149(5):751–6.

52. Bartzela TN, Carels C, Maltha JC. Update on 13 syndromes affecting craniofacial and dental structures. Front Physiol 2017;8:1038.

53. Chang CC, Steinbacher DM. Treacher collins syndrome. Semin Plast Surg 2012; 26(2):83–90.

54. Tanwar R, Iyengar AR, Nagesh KS, et al. Crouzons syndrome: a case report with review of literature. J Indian Soc Pedod Prev Dent 2013;31(2):118–20.

55. Tripathi T, Srivastava D, Bhutiani N, et al. Comprehensive management of Crouzon syndrome: a case report with three-year follow-up. J Orthod 2022;49(1):71–8.

56. Ehizele A, Ojehanon P, Akhionbare O. Nutrition and oral health. Benin J Postgrad Med 2009;11(1):76–82.

57. Psoter WJ, Reid BC, Katz RV. Malnutrition and dental caries: a review of the literature. Caries Res 2005;39(6):441–7.

58. Russell SL, Psoter WJ, Jean-Charles G, et al. Protein-energy malnutrition during early childhood and periodontal disease in the permanent dentition of Haitian adolescents aged 12-19 years: a retrospective cohort study. Int J Paediatr Dent 2010;20(3):222–9.

59. Sheetal A, Hiremath VK, Patil AG, et al. Malnutrition and its oral outcome - a review. J Clin Diagn Res 2013;7(1):178–80.

60. Gilbert C. What is vitamin A and why do we need it? Community. Eye Health 2013; 26(84):65.

61. Touyz LZ. Vitamin C, oral scurvy and periodontal disease. S Afr Med J 1984; 65(21):838–42.

62. Hildebolt CF. Effect of vitamin D and calcium on periodontitis. J Periodontol 2005; 76(9):1576–87.

63. Scardina GA, Messina P. Good oral health and diet. J Biomed Biotechnol 2012; 2012:720692.

64. Arias OR, Marquez-Orozco MC. Aspirin, acetaminophen, and ibuprofen: their effects on orthodontic tooth movement. Am J Orthod Dentofacial Orthop 2006; 130(3):364–70.

65. Tyrovola JB, Spyropoulos MN. Effects of drugs and systemic factors on orthodontic treatment. Quintessence Int 2001;32(5):365–71.

66. Igarashi K, Mitani H, Adachi H, et al. Anchorage and retentive effects of a bi-sphosphonate (AHBuBP) on tooth movements in rats. Am J Orthod Dentofacial Orthop 1994;106(3):279–89.
67. Butterworth C, Chapple I. Drug-induced gingival overgrowth: a case with auto-correction of incisor drifting. Dent Update 2001;28(8):411–6.
68. Kumar IG, Raghunath N, Jyothikiran H, et al. Influence of chronic congenital systemic disorder effects in orthodontic treatment. Int J Orthod Rehabil 2020;11: 123–35.
69. Maurya SK, Tikku T, Verma SL, et al. Scholars Journal of Dental Sciences (SJDS) ISSN 2394-4951 (Print).
70. Franco G, Franco F. Bernardino Ramazzini: the father of occupational medicine. Am J Public Health 2001;91(9):1382.
71. Ayatollahi J, Ayatollahi F, Ardekani AM, et al. Occupational hazards to dental staff. Dent Res J 2012;9(1):2–7.
72. Gerberding JL. Clinical practice. Occupational exposure to HIV in health care settings. N Engl J Med 2003;348(9):826–33.
73. Lanphear BP, Linnemann CC Jr, Cannon CG, et al. Hepatitis C virus infection in healthcare workers: risk of exposure and infection. Infect Control Hosp Epidemiol 1994;15(12):745–50.
74. Mitsui T, Iwano K, Masuko K, et al. Hepatitis C virus infection in medical personnel after needlestick accident. Hepatology 1992;16(5):1109–14.
75. Puro V, Petrosillo N, Ippolito G. Risk of hepatitis C seroconversion after occupational exposures in health care workers. Italian Study Group on Occupational Risk of HIV and Other Bloodborne Infections. Am J Infect Control 1995;23(5):273–7.
76. Younai FS. Health care-associated transmission of hepatitis B & C viruses in dental care (dentistry). Clin Liver Dis 2010;14(1):93–104, ix.
77. Zuckerman J, Clewley G, Griffiths P, et al. Prevalence of hepatitis C antibodies in clinical health-care workers. Lancet 1994;343(8913):1618–20.
78. Pandis N, Pandis BD, Pandis V, et al. Occupational hazards in orthodontics: a review of risks and associated pathology. Am J Orthod Dentofacial Orthop 2007; 132(3):280–92.
79. Roll EMB, Jacobsen N, Hensten-Pettersen A. Health hazards associated with curing light in the dental clinic. Clin Oral Investig 2004;8(3):113–7.
80. Farrier S, Farrier J, Gilmour A. Eye safety in operative dentistry—a study in general dental practice. British Dent J 2006;200(4):218–23.
81. Miller C. Make eye protection a priority to prevent contamination and injury. RDH 1995;15(10):40–2.
82. Szymańska J. Work-related vision hazards in the dental office. Ann Agric Environ Med 2000;7(1):1–4.
83. Garner G, Federman J, Johnson A. Noise induced hearing loss in the dental environment: an audiologist's perspective. J Georgia Dent Assoc 2002;15:9–17.
84. Rubel DM, Watchorn RB. Allergic contact dermatitis in dentistry. Australas J Dermatol 2000;41(2):63–71.
85. Stoeva L. The prevalence of latex gloves-related complications among dental student. J IMAB 2011;17(1):91–2.
86. Contrada F, Causone F, Allab Y, et al. A new method for air exchange efficiency assessment including natural and mixed mode ventilation. Energy Build 2022; 254:111553.
87. Srivastava S, Zhao X, Manay A, et al. Effective ventilation and air disinfection system for reducing coronavirus disease 2019 (COVID-19) infection risk in office buildings. Sustain Cities Soc 2021;75:103408.

88. McNamara Jr JA, Bagramian RA. Prospective survey of percutaneous injuries in orthodontic assistants. Am J Orthod Dentofacial Orthop 1999;115(1):72–6.
89. Fish DR, Morris-Allen DM. Musculoskeletal disorders in dentists. N Y State Dent J 1998;64(4):44.
90. Rundcrantz B, Johnsson B, Moritz U. Pain and discomfort in the musculoskeletal system among dentists. A prospective study. Swedish Dent J 1991;15(5):219–28.
91. Myers H, Myers L. 'It's difficult being a dentist': stress and health in the general dental practitioner. Br Dent J 2004;197(2):89–93.

Systemic Factors Affecting Pain Management in Dentistry

Davis C. Thomas, BDS, DDS, MSD, MSc Med, MSc[a,b],
Junad Khan, DDS, MSD, MPH, PhD[b],
Sowmya Ananthan, BDS, DMD, MSD[a], Mythili Kalladka, BDS, MSD[b,*]

KEYWORDS

- Systemic factors • Pain • Nutrition and orofacial pain • Hormones and orofacial pain
- Infections and orofacial pain • Autoimmune and orofacial pain • Dental pain

KEY POINTS

- Systemic factors may have a significant impact on pain management in dentistry.
- Many systemic factors can predispose, cause, perpetuate, and worsen dental and orofacial pain.
- Hormonal, nutritional, systemic infections, neurodegenerative, and autoimmune are the most robust factors affecting dental and orofacial pain.
- Dental clinicians should consider screening patients for systemic factors that affect their pain experience.

INTRODUCTION

Pain as defined by the International Association for the Study of Pain (IASP) is an unpleasant sensory and emotional experience associated with or resembling that associated with actual or potential damage (IASP 2020).[1] Acute pain, if diagnosed and treated optimally, resolves with no long-lasting consequences. Acute pain serves as a warning signal and is typically protective. On the other hand, chronic pain does not have any protective functions and is considered to be a disease in itself.[2]

Orofacial pain as defined by the International Classification of Orofacial Pain (ICOP 2020)[3] is pain in the head that occurs below the orbitomeatal line, anterior to the pinnae, and above the neck, including the structures in the oral cavity. The ICOP

[a] Center for Temporomandibular Disorders and Orofacial Pain, Rutgers School of Dental Medicine, 110 Bergen Street, Newark, NJ 07103, USA; [b] Orofacial Pain and Temporomandibular Disorders, Eastman Institute of Oral Health, Rochester, NY 14620, USA
* Corresponding author. Orofacial Pain and Temporomandibular Disorders, Eastman Institute for Oral Health, 625 Elmwood Avenue, Rochester, NY 14620.
E-mail address: dr.mythili@gmail.com

Dent Clin N Am 68 (2024) 725–737
https://doi.org/10.1016/j.cden.2024.07.004
0011-8532/24/© 2024 Elsevier Inc. All rights reserved, including those for text and data mining, AI training, and similar technologies.
dental.theclinics.com

classifies orofacial pain into 7 categories: orofacial pain attributed to disorders of den-toalveolar and anatomically related structures, myofascial orofacial pain, temporo-mandibular joint (TMJ) pain, orofacial pain attributed to lesion or disease of the cranial nerves, orofacial pains resembling presentations of primary headaches, idio-pathic orofacial pain, and psychosocial assessment of patients with orofacial pain.[3]

Patients described as pro-nociceptive and/or having a possible genetic predisposi-tion may be requiring additional or adjunct/alternative pain management modalities.[4,5] A specific example of a pain management issue in this regard may be congenital insensitivity to pain, where the pain presentation may be disproportionate to the de-gree of tissue damage or destruction.[6] Also, are patients who may be "nonre-sponders" to conventional pain management modalities. Clinicians also must consider the possibility of patients misusing/abusing medications or those who are already on long-term analgesic treatments.

There are several factors that affect a patient's experience of pain. These include both local and systemic factors. Dental pain is mostly of inflammatory origin. There can be a number of systemic factors that can affect and modify the process of inflam-mation, the pain pathways and, consequently, the pain experience. The systemic fac-tors that affect patients' dental and orofacial pain experience include, but not limited to, hormonal, nutritional, systemic infections, neurodegenerative, and autoimmune, among others.[7]

HORMONAL
Thyroid Disorders

Disorders of the thyroid gland occur in the majority of cases due to insufficiency or excess of thyroid hormones (triiodothyronine; T3) and thyroxine (T4).[8] These can be secondary to multiple causes such as congenital, autoimmune, and iodine defi-ciency.[9] Thyroid hormones play an important role in development of tissues, basal metabolic energy processes, contraction, regeneration, and myogenesis in skeletal muscles. Muscle fatigue and weakness are frequently encountered in hypothyroidism and hyperthyroidism.[8,10] Peripheral neuropathy symptoms such as weakness of prox-imal muscles, delayed muscle relaxation/contraction, paresthesias, anesthesia, and hypoesthesia are encountered in hypothyroidism. Peripheral polyneuropathy is gener-ally secondary to defects in neurons resulting in functional deficits.[8] Growing evidence also suggests that lack of thyroid hormones may be involved in the process of sarco-penia (reduction in quality/mass of skeletal muscle in the aging process). Alterations in thyroid hormone levels may worsen existing myopathies, for instance, muscular dys-trophy.[10] Variety of rheumatologic manifestations may accompany autoimmune thyroiditis.[11]

The hypothalamic pituitary thyroid axis plays an important role in regulating serum levels of thyroid hormones.[12] Thyroid hormones may play a role in specialization and maturation of taste buds and have been implicated in dysgeusia, secondary burning mouth.[13,14] Both instances of hypothyroidism and Hashimoto's thyroiditis have been implicated in the genesis of secondary burning mouth symptoms.[15,16] Thyroid hormones play a role in tissue development, regulating the functions of the nervous system, and may play a role in peripheral, central neuropathies as well.[8,13]

The Hypothalamic–Pituitary–Adrenal Axis

Stress plays an important role in activating biophysiological, behavioral, and neuroen-docrine responses thus activating an individual's adaptive responses to restore ho-meostasis. Neuroendocrine responses of hypothalamic–pituitary–adrenal (HPA) axis involve hormones secreted by 3 organs namely adrenal cortex (cortisol and glucocorticoid hormones), pituitary (adrenocorticotropic hormone), and hypothalamus (corticotropin-releasing hormone) under circadian rhythm modulation. Patients undergoing dental treatment frequently report anxiety and stress that may in turn affect the prognosis of dental treatment by impacting patient compliance.[17] A systematic review concluded low-level evidence for the role of perceived stress and life stressors in the development of chronic musculoskeletal pain disorders such as arthritis and suggested future research.[18] Full description of the HPA axis is discussed elsewhere in this special edition.

Diabetes Mellitus

It is a chronic disorder that develops due to either an inability to produce or to effectively utilize insulin by the pancreas. The polyol pathway and formation of end products in advanced glycosylation may affect various organs and are primarily responsible for the numerous complications associated with diabetes.[19] Diabetic peripheral neuropathy mostly starts peripherally and moves centrally as contrast to central neuropathies starting axially and moving peripherally. Diabetes mellitus (DM) is associated with a higher prevalence of dental caries, periapical lesions,[20] and periodontal disease.[19,21] A recent systematic review reported that DM increases degeneration/inflammation in the dental pulp, and this may predispose patients to develop increased pain, particularly following dental treatment.[22] Patients with diabetes have a higher prevalence of taste disorders, xerostomia, burning mouth, candidiasis, fissured/geographic tongue, higher incidence of infections, and delayed wound healing.[19,23–25]

MUSCLE ISCHEMIA

Skeletal muscles are richly supplied by blood vessels to meet the demands of exercise or usage at relatively short notice.[26] Ischemia could be qualitative or quantitative. In quantitative ischemia, the muscle is actually devoid of sufficient/optimal blood supply by volume. Qualitative ischemia occurs when the volume of blood is relatively sufficient, but the "quality" is less than ideal. This can result in inadequate oxygenation and nutrition, conceivably causing tissue damage. Symptoms may include pain, muscle weakness, involuntary muscle contractions, and sensory disturbances.[27]

NUTRITIONAL DEFICIENCIES
Iron Deficiency Anemia

The condition could be primarily due to impairment in the dietary sources of iron, or of absorption or of iron processing in the body. There is inadequate iron in the body to form hemoglobin. Hemoglobin is needed to carry oxygen in the erythrocytes. In iron deficiency anemia, when there is less oxygenation to the muscles, this can lead to muscle fatigue and pain.[28] In addition, iron deficiency may play a role in the inflammatory pathways, which may lead to increased muscle pain. When there is reduced oxygenation, muscles resort to anaerobic metabolism, which results in lactic acid accumulation leading to pain and discomfort.

Management of iron deficiency may result in improvement in symptoms. Iron deficiency has been shown to have an independent association with chronic daily headaches.[29]

The condition is also associated with glossodynia.[30] The effect of iron deficiency anemia on the severity of associated fatigue has been clinically compared to that of severe abdominal pain.[31] The same literature also confirms the strong association of this condition with chronic inflammatory systemic diseases. Anemia has also been shown to be associated with the pain of events involving vaso-occlusion.[32] Iron deficiency has also been reported in the literature as a perpetuating factor for myalgia.[33] The condition has also been shown to be associated with menstrually related migraine; additionally, the deficiency of ferritin was related to pain severity in migraine.[34] The clinician dealing with temporomandibular disorder (TMD)-associated myalgia, glossodynia, and myofascial pain should consider screening for iron deficiency in clinically appropriate cases. The astute clinician may be able to associate the coexistence of one or more systemic inflammatory conditions in their patients and constitute screening and prompt referral, thereby facilitating optimal pain management.

Vitamin B Deficiencies

Folate, also known as vitamin B9, is crucial for DNA synthesis, repair, methylation, and red blood cell production. It is vital for proper nervous system function. Folate deficiency can cause megaloblastic anemia; this can reduce the oxygen-carrying capacity of the muscles, which can lead to muscle weakness and pain. Folate is also proposed to be essential in myogenesis, proper muscle function, and its deficiency has been linked to sarcopenia.[35]

Vitamin B12 is essential for myelin production and red blood cell formation. A deficiency can lead to anemia, which reduces the oxygen supply to muscles, leading to muscle pain and weakness. A deficiency can also lead to neuropathy, which can present as muscle pain, tingling, or numbness, especially in the extremities. Peripheral neuropathies were associated with deficiencies of vitamin B12 and administration of B vitamins in general improved symptoms.[36] Supplementation of this vitamin was also found to be associated with early healing, lesser recurrence rate, and shorter treatment time for the management of oral ulcers.[37]

Vitamin C Deficiency

Vitamin C (ascorbic acid) has gained more momentum in the more recent literature as a key component in optimal wound healing, pain perception, and anti-inflammation, among others.[38] Vitamin C has been implicated in the synthesis of crucial neurotransmitters such as serotonin, glutamate, and dopamine. Further, recent literature points in the direction of vitamin C having a role in the synthesis of endorphins, essential for the pain modulatory system. Animal studies are showing that vitamin C supplementation leads to reduction of opioid drug tolerance and dependency. It may also have properties of improving the efficacy of analgesics. From the available literature, it appears that supplementation of vitamin C may enhance healing, reduce postoperative pain, and facilitate optimal pain management.[38]

Vitamin D Deficiency

The major health problem associated with vitamin D deficiency was rickets. However, vitamin D deficiency continues to be a problem in both the pediatric and adult populations.[39] A deficiency of vitamin D can affect calcium metabolism, leading to impaired muscle function, weakness, and fatigue culminating in pain upon physical activity.[40] Individuals with fibromyalgia syndrome show lower circulating levels of 25 hydroxy vitamin D (25-OH D) as this may lead to impairment of tissue structure and function. Supplementation with vitamin D can reduce musculoskeletal pain and improve the quality of life in patients with vitamin D deficiency.[40] Vitamin D receptors have been proposed to have interaction with the gene and opioid pathways.[41] Emerging literature points to the potential role in pain modulation by virtue of these pathways.

Vitamin D deficiency is proposed to be contributing to neurologic disorders and supplementation associated with mitigation of the effects/symptoms of neurologic disorders.[42] Studies have shown that vitamin D supplementation improved pain scores in chronic widespread pain.[43] It has also been shown to significantly reduce pain scores in patients with chronic pain.[44] The clinician managing pain may want to consider the vitamin D deficiency as contributing and/or perpetuating chronic pain. Therefore, mitigating these effects may involve appropriate supplementation.

Micronutrient Deficiencies

Zinc is an essential trace element that is required for the metabolic activity of many enzymes in the human body. Even a small deficiency can affect tissue growth, wound healing, taste acuity, connective tissue growth, and maintenance among others. Since zinc is essential for protein synthesis, cell division, and tissue repair, without adequate zinc levels, this can lead to muscle weakness and pain.[45]

Magnesium is a crucial mineral involved in various bodily functions, including muscle and nerve function. Magnesium acts as a natural calcium blocker, helping muscles relax after contraction.

Magnesium deficiency can cause muscle cramps, spasms, weakness, fatigue, and pain.[46]

Sodium is essential for maintaining proper muscle function, nerve impulse transmission, and fluid balance within the body. When sodium levels are deficient, it can lead to muscle-related symptoms such as muscle cramps or weakness. Hyponatremia can be dangerous where seizures, coma, or even death can occur, if left untreated. These conditions can vary from excessive water intake, using certain medications, medical conditions such as heart failure, kidney disease, or conditions such as syndrome of inappropriate antidiuretic hormone secretion, hormonal imbalances such as Addison's disease and hypothyroidism.[47]

Calcium plays a critical role in muscle function, and an imbalance can lead to muscle pain.

Calcium ions are essential for muscle contraction and for neurotransmitter release at the neuromuscular junction. Hypocalcemia can lead to muscle cramps and spasms as normal muscle contractions and nerve function is impaired. Calcium imbalance is also closely linked with hypoparathyroidism and vitamin D deficiency. Hyperparathyroidism results in insufficient production of parathyroid hormone leading to low calcium levels and associated muscle pain.[48–50]

Alpha lipoic acid (ALA) is an antioxidant that can reduce oxidative stress, which is linked to muscle pain and inflammation. ALA may reduce muscle soreness secondary to neuropathic pain and improve recovery, but more research is needed to explore this further.[51]

INFECTIONS
Lyme and Lyme-like Diseases

A tick-borne spirochete, *Borrelia burgdorferi*, is considered one of the major causes for Lyme disease (LD). Early stages following the tick bite are often asymptomatic but later stages can result in arthritis, pain, and joint swelling.[52] In the orofacial region, LD can lead to facial nerve palsy, altered taste, myalgias, dry mouth, neck pain, sore throat, paresthesia, headaches, and TMJ disorders. Some of the common orofacial presentations include headaches, facial and/or neck rash, oculomotor, vestibular, and/or facial palsy, TMJ arthralgia, altered taste, stiff neck, and sore throat. Neuropathy presenting as dental pain has been reported in patients with LD. Other studies have reported the presentation of LD as TMJ disorders, trigeminal neuralgia/neuropathy, toothache, dizziness, tinnitus, and hearing loss.[53–56] Lyme can affect multiple organs and can be difficult to detect especially in the early stages. LD should be a diagnostic consideration in patients presenting in endemic Lyme areas with orofacial pain inconsistent with dental findings.

Epstein–Barr Virus and Cytomegalovirus

Epstein–Barr virus (EBV) belongs to the gamma herpes virus family and is a double-stranded DNA virus. Studies have shown an increase in daily persistent headaches with the virus.[57,58] Studies have reported excessive sleeping, fatigue, and idiopathic hypersomnia in infected patients.[59] EBV has been suggested to be linked to the pathophysiology of rheumatoid arthritis (RA). Anti-EBV titers are elevated in patients with RA.[60] Studies have also shown a higher frequency of periodontal disease and EBV detection.[61] Cytomegalovirus (CMV) is a common double-stranded DNA virus belonging to the herpes viridae family. Oral ulceration in the soft and hard palate can be found in patients infected with human CMV and prevalent in immunocompromised individuals. In immunosuppressed adults, upon reactivation of the virus, it can lead to xerostomia, salivary dysfunction, and sialadenitis.[62]

Coronavirus Disease

Coronavirus is a single-stranded RNA virus and is part of the coronaviridae family. Some patients can present with loss of taste and smell, and it usually subsides in 3 to 4 weeks. However, as the pandemic is over, the long-term effects of the disease are being reported. Long-haul coronavirus disease (COVID) can impact multiple systems and present with a challenge in management. The prevalence of anosmia and dysgeusia has approximately been reported as 40%.[63] A study reported about 21% patient reporting of tooth pain, whereas 19% reporting in gingival pain accompanied with bleeding.[64] The exact mechanism is poorly understood but an interaction between the spike protein of the virus and cell surface protease transaminase protease serine 2 receptor has been postulated.[65] Studies have shown patients with COVID-19 developing a higher incidence of generalized body pain, facial pain, and headaches.[66] As a health care provider, it is important to distinguish various orofacial pain conditions and the long-term effects of the disease to prevent unnecessary treatment, financial burden, and time-loss.

Dengue

Dengue virus is an RNA virus and transmitted via mosquito bite and can lead to dengue fever. Many patients will be asymptomatic, but if the infection progresses, it can have severe health consequences. Dengue infection can result in a variety of symptoms including fever, loss of appetite, metallic taste, headaches, muscle and joint pain, rash generalized weakness and fatigue, muscle aches, bleeding gums, and vomiting. Headaches resembling migraines are reported in infected individuals.[67,68]

Chikungunya Virus

Chikungunya virus (CHIKV) is an arthropod-borne virus predominantly affecting populations in temperate climates.[69] The disease is usually self-limiting; however, in about 10% to 60% some symptoms may persist over years. Complications (in acute stage?) may involve hemorrhage as well as the involvement of the central nervous system, causing meningoencephalitis, Guillain–Barré syndrome, cranial nerve palsies, or neuropathies.[70] Musculoskeletal pain and neuropathy are often seen in the chronic phase (>90 days).[71–75] At this phase, clinical and radiographic features of CHIKV infection can mimic those of rheumatic disease, such as RA.[76] In the orofacial region, TMJ arthralgia and pain with neuropathic features have been documented, but rarely in the chronic phase.[77] The risk factors for chronification of the disease include age above 35 years, preexisting arthralgia, and severity of the acute phase (greater number of joints involved, joint swelling, and high-grade fever).[78]

FIBROMYALGIA

Fibromyalgia is a chronic condition with widespread/global pain. It can be accompanied by fatigue, anxiety, joint and muscle stiffness, mood disorders, depression, sleep disturbances, and other cognitive and somatic symptoms.[79] It is generally agreed that the condition is an example of central sensitization, and the etiology may be multifactorial. Patients often display a lower pain threshold and show clinical presentation of allodynia and hyperalgesia.[80,81] Studies have shown xerostomia, dysgeusia, glossodynia, oral ulcerations, dysphagia, and orofacial pain to be prevalent in patients with fibromyalgia. The prevalence of TMDs has been reported in 75% of the patients. Patients often report jaw stiffness, myalgia, and headaches. Chronic migraines and tension-type headaches have also been reported to be highly prevalent in patients with fibromyalgia.[82–84] When patients present with TMD and concomitant fibromyalgia, an approach to address both the peripheral and central components of pain may be more desirable.

JOINT HYPERMOBILITY SYNDROMES

Patients with joint hypermobility are highly prone to TMDs and often present pain, clicking, jaw locking, and crepitations. The oral mucosa is thin and can lead to bleeding and ulceration. It is important to manage these patients with an interdisciplinary approach to avoid complications and have a successful outcome.[85–87] Global pain, psychological, and other systemic comorbidities are common in joint hypermobility syndromes. The clinician should recognize the possible vulnerability of these patients to joint hyperextensions and possible injury, as that may occur during dental procedures necessitating prolonged mouth opening. These patients also present with fibromyalgia and other central sensitization syndromes.

MEDICATIONS AFFECTING PAIN MANAGEMENT

The concept of preemptive analgesia (using analgesics, anesthetics, or other classes of medications) has gained momentum in the pain management field.[88] Most of the dental procedure and pathology-related pain are of inflammatory origin. Conceivable, drugs with predominantly anti-inflammatory properties are appropriate for optimal dental-related pain management. The prime classes of medications that exhibit these anti-inflammatory qualities are nonsteroidal anti-inflammatory drugs (NSAIDs) and steroids. Among the factors that may preclude NSAIDs are conditions such as gastritis, hyperacidity, gastric/duodenal ulcers, gastroesophageal reflux disease, hypertension, cardiovascular morbidities, among others.[89] Conditions such as diabetes, immunosuppression, glaucoma, osteoporosis among others may form a relative contraindication for steroids.[90,91]

Long-term antithyroid medication use may be associated with minor complications such as arthralgia and myalgia.[91] Statins may induce myalgias and use of certain statins may be associated with statin-induced necrotizing autoimmune myopathy as a rare side effect.[92] Long-term use of statins may be associated with proximal myopathies.[93] When patients on any drugs, including statins, present with myalgia, a proper history regarding the initiation of the medication, dosage adjustment history, possible drug and food interactions, and the temporal relationship to the pain should be explored.[7]

AUTOIMMUNE DISORDERS

Several autoimmune disorders may affect the pain in the orofacial region and thereby modify pain management in dentistry. The prototype of these disorders is RA and systemic lupus erythematosus (SLE). RA affects the hard and soft tissue structures of joints, including those associated with the TMJ.[7,94] The prevalence of RA in the general population is approximately 1.5%.[7] These patients may present to the clinician with complaints of muscle and/or joint pain. It may also manifest as patient's complaints of jaw tiredness and ache upon opening the mouth for dental procedures. The savvy clinician should be able to screen the patient for these entities when a higher suspicion is raised on the probability of these diseases. The orofacial and TMJ involvement in SLE have been well documented in the literature. These include global myalgia, joint pains, pain on chewing, and "stuck" feeling in the jaw.[7] Identification and prompt referral to the appropriate medical specialist are crucial for optimal care of these patients.

NEURODEGENERATIVE DISORDERS

The neurodegenerative disorders of interest to the dental clinician in terms of pain management in dentistry include Parkinsonism syndromes (including Parkinson's disease, [PD]), Alzheimer's disease, and multiple sclerosis, among others. Pain is one of the chief non-motor symptoms of PD.[95] Oral burning sensations and painful TMDs contribute to the reduced quality of life in PD.

SUMMARY

Several local and systemic factors may play an important role in pain management during dental procedures. The savvy clinician should be able to screen the patient for these entities when a higher suspicion is raised on the probability of these diseases and refer them to appropriate specialists for successful interdisciplinary management.

CLINICS CARE POINTS

- Comprehensive medical history is essential to delineate any possible systemic factors affecting pain experience.
- A thorough review of systems should form the foundation of pain management, since multiple factors can affect the prognosis of pain management in dentistry and orofacial pain.
- This would facilitate early recognition and trigger prompt referrals to the appropriate medical professionals.
- These succinct steps help to reduce the health care burden and form the scaffolding for interdisciplinary pain management.

DISCLOSURE

The authors declare that there are no commercial or financial conflicts of interest and any funding sources for all authors.

REFERENCES

1. Merskey H., Bogduk N., Updated terminology from "part III: pain terms, a current list with definitions and notes on usage", In: Merskey H., Bogduk N., editor. *Classification of chronic pain*, IASP task force on taxonomy, 2nd edition, 1994, IASP Press; Seattle (WA), 209–214, Available at: https://www.iasp-pain.org/resources/terminology/#pain.

2. Khan J, Zusman T, Wang Q, et al. Acute and chronic pain in orofacial trauma patients. Dent Traumatol 2019;35(6):348–57.

3. International Classification of Orofacial Pain, 1st edition. Cephalalgia 2020;40(2): 129–221 (ICOP).

4. Kalladka M, Young A, Khan J. Myofascial pain in temporomandibular disorders: Updates on etiopathogenesis and management. J Bodyw Mov Ther 2021;28: 104–13.

5. Khan J, Singer SR, Young A, et al. Pathogenesis and Differential Diagnosis of Temporomandibular Joint Disorders. Dent Clin North Am 2023;67(2):259–80.

6. Butler J, Fleming P, Webb D. Congenital insensitivity to pain–review and report of a case with dental implications. Oral Surg Oral Med Oral Pathol Oral Radiol Endod 2006;101(1):58–62.

7. Thomas DC, Eliav E, Garcia AR, et al. Systemic Factors in Temporomandibular Disorder Pain. Dent Clin North Am 2023;67(2):281–98.

8. Gupta N, Arora M, Sharma R, et al. Peripheral and Central Nervous System Involvement in Recently Diagnosed Cases of Hypothyroidism: An Electrophysiological Study. Ann Med Health Sci Res 2016;6(5):261–6.

9. Fariduddin MM, Haq N, Bansal N. Hypothyroid Myopathy. In: StatPearls [internet]. Treasure island (FL): StatPearls Publishing; 2024.

10. Bloise FF, Oliveira TS, Cordeiro A, et al. Thyroid Hormones Play Role in Sarcopenia and Myopathies. Front Physiol 2018;9:560.

11. Punzi L, Betterle C. Chronic autoimmune thyroiditis and rheumatic manifestations. Joint Bone Spine 2004;71(4):275–83.

12. Ortiga-Carvalho TM, Chiamolera MI, Pazos-Moura CC, et al. Hypothalamus-Pituitary-Thyroid Axis. Compr Physiol 2016;6(3):1387–428.

13. Egido-Moreno S, Valls-Roca-Umbert J, Perez-Sayans M, et al. Role of thyroid hormones in burning mouth syndrome. Systematic review. Med Oral Patol Oral Cir Bucal 2023;28(1):e81–6.

14. Brosvic GM, Doty RL, Rowe MM, et al. Influences of hypothyroidism on the taste detection performance of rats: a signal detection analysis. Behav Neurosci 1992; 106(6):992–8.

15. Talattof Z, Dabbaghmanesh MH, Parvizi Y, et al. The Association between Burning Mouth Syndrome and Level of Thyroid Hormones in Hashimotos Thyroiditis in Public Hospitals in Shiraz, 2016. J Dent (Shiraz) 2019;20(1):42–7.

16. Femiano F, Lanza A, Buonaiuto C, et al. Burning mouth syndrome and burning mouth in hypothyroidism: proposal for a diagnostic and therapeutic protocol. Oral Surg Oral Med Oral Pathol Oral Radiol Endod 2008;105(1):e22–7.

17. Herman JP, McKlveen JM, Ghosal S, et al. Regulation of the Hypothalamic-Pituitary-Adrenocortical Stress Response. Compr Physiol 2016;15(6 2):603–21.

18. Buscemi V, Chang WJ, Liston MB, et al. The Role of Perceived Stress and Life Stressors in the Development of Chronic Musculoskeletal Pain Disorders: A Systematic Review. J Pain 2019;20(10):1127–39.

19. Mauri-Obradors E, Estrugo-Devesa A, Jané-Salas E, et al. Oral manifestations of Diabetes Mellitus. A systematic review. Med Oral Patol Oral Cir Bucal 2017;22(5): e586–94.

20. Wang Y, Xing L, Yu H, et al. Prevalence of dental caries in children and adolescents with type 1 diabetes: a systematic review and meta-analysis. BMC Oral Health 2019;19(1):213.

21. Zainal Abidin Z, Zainuren ZA, Noor E, et al. Periodontal health status of children and adolescents with diabetes mellitus: a systematic review and meta-analysis. Aust Dent J 2021;66(Suppl 1):S15–26.

22. Pimenta RMN, Dos Reis-Prado AH, de Castro Oliveira S, et al. Effects of diabetes mellitus on dental pulp: A systematic review of in vivo and in vitro studies. Oral Dis 2024;30(2):100–15.

23. Khan J, Anwer M, Noboru N, et al. Topical application in burning mouth syndrome. J Dent Sci 2019;14(4):352–7.

24. Khan J, Noma N, Kalladka M. Taste changes in orofacial pain conditions and coronavirus disease 2019: a review. Front Oral Maxillofac Med 2021;3:5.

25. Thomas DC, Chablani D, Parekh S, et al. Dysgeusia: A review in the context of COVID-19. J Am Dent Assoc 2022;153(3):251–64.

26. Harriman DG. Ischaemia of peripheral nerve and muscle. J Clin Pathol Suppl (R Coll Pathol) 1977;11:94–104.

27. Rubin BB, Romaschin A, Walker PM, et al. Mechanisms of postischemic injury in skeletal muscle: intervention strategies. J Appl Physiol 1985;80(2):369–87.

28. Elstrott B, Khan L, Olson S, et al. The role of iron repletion in adult iron deficiency anemia and other diseases. Eur J Haematol 2020;104(3):153–61.

29. Singh RK, Kaushik RM, Goel D, et al. Association between iron deficiency anemia and chronic daily headache: A case-control study. Cephalalgia 2023;43(2). 3331024221143540.

30. Osaki T, Ueta E, Arisawa K, et al. The pathophysiology of glossal pain in patients with iron deficiency and anemia. Am J Med Sci 1999;318(5):324–9.

31. Cacoub P, Choukroun G, Cohen-Solal A, et al. Iron deficiency screening is a key issue in chronic inflammatory diseases: A call to action. J Intern Med 2022; 292(4):542–56.

32. Kassebaum NJ, GBD 2013 Anemia Collaborators. The Global Burden of Anemia. Hematol Oncol Clin North Am 2016;30(2):247–308.

33. Gerwin RD. A review of myofascial pain and fibromyalgia–factors that promote their persistence. Acupunct Med 2005;23(3):121–34.

34. Sari US, Kama Başci Ö. Association between anemia severity and migraine in iron deficiency anemia. Eur Rev Med Pharmacol Sci 2024;28(3):995–1001.

35. Hwang SY, Sung B, Kim ND. Roles of folate in skeletal muscle cell development and functions. Arch Pharm Res 2019;42(4):319–25.

36. Stein J, Geisel J, Obeid R. Association between neuropathy and B-vitamins: A systematic review and meta-analysis. Eur J Neurol 2021;28(6):2054–64.

37. Shi J, Wang L, Zhang Y, et al. Clinical efficacy of vitamin B in the treatment of mouth ulcer: a systematic review and meta-analysis. Ann Palliat Med 2021; 10(6):6588–96.

38. Zelfand E. Vitamin C, Pain and Opioid Use Disorder. Integr Med (Encinitas) 2020; 19(3):18–29.

39. Holick MF. Vitamin D deficiency. N Engl J Med 2007;357(3):266–81.

40. Lombardo M, Feraco A, Ottaviani M, et al. The Efficacy of Vitamin D Supplementation in the Treatment of Fibromyalgia Syndrome and Chronic Musculoskeletal Pain. Nutrients 2022;14(15):3010.

41. Habib AM, Nagi K, Thillaiappan NB, et al. Vitamin D and Its Potential Interplay With Pain Signaling Pathways. Front Immunol 2020;11:820.
42. Moretti R, Morelli ME, Caruso P. Vitamin D in Neurological Diseases: A Rationale for a Pathogenic Impact. Int J Mol Sci 2018;19(8):2245.
43. Yong WC, Sanguankeo A, Upala S. Effect of vitamin D supplementation in chronic widespread pain: a systematic review and meta-analysis. Clin Rheumatol 2017; 36(12):2825-33.
44. Wu Z, Malihi Z, Stewart AW, et al. Effect of Vitamin D Supplementation on Pain: A Systematic Review and Meta-analysis. Pain Physician 2016;19(7):415-27.
45. Roohani N, Hurrell R, Kelishadi R, et al. Zinc and its importance for human health: An integrative review. J Res Med Sci 2013;18(2):144-57.
46. Shin HJ, Na HS, Do SH. Magnesium and Pain. Nutrients 2020;12(8):2184.
47. Buffington MA, Abreo K. Hyponatremia: A Review. J Intensive Care Med 2016; 31(4):223-36.
48. Bove-Fenderson E, Mannstadt M. Hypocalcemic disorders. Best Pract Res Clin Endocrinol Metabol 2018;32(5):639-56.
49. Peacock M. Calcium metabolism in health and disease. Clin J Am Soc Nephrol 2010;5(Suppl 1):S23-30.
50. Oberger Marques JV, Moreira CA. Primary hyperparathyroidism. Best Pract Res Clin Rheumatol 2020;34(3):101514.
51. Salehi B, Yılmaz BY, Antika G, et al. Insights on the Use of α-Lipoic Acid for Therapeutic Purposes. Biomolecules 2019;9(8):356.
52. Arvikar SL, Steere AC. Diagnosis and treatment of Lyme arthritis. Infect Dis Clin North Am 2015;29(2):269-80.
53. Bradshaw BT, Jones KM, Westerdale-McInnis JM, et al. Orofacial manifestations of lyme disease: a systematic review. American Dental Hygienists' Association 2021;95(4):23-31.
54. McEntire CR, Chwalisz BK. Cranial nerve involvement, visual complications and headache syndromes in Lyme disease. Curr Opin Ophthalmol 2024;35(3):265-71.
55. Cameron DC-D. Study finds hearing loss and tinnitus common in patients with tick-borne diseases. Otolaryngol Pol 2018;72(1):30-4.
56. Mello I, Peters J, Lee C. Neuropathy mimicking dental pain in a patient diagnosed with Lyme disease. J Endod 2020;46(9):1337-9.
57. Diaz-Mitoma F, Vanast WJ, Tyrrell DL. Increased frequency of Epstein-Barr virus excretion in patients with new daily persistent headaches. Lancet 1987;1(8530):411-5.
58. Quearney J. Burkitt lymphoma-no ordinary toothache. Br Dent J 2023;234(10):712.
59. Sforza E, Hupin D, Roche F. Mononucleosis: A Possible Cause of Idiopathic Hypersomnia. Front Neurol 2018;9:922.
60. Maulani C, Auerkari EI, SL CM, et al. Association between Epstein-Barr virus and periodontitis: A meta-analysis. PLoS One 2021;16(10):e0258109.
61. Toussirot E, Roudier J. Pathophysiological links between rheumatoid arthritis and the Epstein-Barr virus: an update. Joint Bone Spine 2007;74(5):418-26.
62. Greenberg MS, Glick M, Nghiem L, et al. Relationship of cytomegalovirus to salivary gland dysfunction in HIV-infected patients. Oral Surgery, Oral Medicine, Oral Pathology, Oral Radiology, and Endodontology 1997;83(3):334-9.
63. Ibekwe TS, Fasunla AJ, Orimadegun AE. Systematic Review and Meta-analysis of Smell and Taste Disorders in COVID-19. OTO Open 2020;4(3). 2473974X20957975.

64. Kim S-Y. Lifestyle Changes Caused by COVID-19 Pandemic Increase Oral Disease Symptoms. Asia Pac J Publ Health 2024. 10105395231225325.
65. Hoffmann M, Kleine-Weber H, Schroeder S, et al. SARS-CoV-2 Cell Entry Depends on ACE2 and TMPRSS2 and Is Blocked by a Clinically Proven Protease Inhibitor. Cell 2020;181(2):271–280 e8.
66. Fan Y, Liang X. Causal relationship between COVID-19 and chronic pain: A mendelian randomization study. PLoS One 2024;19(1):e0295982.
67. Domingues R, Kuster G, de Castro FO, et al. Headache features in patients with dengue virus infection. Cephalalgia 2006;26(7):879–82.
68. Bhardwaj VK, Negi N, Jhingta P, et al. Oral manifestations of dengue fever: A rarity and literature review. European Journal of General Dentistry 2016;5(02):95–8.
69. de Lima Cavalcanti TYV, Pereira MR, de Paula SO, et al. A Review on Chikungunya Virus Epidemiology, Pathogenesis and Current Vaccine Development. Viruses 2022;14(5):969.
70. Murillo-Zamora E, Mendoza-Cano O, Trujillo-Hernandez B, et al. Persistent arthralgia and related risks factors in laboratory-confirmed cases of Chikungunya virus infection in Mexico. Rev Panam Salud Publica 2017;41:e72.
71. Paixão ES, Rodrigues LC, Costa MDCN, et al. Chikungunya chronic disease: a systematic review and meta-analysis. Trans R Soc Trop Med Hyg 2018;112(7): 301–16.
72. Rodríguez-Morales AJ, Cardona-Ospina JA, Fernanda Urbano-Garzón S, et al. Prevalence of Post-Chikungunya Infection Chronic Inflammatory Arthritis: A Systematic Review and Meta-Analysis. Arthritis Care Res (Hoboken) 2016;68(12): 1849–58.
73. Edington F, Varjão D, Melo P. Incidence of articular pain and arthritis after chikungunya fever in the Americas: A systematic review of the literature and meta-analysis. Joint Bone Spine 2018;85(6):669–78.
74. de Andrade DC, Jean S, Clavelou P, et al. Chronic pain associated with the Chikungunya Fever: long lasting burden of an acute illness. BMC Infect Dis 2010; 10:31.
75. Assunção-Miranda I, Cruz-Oliveira C, Da Poian AT. Molecular mechanisms involved in the pathogenesis of alphavirus-induced arthritis. BioMed Res Int 2013;2013:973516.
76. Amaral JK, Bilsborrow JB, Schoen RT. Chronic Chikungunya Arthritis and Rheumatoid Arthritis: What They Have in Common. Am J Med 2020;133(3):e91–7.
77. Brostolin da Costa D, De-Carli AD, Probst LF, et al. Oral manifestations in chikungunya patients: A systematic review. PLoS Negl Trop Dis 2021;15(6):e0009401.
78. Murillo-Zamora E, Mendoza-Cano O, Trujillo-Hernández B, et al. Persistent arthralgia and related risks factors in laboratory-confirmed cases of Chikungunya virus infection in Mexico. Rev Panam Salud Publica 2017;41:e72.
79. Duschek S, de Guevara CML, Serrano MJF, et al. Variability of reaction time as a marker of executive function impairments in fibromyalgia. Behav Neurol 2022; 5(2022):1821684.
80. Malatji BG, Mason S, Mienie LJ, et al. The GC–MS metabolomics signature in patients with fibromyalgia syndrome directs to dysbiosis as an aspect contributing factor of FMS pathophysiology. Metabolomics 2019;15:1–13.
81. O'Brien AT, Deitos A, Pego YT, et al. Defective endogenous pain modulation in fibromyalgia: a meta-analysis of temporal summation and conditioned pain modulation paradigms. J Pain 2018;19(8):819–36.
82. Rhodus NL, Fricton J, Carlson P, et al. Oral symptoms associated with fibromyalgia syndrome. J Rheumatol 2003;30(8):1841–5.

83. Plesh O, Wolfe F, Lane N. The relationship between fibromyalgia and temporomandibular disorders: prevalence and symptom severity. J Rheumatol 1996; 23(11):1948–52.
84. De Tommaso M. Prevalence, clinical features and potential therapies for fibromyalgia in primary headaches. Expert Rev Neurother 2012;12(3):287–96.
85. Willich L, Bohner L, Köppe J, et al. Prevalence and quality of temporomandibular disorders, chronic pain and psychological distress in patients with classical and hypermobile Ehlers-Danlos syndrome: an exploratory study. Orphanet J Rare Dis 2023;18(1):294.
86. Létourneau Y, Pérusse R, Buithieu H. Oral manifestations of Ehlers-Danlos syndrome. J Can Dent Assoc 2001;67(6):330–4.
87. Abel MD, Carrasco LR. Ehlers-Danlos syndrome: classifications, oral manifestations, and dental considerations. Oral Surgery, Oral Medicine, Oral Pathology, Oral Radiology, and Endodontology 2006;102(5):582–90.
88. Bhavaraju SA, Vorrasi JS, Talluri S, et al. Pre-emptive administration of gabapentinoids to reduce postoperative pain and opioid usage following oral and maxillofacial surgical procedures. Oral Surg 2022;15:106–15.
89. Camu F, Lauwers MH, Vanlersberghe C. Side effects of NSAIDs and dosing recommendations for ketorolac. Acta Anaesthesiol Belg 1996;47(3):143–9.
90. Šimurina T, Mraović B, Župčić M, et al. LocalAnesthetics and steroids: contraindications and complications - Clinical update. Acta Clin Croat 2019;58:53–61.
91. Azizi F, Malboosbaf R. Safety of long-term antithyroid drug treatment? A systematic review. J Endocrinol Invest 2019;42(11):1273–83.
92. Somagutta MKR, Shama N, Pormento MKL, et al. Statin-induced necrotizing autoimmune myopathy: a systematic review. Reumatologia 2022;60(1):63–9.
93. Rao A, Nawaz I, Arbi FM, et al. Proximal myopathy: causes and associated conditions. Discoveries (Craiova) 2022;31(10 4):e160.
94. Thomas DC, Kohli D, Chen N, et al. Orofacial manifestations of rheumatoid arthritis and systemic lupus erythematosus: a narrative review. Quintessence Int 2021;52(5):454–66.
95. Verhoeff MC, Eikenboom D, Koutris M, et al. Parkinson's disease and oral health: A systematic review. Arch Oral Biol 2023;151:105712.

Psychological Factors Determining Prognosis of Dental Treatments

Mythili Kalladka, BDS, MSD[a],*, Stanley Markman, DDS, DABOP, FOFP[b],
Kartik R. Raman, BDS, MDS, FOFP[c], Asher Mansdorf, DDS, MA[d]

KEYWORDS

- Dental fear • Dental anxiety • Dental phobia • Psychological factors
- Dental treatment

KEY POINTS

- Psychological factors may have a significant impact on the prognosis of dental treatment.
- Dental anxiety, fear/phobia, occlusal dysesthesia, body dysmorphia disorders are important patient-related psychological factors affecting the prognosis of dental treatment.
- Empathy, good listening skills, clear communication, comprehensive documentation, informed consent, and setting patient-based realistic expectations/goals for treatment by the physician are pivotal prior to initiation of dental treatment.
- Pharmacologic, non-pharmacologic, and alternative therapies may be used for management of the psychological factors to ensure success of dental treatment.

INTRODUCTION

Psychological factors may present a significant impediment to dental care and affect the prognosis of dental treatment.[1] Practitioners periodically experience disappointment when a treatment plan outcome fails to meet their patient's expectations.[2] When discussing factors that may determine the prognosis of dental treatment in general, it is necessary to be cognizant of the fact that the patient represents a psychological aggregation of experiences, thoughts, concerns, and a variety of mild fears which collectively is best described as personality.[3] It includes distinctive internal

[a] Diplomate American Board of Orofacial Pain, Eastman Institute for Oral Health, 625 Elmwood Avenue, Rochester, NY 14642, USA; [b] Orofacial Pain, Rutgers School of Dental Medicine, 110 Bergen Street, Newark, NJ 07103, USA; [c] CSMSS Dental College Aurangabad, Plot No. G48, Sector N4, CIDCO, Aurangabad, Maharashtra 431003, India; [d] Board Certified Orofacial Pain, Board Certified Dental Anesthesia, Touro College of Dental Medicine, 858 Bryant Street, Woodmere, NY 11598, USA
* Corresponding author. 64, Vaishnavi, Halasahalli, Ginjur, Varthur, Bangalore-560087, Karnataka, India.
E-mail address: dr.mythili@gmail.com

Dent Clin N Am 68 (2024) 739–750
https://doi.org/10.1016/j.cden.2024.05.006
0011-8532/24/© 2024 Elsevier Inc. All rights are reserved, including those for text and data mining, AI training, and similar technologies.

dental.theclinics.com

design of long-standing traits, uniqueness, and interaction with other individuals and the world. The patient's personality will reveal whether the patient is expressive, shy, or reticent, their dental and health care priorities. Personality is thought to be long term and likely unchangeable. The dentist's personality will contribute or be a factor affecting the prognosis of dental treatment. It is important for a practitioner to evaluate and understand the patient's personality and develop a patient-focused treatment plan for the best prognosis.

Many factors influence a treatment plan's development including the degree of dental disease. Dentistry, being a biomechanical specialty, must allow for treatment of the disease process and the mechanics of tooth and occlusal restoration. As a result, the practitioner must manage both active disease and the mechanical result of the diseased teeth and soft tissues. The treatment prognosis represents an educated prospectus of how the plan may turn out, with a realistic expectation of what is possible to achieve. That is envisioned as an anticipated outcome. The dental history and examination, including radiographs and laboratory tests, are used to develop a treatment plan which will culminate in an anticipated result. All the aspects related to the examination produce the data used to determine the pathways that may be used to correct disease.[4] Understanding a patient's expectations prior to finalizing the treatment plan can be a factor in the prognosis for the treatment plan.

Our discussion will focus on the dentist's perception of the patient's fear, anxiety, avoidance behavior, noncompliance, as well as the dentist's reaction to those factors and briefly dwell on other pathophysiologic considerations and management.

FACTORS AFFECTING THE PROGNOSIS OF DENTAL TREATMENT
The Dentist

Unwittingly, the dentist is a factor in affecting the prognosis of dental care. Empathy is the foundation for a therapeutic physician–patient relationship. A precise definition of empathy may be lacking. Its meaning should be found within a physician's psychology to help evaluate a patient's feelings, circumstances, and health perspectives to offer competent management or therapeutic treatment in an understanding manner.

Empathy has been reported to improve patient compliance, satisfaction, reduce anxiety and stress levels, improve diagnostics, treatment prognosis, and outcomes.[5]

A previous study reported that more than 80% of the patients are likely to recommend an empathetic physician.[6] Empathy has a neurobiological basis. Functional magnetic resonance imaging (FMRI) studies have confirmed the involvement of mirror neuron system (parietal area, ventral premotor cortex, somatosensory areas, limbic and paralimbic structures connected by insula).[7] It encompasses 3 components: affective (attitude), behavioral, and cognitive (competency) aspect.[5]

Attitude describes the moral standards developed in a physician's mind through medical training, knowledge, personal experiences, and socialization. It encompasses virtues such as respect of authenticity, interest in the other person, receptivity, and impartiality.[5] An attitude of arrogance can erode and destroy dentist–patient trust relationships when the patient senses personal disrespect. When combined with poor listening skills, wherein the dentist hears only words and not the emotional context of what is being said, communications become short-circuited. Arrogance can lead to a condition in which the patient is viewed not as an individual but only as a procedure to be executed in a cost-effective manner.[8] A substandard professional attitude results in deficient patient trust often influencing dental outcomes.[9] When a practitioner behaves in an arrogant manner, it is done at the patient's expense; the patient feels despised and loses trust in the treating professional, eroding a healthy communication between the two.[10,11] A systematic review concluded that professional skills, attitude of health care professionals, and physician–patient trust are the cardinal factors influencing patient satisfaction.[8] Sources of physician bias may include belief, knowledge, training/education, and speciality.[12] In a study that discussed the many ways medical errors may occur in hospitals, the authors pointed out that physician's errors occur because of the fears of the physician including the risk of liability, fear of punishment, fear to change systems, and the fear of disclosure or humiliation.[13,14]

Competency comprises skills to build empathy, communication, and mutual trust with the patient. Behavior includes an affective and a cognitive part. The cognitive part comprises nonverbal and/or verbal skills. Empathy is of prime importance and is a backbone of patient–physician communication in building dentist–patient trust. Anything that blocks physician–patient communication will interfere with the prognosis. Many dysfunctional physician attributes, including poor communication, listening, patient interaction skills, and lack of empathy, often lead to patient dissatisfaction.[5,15] Competency ensures fruitful communication and development of longstanding trust with the patient. Recognition and identification, relating to the perception and emotions of patient's concerns, may result in behavioral changes and better communication by the physician.

Treatment outcomes may also fail due to differences in dentist expectations/goals versus patient-expected outcomes. Many dentists are less candid than they should be about aggressive treatments used to achieve cosmetic dental accomplishments and the possible side effects in planned cosmetic procedures.[15] Expectations regarding treatment outcomes need to be modulated and realistic goals set with good communications skills.

The Patient

A new patient, with a skeptical personality trait, may question or challenge professional explanations. Patients' concerns and questions may include fear, treatment costs, the number of visits required, days of loss of work, insurance cover, elimination of pain, restoration of function, and esthetics. While those issues will affect the final treatment plan and the prognosis, the following are some additional psychological factors that play an important role in determining prognosis of dental treatment. The various psychological factors have been described in **Table 1**.

Expectations

Esthetics and improvement in oral function are primary motives for seeking treatment in majority of the cases.[16] The dental public health related to cosmetic dentistry is considerable and there may be possible psychological and physiologic harm to patients considering such procedures.[15,17] The dentists may be extremely satisfied with the dental outcome only to learn that the patient is very unhappy. Duration of treatment, postsurgical dysfunction, and omission of explanation of possible/less anticipated side effects have been suggested as negative prognostic indicators.[18] Unhappiness can be expressed in a variety of ways, including a request for a refund, a letter of complaint to the state dental association, and the threat of a suit. When the dentist alerts his/her cosmetic patient to the potential negative aspects of some cosmetic procedures, a treatment plan is likely to be altered with better prognosis and patient acceptance.

A systematic review concluded that 20% to 86% of the patients could recollect and 27% to 85% could comprehend an informed consent. In addition, some patients firmly denied receiving related information and only minority of the patients could recollect complications from treatment procedures.[19] Clear documentation, informed consent, and candid discussion of the procedure and possible side effects are critical.

Table 1		
The various psychological factors that may affect the prognosis of dental treatment		
SI No	Psychological Factor	Description
1	Empathy	A precise definition of empathy may be lacking, its meaning should be found within a physician's psychology to help evaluate a patient's feelings, circumstances, and health perspectives to offer competent management or therapeutic treatment in an understanding manner
2	Anxiety	Avoidance of anticipated activities because of exaggerated worry including unrealistic expectations about everyday outcomes
3	Fear	Fear is associated with specific perceived threat and particular stimulus
4	Phobia	Continuous, unrealistic, extreme terror, irrational fear, hypertension, trepidation accompanied by uneasiness toward dental treatment resulting in complete avoidance
5	Occlusal Dysesthesia	Preoccupation with their occlusion, complain of uncomfortable, persistent bite changes and are inability to continually adapt to altered occlusion in spite of treatments to alter occlusion, intra and extra oral structures
6	Body Dysmorphia	A condition involving patient self-absorption in perceived body defects

The table describing various psychological factors affecting prognosis of dental treatment.

Dental Fear and Anxiety and Phobia

Despite advancements in dental equipment, pain management during dental procedures, and the growing emphasis on establishing trusting relationships between dentists and patients, dental fear and anxiety (DFA) and phobia continue to be a significant concern for both dentists and their patients and are significant indicators to pain experienced prior to, during, and subsequent to different types of dental treatment procedures.[20,21] It can result in delay, inconsistent, and irregular use of health care service.[22]

Concern or overt concern is not the same as anxiety though the former may lead to the latter. Anxiety is described as a disorder that begins in early adulthood and includes the avoidance of anticipated activities because of exaggerated worry including unrealistic expectations about everyday outcomes.[23] The worries include all aspects of life's current and future activities. Dental anxiety may represent more than an obstacle or perhaps a significant roadblock toward achieving a quality prognosis. Dental patients have concerns which can be categorized into mild, moderate, severe, and excessive. While a concern may be clear, patients do not think or worry uncontrollably about it. It is likely not to affect one's sleep or energy level during much of any day when compared to anxiety. It has been reported that approximately 15% of the world's population are afraid and experience anxiety about having or contemplating dental treatment.[20]

Previous studies have introduced and provided evidence for the concept of a "vicious circle of dental fear." This theory suggests that individuals with dental anxiety often avoid dental appointments, resulting in worsened oral health and potential dental pain.[24] Avoiding regular dental examinations and necessary treatments can lead to worsening oral health problems overtime, potentially requiring more invasive and uncomfortable procedures later. Manifestations of DFA co-related with invasiveness of the restorative procedure in pediatric patients.[25] In adults, moderate-to-high anxiety levels were associated with oral surgical procedures and nonsurgical root canal treatments.[26] Factors associated with DFA include age, gender, marital status, siblings, previous negative experience of self or siblings, parenting style, anxiety propensity, patient expectation, previous experience, type of procedure, level of difficulty, disturbance during the dental procedure, local anesthesia use, anticipation, a continuous, unrealistic, extreme terror, irrational fear, hypertension, and trepidation accompanied by uneasiness toward dental treatment resulting in complete avoidance and pain experience.[27–29]

While DFA may have common elements, fear is associated with specific perceived threat while anxiety is diffuse and can occur in absence of the stimulus.[30] Fear is a significant component that will also affect restorative plans especially when a patient is gripped with dental phobia. Dental fear can develop at different life stages, including childhood, adolescence, and adulthood.[31] Research shows a wide-ranging prevalence of dental fear among adults, with rates spanning from 4% to exceeding 50%.[20] Odontophobia is a continuous, unrealistic, extreme terror, irrational fear, hypertension, trepidation accompanied by uneasiness toward dental treatment resulting in complete avoidance.[30,32]

While non-modifiable factors like age, gender, siblings, their attitude, experiences and presence of dental fear or anxiety in siblings, maternal anxiety and socioeconomic conditions contribute to DFA[20,30,33–37]; modifiable issues require the attention of dental practitioners. The facility should address past dental experiences, patient education, use of pain control techniques including local anesthesia and contributing environmental elements that have significantly influenced negative emotional development.[20,33]

Other pathophysiological conditions to be considered.

Occlusal Dysesthesia

Terms such as phantom bite syndrome, occlusal neurosis, occlusal hyperawareness, occlusal dysesthesia, and occlusal hypervigilance are used to describe a condition where patients are preoccupied with their occlusion, complain of uncomfortable, persistent bite changes and are unable to continually adapt to altered occlusion despite treatments to alter occlusion, intraoral and extraoral structures. The patients present with extensive dental treatment, objective and subjective mismatch of occlusion and sensory symptoms, focus on occlusion with belief that it is the etiologic factor for their medical symptoms. They often blame previous dentists for the condition, set high expectation for current treatment, and may often place unreasonable demands. They often present with stubborn attitude, strict persistence, psychological/psychosocial distress, and nonspecific bodily symptoms.[38–40] It may be unilateral (often beginning on the side of dental treatment) or bilateral and is often comorbid with psychiatric disorders. Lack of dental trigger at onset and psychological comorbidities are negative prognostic indicators.[41,42] It has been proposed to be a psychosomatic disorder. Both central and peripheral etiologies have been proposed including neuroplasticity, central nervous system dysfunction, and alterations in proprioception.[41,43–47] Often the patients and dentists are frustrated, and it can result in patients attributing the condition to incompetency of the dentist. Early detection and multidisciplinary approach are critical, and it is essential to avoid further dental treatments.

Body Dysmorphia

It is described as a condition involving patient self-absorption in perceived body defects. They often visit multiple health care providers to resolve their issues many of which are primarily cosmetic in nature. The patients are often dissatisfied with the treatment and often undergo multiple procedures with multiple health care providers. The majority of the complaints are focused on the face and teeth. An estimated 5% of patients presenting for cosmetic/orthodontic procedures and 11% to 20% patients undergoing orthognathic surgery have been estimated to have BD. It occurs more frequently in female individuals and comorbidities include depression, anxiety, and substance abuse.[48]

Other Mental Health Disorders

"Mental health disorders (MHD)" is a comprehensive term that includes, but is not limited to, mood, anxiety, substance, eating, intellectual, and personality disorders. In individuals with MHD, it may include a variety of pathophysiological pathways that interact directly or indirectly with environmental factors, psychosocial conditions, and lifestyle factors. Potentially it can act as a risk factor or contribute to the development of oral diseases. These individuals may display changes in behavior, negligent self-care, and fail to adhere to prescribed treatment plans or follow-up appointments. Those behaviors can lead to poor oral health including severe dental and periodontal conditions and negatively impact on treatment outcomes. Substance abuse leads to poor oral hygiene, impaired healing following dental treatments, and may increase the risk of periimplantitis and secondary infections after implant placement. Medications used in the treatment of psychiatric disorders can cause dry mouth (xerostomia). Some can lead to teeth grinding (bruxism), which can in turn affect dental treatment outcomes. Additionally, altered interpersonal skills observed in several intellectual disorders can lead to miscommunication regarding patient treatment expectations.[49]

FACTORS AFFECTING LACK OF PATIENT APPRECIATION TOWARD DENTAL TREATMENT
Unease

A significant and common reason that people dislike seeing a dentist, especially a new one, is the anticipation of pain or discomfort during treatment. This concern often stems from previous negative experiences or stories heard from others.[50,51] As an example, the fear stemming from a child's past traumatic experience, including an unanticipated pain experience during a restoration procedure, may leave an emotional mark that sometimes persists into adulthood. When that adult develops a dental problem, recollections of past negative experience create emotional stress during the contemplation of making an appointment for needed care.

Needles and Fear

Many dental procedures require the use of local anesthesia. The fear of needles can be a significant source of anxiety for many individuals.[51,52] Some faint when viewing a needle or may tremble uncontrollably. This phenomenon is not related to only dental treatment but to any medical condition. Dental manufacturers have developed devices and aid to mitigate the pain of local anesthetic injections. Techniques and equipment for delivering local anesthesia in dentistry have evolved in the attempt to mitigate the pain associated with local anesthetic injections. Good communication is required to obtain a fearful patient's consent and confidence to institute such procedures.

Distress Associated with Control

The loss of control during a treatment procedure is a major contributor to anxiety.[32] Being in a dental chair while an unfamiliar practitioner does an examination or treatment can make some feel vulnerable and as the patient has little control over the environment. Such loss can be stress-inducing, which can be mitigated by the practitioner by the practitioner by, for example, indicating to the patient is to rinse or raise their hand if they feel pain. Implementing a sense of control can be instituted by suggesting that when the patient wishes to communicate with the dentist, a wiggle of the right index finger will cause the dentist to stop treatment.

Unfamiliar Environs

Dental clinics frequently feature unfamiliar apparatuses which can be intimidating for the intimidated patient and includes non-equipment odors. Additionally, dental procedures encompass various sensory experiences, including the sound of the drill, the taste of dental materials, and the sensation of dental instruments in the mouth. These sensations may prove annoying or distressing for certain individuals, leading to anxiety, especially in response to the sounds and appearances of accoutrements like drills and suction devices, as well as the dental chair. All can evoke feelings of confinement or helplessness.[20,33]

History of Negative Dental Experiences

Previous negative dental experiences have been identified as a significant factor contributing to dental apprehensioness.[1,20,53,54] In the context of dental visits, young children are likely to experience some level of fear initially, possibly due to factors such as separation from a parent, unfamiliarity with dental procedures, or unfamiliar procedures. For most children, this fear tends to diminish with repeated dental visits as they become accustomed to the dental surroundings. However, in a minority of cases, this fear may persist into adulthood creating chronic deference wishes.[55]

Studies have linked prior distressing experiences to heightened perceptions of pain and negative thoughts about dental treatment.[1,54] Individuals with high dental anxiety (HDA) tend to report more traumatic past experiences, particularly those related to dental settings, compared to individuals with no dental anxiety. Distressing experiences in dental settings are often the most reported traumatic events, and a significant portion of individuals with HDA exhibit symptoms related to post-traumatic stress disorder, such as insomnia and avoidance behaviors. This underscores that dental trauma does not solely impact oral health but leads to treatment avoidance and having adverse effects on mental health.[54]

What has been outlined is that there are significant psychological factors that may influence the prognosis or treatment plan acceptance. To negate a possible prognosis failure related to psychological factors, it is important to know or understand your patient; to observe his or her facial expressions; to recognize the patient's steadfastness; and to deal with a patient's concerns; and most importantly to recognize that you are dealing with a neurologic factors which constitutes the patient's personality. A patient's concerns, fears that may also be associated with costs, time allocations, insurance coverage, history of painful dental care, low pain thresholds, and expectations, are some of the psychological factors that will affect treatment choices; choices that will affect treatment plan selection, treatment limitations, and hence outcomes.

Good communication is dependent on listening skills, and when the former fails, the prognosis is jeopardized. Communication is the preeminent factor in dealing with and confronting patients' dental fears and concerns. Hospital communication failures have been shown to be responsible for many hospital deaths. The recognition of psychological factors and which are not confronted can easily compromise the prognosis of planned dental care.

MANAGEMENT
Management of Dentist/Health Care Team-Related Factors

The dentist and the entire dental team should be trained in enhancing their communication skills, empathy, and listening prowess, through traditional or blended digital

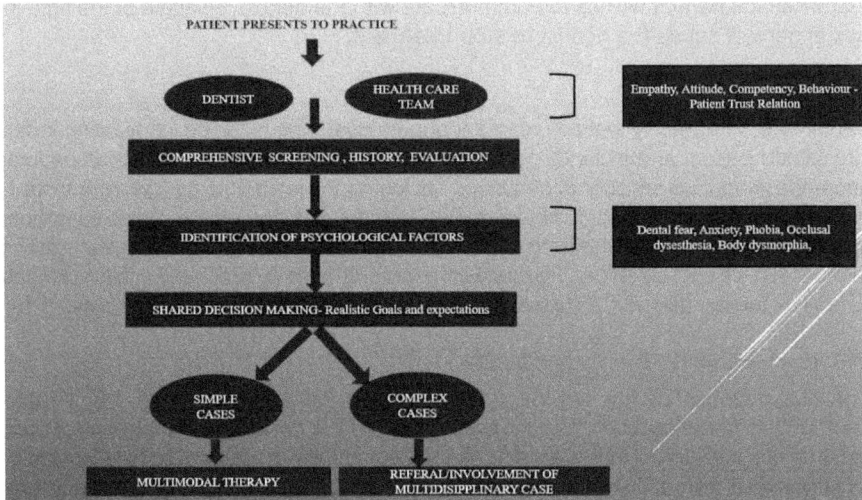

Fig. 1. The management of various psychological factors affecting prognosis of dental treatment. Figure depicting paradigm for management of various psychological factors affecting the prognosis of dental treatment.

training programs.[56,57] Incorporation of communication-skill-interventions (didactic teaching, personalized feedback, role-play) during training may enhance interpersonal communication skills in students.[58–60]

Shared decision-making may also improve treatment outcomes particularly in invasive procedures. Ensuring the patient's comprehension of condition, treatment options, lifestyle, confounding factors, proposing recommended treatment, and finally enabling patients to decide treatment may help in achieving better prognosis. Patients preferred role in decision-making should be solicited and a tailored approach to individual patients may be utilized.[5]

The management of various psychological factors affecting prognosis of dental treatment has been outlined in **Fig. 1**.

Management of Patient-Related Factors

Pharmacologic (sedation, local or general anesthesia),[56] non-pharmacologic methods (cognitive behavioral therapy [CBT], pyscho-therapeutic techniques) and alternative therapies and techniques (hypnotherapy, acupuncture, acupressure, distraction, use of better techniques for pain control, computer-assisted relaxation learning, music, patient education, massage, social support, aromatherapy, nature visual stimuli, nature sounds, and reduction of sensory triggers) may be used for management of DFA and phobia.[61–63]

Pharmacotherapy utilizing nitrous oxide, conscious oral or intravenous sedation may be helpful in patients with dental phobia, uncooperative patients, and patients with special needs. However, careful considerations on possible interactions, side effects, contraindications need to be considered before usage.[63]

Behavior modification techniques involve alteration of unacceptable behavior and progressive muscle relaxation, breathing utilizing guided imagery, biofeedback, CBT, confidence building alone, patient motivation, distraction, acclimatization, systematic desensitization/exposure therapy, enhancing control (tell-show-do, modeling), positive reinforcement, and acupuncture. In severe cases of phobia, neurolinguistic programming skills, hypnosis may be helpful.[30,64–66] Early identification and addressing concerns of patients are critical.

CBT has also been found to be beneficial in personality disorders. Schema therapy and dialectical behavior therapy that are different models in addition to cognitive therapy and behavioral therapy have been found to be beneficial. Pharmacotherapy utilizing tricyclic antidepressants, selective serotonin reuptake inhibitors has also been used in cases of occlusal dysesthesia and body dysmorphia with limited success. Avoidance of further dental treatments/invasive body-altering procedures, psychiatric consultation, and institution of multidisciplinary multimodal treatment is essential.[37,46]

SUMMARY

An effort has been made to demonstrate that in determining the prognosis of dental treatment, there are multiple psychological factors that will affect outcomes. The personality and the moral compass of the dentist is a factor as well as the patient's non-pathologic psychology. Professional attitudes about patients' pain control and empathetic attitudes toward patients represent a significant ingredient. A child's negative dental experiences will affect an adults' dental attitudes including the many possible fears and concerns. The patient has other contending concerns, including the presence or lack of dental insurance, the possible loss of time from work, the length of the treatment time, the cost of treatment, the expected longevity of the recommended treatment, and whether dental care represents a priority in that individual's life. Early identification and prompt management are critical to ensure successful dental treatment and patient satisfaction.

CLINICS CARE POINTS

- Several psychological factors may affect the prognosis of dental treatment.
- Broadly they may be categorised into patient related factors and physician related factors.
- Identifying and modifying these factors may enhance the success of dental treatment.

DISCLOSURE

The authors declare that there is no commercial or financial conflicts of interest and any funding sources for all authors.

REFERENCES

1. de Jongh A. Het beoordelen van het psychisch functioneren van patiënten in de tandartspraktijk [Evaluation of patient's level of functioning in the dental practice]. Ned Tijdschr Tandheelkd 2001;108(11):439–41.
2. El-Haddad C, Hegazi I, Hu W. Understanding Patient Expectations of Health Care: A Qualitative Study. J Patient Exp 2020;7(6):1724–31.
3. Kernberg OF. What is Personality? J Pers Disord 2016;30(2):145–56.
4. Rizzi DA. Medical prognosis–some fundamentals. Theor Med 1993;14(4):365–75.
5. Derksen F, Bensing J, Lagro-Janssen A. Effectiveness of empathy in general practice: a systematic review. Br J Gen Pract 2013;63(606):e76–84.
6. Vedsted P, Heje HN. Association between patients' recommendation of their GP and their evaluation of the GP. Scand J Prim Health Care 2008;26(4):228–34.

7. Kaplan JT, Iacoboni M. Getting a grip on other minds: mirror neurons, intention understanding, and cognitive empathy. Soc Neurosci 2006;1(3–4):175–83.
8. Berger AS. Arrogance among physicians. Acad Med 2002;77(2):145–7.
9. Moore R. Trusting the Dentist-Expecting a Leap of Faith vs. a Well-Defined Strategy for Anxious Patients. Dent J 2022;10(4):66.
10. Armfield JM, Ketting M, Chrisopoulos S, et al. Do people trust dentists? Development of the Dentist Trust Scale. Aust Dent J 2017;62(3):355–62.
11. Li Y, Gong W, Kong X, et al. Factors Associated with Outpatient Satisfaction in Tertiary Hospitals in China: A Systematic Review. Int J Environ Res Public Health 2020;17(19):7070.
12. Le Glaz A, Lemey C, Berrouiguet S, et al. Physicians' and medical students' beliefs and attitudes toward psychotic disorders: A systematic review. J Psychosom Res 2022;163:111054.8.
13. Rodziewicz TL, Houseman B, Hipskind JE. Medical Error Reduction and Prevention. 2023 May 2. In: StatPearls [internet]. Treasure Island (FL): StatPearls Publishing; 2023.
14. Ammi M, Fooken J, Klein J, et al. Does doctors' personality differ from those of patients, the highly educated and other caring professions? An observational study using two nationally representative Australian surveys. BMJ Open 2023;13(4):e069850.
15. Kelleher M. Ethical issues, dilemmas and controversies in 'cosmetic' or aesthetic dentistry. A personal opinion. Br Dent J 2012;212(8):365–7.
16. Yao J, Tang H, Gao XL, et al. Patients' expectations to dental implant: a systematic review of the literature. Health Qual Life Outcomes 2014 29;12:153.
17. Doughty J, Lala R, Marshman Z. The dental public health implications of cosmetic dentistry: a scoping review of the literature. Community Dent Health 2016;33(3):218–24.
18. Pachêco-Pereira C, Abreu LG, Dick BD, et al. Patient satisfaction after orthodontic treatment combined with orthognathic surgery: A systematic review. Angle Orthod 2016 May;86(3):495–508.
19. Moreira NC, Pachêco-Pereira C, Keenan L, et al. Informed consent comprehension and recollection in adult dental patients: A systematic review. J Am Dent Assoc 2016;147(8):605–19.e7.
20. Silveira ER, Cademartori MG, Schuch HS, et al. Estimated prevalence of dental fear in adults: A systematic review and meta-analysis. J Dent 2021;108:103632.
21. Lin CS, Wu SY, Yi CA. Association between Anxiety and Pain in Dental Treatment: A Systematic Review and Meta-analysis. J Dent Res 2017;96(2):153–62.
22. Horenstein A, Heimberg RG. Anxiety disorders and healthcare utilization: A systematic review. Clin Psychol Rev 2020 Nov;81:101894.
23. Penninx BW, Pine DS, Holmes EA, et al. Anxiety disorders. Lancet 2021;397(10277):914–27. Erratum in: Lancet. 2021 6;397(10277):880.
24. Armfield JM, Stewart JF, Spencer AJ. The vicious cycle of dental fear: exploring the interplay between oral health, service utilization and dental fear. BMC Oral Health 2007;7:1.
25. Ladewig NM, Tedesco TK, Gimenez T, et al. Patient-reported outcomes associated with different restorative techniques in pediatric dentistry: A systematic review and MTC meta-analysis. PLoS One 2018;13(12):e0208437.
26. Khan S, Hamedy R, Lei Y, et al. Anxiety Related to Nonsurgical Root Canal Treatment: A Systematic Review. J Endod 2016;42(12):1726–36.
27. Astramskaitė I, Poškevičius L, Juodžbalys G. Factors determining tooth extraction anxiety and fear in adult dental patients: a systematic review. Int J Oral Maxillofac Surg 2016;45(12):1630–43.

28. Pak JG, White SN. Pain prevalence and severity before, during, and after root canal treatment: a systematic review. J Endod 2011;37(4):429–38.
29. Lee DW, Kim JG, Yang YM. The Influence of Parenting Style on Child Behavior and Dental Anxiety. Pediatr Dent 2018;40(5):327–33.
30. Murad MH, Ingle NA, Assery MK. Evaluating factors associated with fear and anxiety to dental treatment-A systematic review. J Family Med Prim Care 2020; 9(9):4530–5.
31. Thomson WM, Broadbent JM, Locker D, et al. Trajectories of dental anxiety in a birth cohort. Community Dent Oral Epidemiol 2009;37(3):209–19.
32. Appukuttan DP. Strategies to manage patients with dental anxiety and dental phobia: literature review. Clin Cosmet Investig Dent 2016;8:35–50.
33. Yildirim TT. Evaluating the Relationship of Dental Fear with Dental Health Status and Awareness. J Clin Diagn Res 2016;10(7):Zc105–Z109.
34. Heidari E, Banerjee A, Newton JT. Oral health status of non-phobic and dentally phobic individuals; a secondary analysis of the 2009 Adult Dental Health Survey. Br Dent J 2015;219(9):E9.
35. Kankaanpää R, Auvinen J, Rantavuori K, et al. Pressure pain sensitivity is associated with dental fear in adults in middle age: Findings from the Northern Finland 1966 birth cohort study. Community Dent Oral Epidemiol 2019;47(3):193–200.
36. Liinavuori A, Tolvanen M, Pohjola V, et al. Longitudinal interrelationships between dental fear and dental attendance among adult Finns in 2000-2011. Community Dent Oral Epidem 2019;47(4):309–15.
37. Talo Yildirim T, Dundar S, Bozoglan A, et al. Is there a relation between dental anxiety, fear and general psychological status? PeerJ 2017;5:e2978.
38. Marbach JJ. Phantom bite syndrome. Am J Psychiatry 1978;135(4):476–9.
39. Clark GT, Tsukiyama Y, Baba K, et al. The validity and utility of disease detection methods and of occlusal therapy for temporomandibular disorders. Oral Surg Oral Med Oral Pathol Oral Radiol Endod 1997;83(1):101–6.
40. Ligas BB, Galang MT, BeGole EA, et al. Phantom bite: a survey of US orthodontists. Orthodontics (Chic.) 2011;12(1):38–47. PMID: 21789289.
41. Watanabe M, Umezaki Y, Suzuki S, et al. Psychiatric comorbidities and psychopharmacological outcomes of phantom bite syndrome. J Psychosom Res 2015; 78(3):255–9.
42. Miyachi H, Wake H, Tamaki K, et al. Detecting mental disorders in dental patients with occlusion-related problems. Psychiatry Clin Neurosci 2007;61(3):313–9.
43. Umezaki Y, Tu TTH, Toriihara A, et al. Change of Cerebral Blood Flow After a Successful Pharmacological Treatment of Phantom Bite Syndrome: A Case Report. Clin Neuropharmacol 2019;42(2):49–51.
44. Toyofuku A. Psychosomatic problems in dentistry. Biopsychosoc Med 2016 30; 10:14.
45. Shinohara Y, Umezaki Y, Minami I, et al. Comorbid depressive disorders and left-side dominant occlusal discomfort in patients with phantom bite syndrome. J Oral Rehabil 2020;47(1):36–41.
46. Toyofuku A, Kikuta T. Treatment of phantom bite syndrome with milnacipran - a case series. Neuropsychiatr Dis Treat 2006;2(3):387–90.
47. Umezaki Y, Watanabe M, Shinohara Y, et al. Comparison of Cerebral Blood Flow Patterns in Patients with Phantom Bite Syndrome with Their Corresponding Clinical Features. Neuropsychiatr Dis Treat 2020;16:2277–84.
48. Dons F, Mulier D, Maleux O, et al. Body dysmorphic disorder (BDD) in the orthodontic and orthognathic setting: A systematic review. J Stomatol Oral Maxillofac Surg 2022;123(4):e145–52.

49. Ball J, Darby I. Mental health and periodontal and peri-implant diseases. Perio-dontol 2000 2022;90(1):106–24.
50. Heft MW, Meng X, Bradley MM, et al. Gender differences in reported dental fear and fear of dental pain. Community Dent Oral Epidemiol 2007;35(6):421–8.
51. van Houtem CM, Aartman IH, Boomsma DI, et al. Is dental phobia a blood-injection-injury phobia? Depress Anxiety 2014;31(12):1026–34.
52. Vika M, Skaret E, Raadal M, et al. Fear of blood, injury, and injections, and its rela-tionship to dental anxiety and probability of avoiding dental treatment among 18-year-olds in Norway. Int J Paediatr Dent 2008;18(3):163–9.
53. Humphris G, King K. The prevalence of dental anxiety across previous distress-ing experiences. J Anxiety Disord 2011;25(2):232–6.
54. Stein Duker LI, Grager M, Giffin W, et al. The Relationship between Dental Fear and Anxiety, General Anxiety/Fear, Sensory Over-Responsivity, and Oral Health Behaviors and Outcomes: A Conceptual Model. Int J Environ Res Public Health 2022;19(4):2380.
55. Shim YS, Kim AH, Jeon EY, et al. Dental fear & anxiety and dental pain in children and adolescents; a systemic review. J Dent Anesth Pain Med 2015;15(2):53–61.
56. Kyaw BM, Posadzki P, Paddock S, et al. Effectiveness of Digital Education on Communication Skills Among Medical Students: Systematic Review and Meta-Analysis by the Digital Health Education Collaboration. J Med Internet Res 2019;21(8):e12967.
57. Levinson W, Hudak P, Tricco AC. A systematic review of surgeon-patient commu-nication: strengths and opportunities for improvement. Patient Educ Couns 2013; 93(1):3–17.
58. Gilligan C, Powell M, Lynagh MC, et al. Interventions for improving medical stu-dents' interpersonal communication in medical consultations. Cochrane Data-base Syst Rev 2021;2(2):CD012418.
59. Chewning B, Bylund CL, Shah B, et al. Patient preferences for shared decisions: a systematic review. Patient Educ Couns 2012;86(1):9–18.
60. Matharu L, Ashley PF. Sedation of anxious children undergoing dental treatment. Cochrane Database Syst Rev 2006;1:CD003877.
61. Weisfeld CC, Turner JA, Dunleavy K, et al. Dealing with Anxious Patients: A Sys-tematic Review of the Literature on Nonpharmaceutical Interventions to Reduce Anxiety in Patients Undergoing Medical or Dental Procedures. J Altern Comple-ment Med 2021;27(9):717–26.
62. De Stefano R, Bruno A, Muscatello MR, et al. Fear and anxiety managing methods during dental treatments: a systematic review of recent data. Minerva Stomatol 2019;68(6):317–31.
63. Hoffmann B, Erwood K, Ncomanzi S, et al. Management strategies for adult pa-tients with dental anxiety in the dental clinic: a systematic review. Aust Dent J 2022;67(Suppl 1):S3–13.
64. Burghardt S, Koranyi S, Magnucki G, et al. Non-pharmacological interventions for reducing mental distress in patients undergoing dental procedures: Systematic review and meta-analysis. J Dent 2018;69:22–31.
65. Gomes HS, Viana KA, Batista AC, et al. Cognitive behaviour therapy for anxious paediatric dental patients: a systematic review. Int J Paediatr Dent 2018. Epub ahead of print.
66. Borrelli B, Tooley EM, Scott-Sheldon LA. Motivational Interviewing for Parent-child Health Interventions: A Systematic Review and Meta-Analysis. Pediatr Dent 2015; 37(3):254–65.

Systemic Factors Affecting Prognosis in Restorative and Prosthetic Dentistry: A Review

Fengyuan Zheng, BDS, PhD[a],
Lovely Muthiah Annamma, BDS, MDS, PhD[b],
Sunil Suresh Harikrishnan, MDS[c], Damian J. Lee, DDS, MS[d],*

KEYWORDS

- Prognosis • Systemic diseases • Diabetes • Removable prosthesis
- Fixed prosthesis • Osteoporosis • Endocrine disorders • Neurologic disorders

KEY POINTS

- Understanding how various systemic factors can affect the prognostic outcome of removable and fixed prosthetic rehabilitation.
- Healing procedures and bone density are affected by many systemic factors such as metabolic, bone, autoimmune, cardiovascular, and endocrine disorders.
- Patients who are suffering from systemic diseases can have negative prognosis outcomes when treated for prosthodontic rehabilitation.

INTRODUCTION

The integrity and health of the oral cavity play a pivotal role in overall health. Fixed, removable, and implant prosthodontics are effective ways to restore partial or complete edentulous arches and rehabilitate oral cavities to restore or improve oral health and esthetics. The restorative and prosthetic dentistry must rely on the retention and support by remaining hard and soft tissue in oral cavities. On the other hand, the remaining hard and soft tissues, as parts of the body, are closely regulated by systemic conditions and medical interventions.[1,2] Therefore, the purpose of this review is to search and summarize published studies on the impact of systemic factors on supporting structures and outcomes of prosthetic treatments.

[a] Advanced Education Program in Prosthodontics, Department of Restorative Sciences, Division of Prosthodontics, University of Minnesota School of Dentistry, 9-176 Moos Tower, 515 Delaware Street Southeast, Minneapolis, MN 55455, USA; [b] College of Dentistry, Ajman University, PO Box 346, University Street Al Jeft 1, Ajman, United Arab Emirates; [c] Private Practice, Flat No. 26, Building No. 16, Street No. 890, Zone 26, Najma, Doha, Qatar; [d] Department of Prosthodontics, Tufts University School of Dental Medicine, 1 Kneeland Street, DHS 220; Boston, MA 02111, USA
* Corresponding author.
E-mail address: damian.lee@tufts.edu

Dent Clin N Am 68 (2024) 751–765
https://doi.org/10.1016/j.cden.2024.05.007
0011-8532/24/© 2024 Elsevier Inc. All rights reserved, including those for text and data mining, AI training, and similar technologies.
dental.theclinics.com

The main factors that may influence hard and soft tissue turnover and healing capabilities were considered in this review, including systemic conditions and behavioral or medical interventions. The systemic conditions include age, gender, diabetes, autoimmune diseases, and osteoporosis, while behavioral or medical interventions include smoking, Parkinson's, Alzheimer's, bisphosphonates, radiotherapy, and chemotherapy.[1,2] Relevant articles regarding systemic factors affecting restoration, removable and fixed prostheses excluding implants were selected for the review (**Fig. 1**).

General Factors

Age

While considering prosthodontic treatment, the longevity of the restorations is of a major concern to the patients and the clinicians. The prognosis of the treatment depends on multiple factors. Among them, age, gender, and other socio-economic factors play important roles.[3,4] It is a known fact that the integrity and function of the stomatognathic system are affected by the natural aging process. As age advances, teeth develop caries resistant sclerotic dentin but risk of root caries do prevail.[5,6] Increase in caries incidence in the elderly can be attributed to the alterations in the rate of salivary flow induced by hypo-function of the salivary glands or medication.[3] Also in aged dentin, fracture toughness is decreased and crack propagation is more common due to an internal rearrangement of its structure. Finally, reduced motor capacity is also seen with the older individuals, leading to reduced ability to maintain satisfactory oral hygiene and lesser adaptability to prostheses.[7,8] All the aforementioned changes seen in the aging population may affect the prognosis and longevity of tooth supported fixed prosthetic restorations and therefore increased age may pose a risk factor for success.

There are conflicting results in the literature regarding the influence of patients' age on the longevity of fixed restorations. A systematic review article by G. Ioannidis and colleagues showed that middle aged individuals may present with higher failure rates and the reason attributed to early onset of dental disease.[3] De Backer and colleagues in their 18 to 20 year follow-up study (2007) showed that the patients receiving first

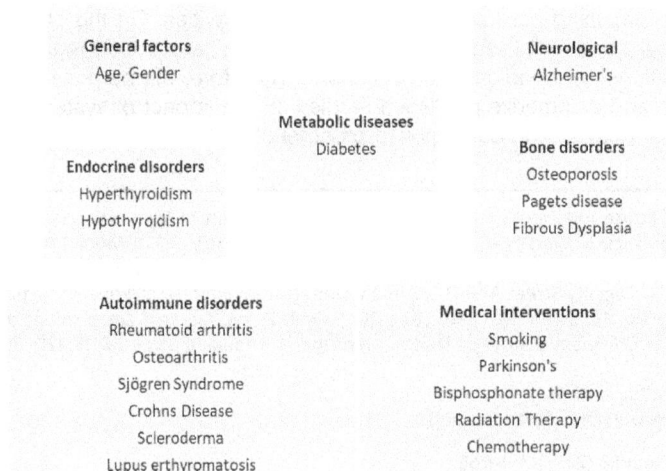

General factors
Age, Gender

Neurological
Alzheimer's

Metabolic diseases
Diabetes

Endocrine disorders
Hyperthyroidism
Hypothyroidism

Bone disorders
Osteoporosis
Pagets disease
Fibrous Dysplasia

Autoimmune disorders
Rheumatoid arthritis
Osteoarthritis
Sjögren Syndrome
Crohns Disease
Scleroderma
Lupus erthyromatosis

Medical interventions
Smoking
Parkinson's
Bisphosphonate therapy
Radiation Therapy
Chemotherapy

Fig. 1. Common systemic factors affecting prognosis in fixed and removable prosthesis.

restorations at an older age show more failures than individuals receiving their first at a much younger age, regardless complete crowns, 3 unit fixed partial dentures (FPDs), or other fixed prostheses.[9]

In terms of direct restorations, on the other hand, van de Sande and colleagues in a systematic review articles showed that adolescents have more failure rates than younger children in relation to Class I & II composite restorations; individuals around 30 years no significance; people older than 30 years showed lower survival for amalgam restorations; and group between 41 and 45 years had higher failures than older age groups.[10,11]

For complete dentures, the majority of studies showed that age is of no prognostic value in determining the denture success.[7,12,13] Other studies (Diehl [1996], Allen [2003], Zarb [1982]) showed that patients over 60 years of age have difficulty in adapting to dentures, probably due to decreased muscle adaptability and lack of new reflex arcs.[8,14,15]

Gender

Previous studies have shown that no significant correlation between gender and fixed prostheses longevity has been found; nevertheless, higher failure rates on direct restorations among men have been reported.[9,11,16–18] While the stronger occlusal force was considered to be a contributing factor for fatigue of the material, fracture, or debonding, some have reported that that women make regular follow-up visits than men and hence, men show more failures.[19,20]

In terms of complete dentures, there were no studies showing notable correlation between complete denture longevity and gender. However, a far less acceptance rate was found in postmenopausal women due to decreased muscle adaptability and lack of formation of new reflex arcs.[21]

Diabetes

Diabetes mellitus (DM) is a prevalent systemic disease among adults, especially those over the age of 40. Usually the adult-onset type 2 DM has been associated with having a higher prevalence of developing periodontal disease,[22–24] caries,[5,6,25-] diminished masticatory efficiency,[26] and even oral candidiasis associated with removable prostheses,[27] but not research directly related to prosthodontic outcome is scarce. Study by Azogui-Levy and colleagues showed that subjects with DM were more likely to have dental problems, as well as use a form of partial or complete denture.[28] A study by Ambikathanaya and colleagues showed that impact of using a removable partial denture (RPD) may be lessened on developing caries with good oral hygiene, proper RPD instructions, and regular dental visits, regardless of the patient being diabetic.[25] As for fixed prosthodontic patients, diabetic patients were correlated with deeper periodontal pockets, bleeding on probing and increased bone loss with higher values associated with inflammatory markers.[29] A study by Elsalhin and colleagues showed that there was also a higher incidence of deep pockets and gingival recession around FPDs and emphasized on making the design of fixed partial denture more accessible for hygiene for diabetic patients.[30] Because prosthodontic therapy is very dependent on the health of supporting tissues, the bidirectional relationship between DM and oral health and its sequelae must be educated to our patients.[31] Several studies have advocated for patients to understand the nature of DM and being familiar with the clinical manifestation so that patients along with an oral health care provider can work toward preserving oral health, rather than focusing on replacing missing teeth from ongoing exacerbation of DM.[32–34]

Autoimmune Disorders

Autoimmune disorders cause immunosuppression. The most common systemic auto-immune disorders that can affect the outcome of prosthodontic treatment include rheumatoid arthritis, Sjögren Syndrome, and Crohn's disease.[35] Many of the autoimmune disorder patients will be on steroid drugs which in turn can negatively affect bone metabolism causing steroid osteoporosis.[36] Autoimmune disorders can have oral manifestations such as Sjögren Syndrome, epidermolysis bullosa, and oral lichen planus. These patients are prone to hyposalivation and gingival bleeding.[37] Patients suffering from autoimmune diseases wearing removable prostheses are prone to dry mouth and oral ulcers causing unpleasant burning sensations. Hence, the removable prosthesis prognosis is poor for such patients as they are often unable to wear them. The preferred option for these patients is implant retained prosthesis.[38] Other autoimmune disorders such as systemic sclerosis cause stiffening of connective tissues resulting in reduced mouth opening, with subsequent problems such as difficulty in food intake, chewing, swallowing, and dental hygiene.[39] Due to the consequent effects of these disorders, there is a poor outcome of the removable prosthesis and hence, a fixed prosthesis is the preferred treatment option for patients suffering from systemic sclerosis.[40]

Treatment Management

Removable prosthesis requires multiple visits and most of the autoimmune disorders affect the temporomandibular joint movement thereby restricting jaw movement. This causes difficulty in jaw relation procedures.[41] Hyposalivation can also result in *Candida albicans*, seen as erythema of the oral mucosa, and inflamed fissures at the corners of the mouth.[42] A removable prosthesis can cause excessive soreness and ulcerations due to adverse mucosal conditions. In most autoimmune disorders, such as Sjogren's syndrome, implant prosthesis is preferred. An artificial salivary reservoir denture can be used in cases where the implant prosthesis is contraindicated.[43,44]

Osteoporosis

Osteoporosis is a systemic disorder causing a reduction of bone strength due to a reduction in the density of bone.[45] Any decrease in bone loss systemically affects the jawbone causing excessive bone resorption and periodontitis. Periodontitis is a local progressive and persistent inflammatory response of supporting tissues of teeth leading to loss of clinical attachment, alveolar bone loss, and periodontal pocket formation.[46] Osteoporosis commonly occurs in older people, especially women,[47] and periodontal disease in adults with more prevalence in men.[4] Any systemic disorders affecting the bone can, in turn, affect the supporting tooth and edentulous area, because of bone resorption or periodontitis. Patients with bone disorders wearing partial or complete dentures require constant monitoring and adjustments in dentures.[48] The reasons for this are that an existing systemic disease can aggravate the severity of periodontal disease due to the higher level of cytokines and inflammatory mediators present.[49] The prognosis outcomes of rehabilitating patients with bone disorders can lead to deterioration of periodontal status or excessive bone resorption coupled with osteoporosis and other risk factors such as habits, estrogen deficiency, osteopenia, Vitamin D, and calcium deficiency.[50–53]

Most bone disorders affect the prosthodontic treatment outcome due to the loss of supporting structures such as teeth and bone. If the tooth that is affected is an abutment then the retainer component fails causing failure in fixed and partial removable prosthesis. Bone resorption can cause loosening of dentures leading to repeated relining procedures. The reason for bone resorption is that systemic diseases such as osteoporosis increase the levels of pro-inflammatory cytokines causing osteoclastic activity.[54]

Bisphosphonates

Antiresorptive medications such as bisphosphonates and denosumab, and RANK ligand inhibitors are used to prevent bone resorption in systemic bone disorders.[55] Bisphosphonates cause increased activity of osteoclasts and osteoblasts, while denosumab reduces osteoclast activity.[56,57]

Many bone disorders such as fibrous dysplasia, osteitis deformans, and arthritis are treated by bisphosphonates, which in turn can cause osteoradionecrosis of the jaw.[58] The therapy with bisphosphonates when continued for more than 4 years orally or via intravenous injections the chances of osteoradionecrosis in such patients are high.[59,60] Regarding prosthodontic outcome, the complications in such patients taking bisphosphonates arise when an ill-fitting denture causing ulceration can trigger medication-related necrosis.[61]

Treatment planning for patients with bone disorders

For the success of the RPD, the treatment planning to the design needs a thorough analysis. The treatment planning and designing should be considered to protect the tooth and tissue structures preventing further deterioration in bone resorption and periodontal involvement. Post-operative instructions and dietary guidance with calcium supplements can improve the prognosis. The recommended calcium intake for an average person is 800 mg per day and 1500 mg for a postmenopausal woman.[45]

Neurologic Disease

Direct relationship between neurologic diseases on the treatment outcome for prosthodontic patients may not be very well-documented. Previous studies have suggested that loss of occlusal support may be a risk factor for neurologic disease where it can lead to cognitive dysfunction through the "reduction of chewing-related stimuli, aggravation of nerve damage, and long-term inflammatory stress".[62,63] Alzheimer's disease is a degenerative disease of the brain that may have some detrimental effect on the prosthodontic therapy and its outcome. Previous studies have described the oral health deterioration due to the onset of Alzheimer's disease (Marchini, Campos CH) where mandibular movements, bite force, and masticatory efficiency, as well as quality of life has been affected.[64–67]

Parkinson's disease is a degenerative disease where this happens and that happens. Previous studies have described the impact of Parkinson's disease on the oral health with reduced oral sensorimotor ability such as range of motion in eccentric movements, tongue pressure, dysphagia, and impaired masticatory function.[68–72] Impaired motor function may have negative effect on oral hygiene from increased biofilm formation.[69–72]

Emphasizing good oral health throughout the disease progression and customized plan to address the individual needs are essential in preventing the decline in oral health quality of life.[64]

Cancer and Radiation

Radiation therapy is widely applied to head and neck cancer treatment and the effect of radiation on different types of cells and tissues have been well-studied.[73] Xerostomia, dysgeusia, mucositis, radiation caries, are osteoradionecrosis are the main adverse effects from the radiation therapies.[74–79]

Table 1
Summary of systemic factors and likely prosthodontic complications with reasons

Systemic Factors	Complications Likely to Cause Failures in Prosthodontic Outcome	Reasons for the Poor Diagnostic Outcome
Age *Above 65 ys more complaint*	• Oral stomatitis/burning mouth syndrome • Mucosal lesions • Angular cheilitis, superimposed infection • Hyperplasia, mandibular dysfunction	Older patients with cognitive impairment, frailty multiple chronic diseases have side effects from medications.[87,88]
Gender	Women of menopausal experience more difficulty in adapting to dentures than those in the younger age group	Due to the physical and emotional changes during and after menopause[21]
Smoking and chewing tobacco.	• Median rhomboid glossitis • Chewer's mucositis • Leukoplakia • Oral squamous cell carcinoma • Oral submucous fibrosis	Aggravated by local proliferation of *Candida albicans* on the dorsum of the tongue.[89,90]
Metabolic disorders *Diabetes*	Xerostomia cause difficulty in wearing complete dentures due to soreness and ulceration. Denture retention may be affected by lack of saliva.	Xerostomia in diabetes mellitus is thought to be caused by the polyurea of the disease while drugs like diuretics used in the treatment of hypertension are possible causes of xerostomia.[91,92]
Autoimmune Disorders		
Rheumatoid Arthritis	Jaw movement restrictions	Difficulty in making jaw relations and impressions. Rheumatoid Arthritis decreases masticatory function and maximum bite force.[93,94]
Osteoarthritis	Mandibular movements are painful.	Shorter appointments due to difficulty in opening the mouth for a longer period. Preference for removable prosthesis over the fixed. It is difficult to record and repeat jaw relation records.[95]
Sjögren Syndrome	Hyposalivation, high caries rate, burning sensation, early tooth loss, and repeated failure of restorations	Difficulty in wearing a removable prosthesis which irritates mucosa and causes painful ulcerations. Implant treatment is the preferred choice.[38]

Crohn's Disease	Oral manifestations, possible hyposalivation, gum bleeding, ulceration in mouth, canker sores, thick mucus, and increased caries	Implant treatment is preferred.[96]
Systemic Sclerosis	Reduced mouth opening, preference for fixed prosthesis	Patients with microstomia can have difficulties in inserting and removing their dentures from the mouth.[39]
Bisphosphonates/Bone Disorders		*Prosthodontic Complications*
Osteoporosis	Bone resorption Lack of denture retention, gingival attachment loss Interproximal bone loss	Increased osteoclastic activity causing denture loosening Preservation of underlying tissue structure by: i. Mucostatic or open mouth impression technique is recommended ii. Use of non- or semi-anatomic acrylic teeth with narrow buccolingual width is advised iii. Extended tissue rest from dentures is advised for at least 10 hs per day iv. Optimal use of soft liners may be considered and v. Frequent relining of dentures is often required.[97]
Fibrous Dysplasia	Malocclusion, craniofacial defects, growth of the jaw, tooth abnormalities, and high caries index	Frequent recalls are required to redo prostheses and failed restorations.[98]
Osteitis Deformans/Paget's Disease	Affects the jaws	• Prosthesis failures are quite common and need frequent refabrication.[99]
Endocrine Disorders		
Hypothyroidism	Macroglossia, glossitis, enamel hypoplasia, anterior open bite, and micrognathia	Congenital hypothyroidism is reported to have a hypodontia mandible delayed eruption and retained deciduous tooth. These patients will need removable prostheses from a young age with constant relining and rebasing.[100–102]
Hyperthyroidism	Increase caries susceptibility, periodontal disease, burning mouth syndrome, osteoporosis, Sjogren's syndrome, and systemic lupus erythematosus	Can cause failure of abutment tooth in removable cast partial dentures.[103]

(continued on next page)

Table 1
(continued)

Systemic Factors	Complications Likely to Cause Failures in Prosthodontic Outcome	Reasons for the Poor Diagnostic Outcome
Parkinson's disease (PD)	PD-related rigidity, tremors, and dyskinesia. Also cause cracked teeth, tooth wear, changes in the fit and wear of dentures, and tooth grinding.	Hard to brush one's teeth. Hence oral hygiene maintenance is difficult. Swallowing and speech can also be affected. A well-fitting prosthesis is required but recording of jaw relation to final clinical procedures is difficult depending on the severity of the disease.[104]

The direct effect of radiation therapy on restorative and prosthodontic treatment remains unclear. However, due to the adverse effects on salivary glands, soft tissue, and bone, the risk assessment must be carefully considered when removable or fixed prostheses are planned in conjunction with remaining hard and soft tissue. Xerostomia has been known for high caries risk for remaining dentition and lack of retention for complete denture employment. The increased caries risk associated with RPDs can be aggravated by xerostomia.[80,81] Patients' diligent personal care must be emphasized and closely monitored if such a combination has to be planned and executed. Removable dental prostheses, including complete dentures and partial dentures, that rely on mucosa support may predispose ulcerations and lead to osteonecrosis. Therefore, care must be given meticulous attention to tissue surface adaptation and tissue conditioning to assure well-functioning prostheses.

The self-etch adhesive has shown to be affected by gamma irradiation.[82] Gamma irradiation resulted in reduced fracture resistance of intact teeth and increased cusp strain.[83] The bonding between fiber post and irradiated endodontically-treated teeth dentin resulted in significantly lower bond strength than non-irradiated teeth. Etch-and-rinse showed significantly higher bond strength than self-etch approaches.[84] In terms of adhesive restorative materials, glass ionomer provide clinical caries inhibition but erode easily, while composite resin provides great structural integrity.[85] The radiation therapy, depending on the dosage and location, indirectly adversely affects function and longevity of removable, fixed, and direct restorations. A careful pretreatment planning, maintenance during radiotherapy, dental treatment, and follow-up post-radiotherapy are critical for optimal outcome of dental treatment for patients who have undergone radiotherapies.

Smoking

There are not many studies available relating smoking to prostheses longevity directly; however, mainly describing the effects of smoking on wound healing or periodontal disease. A study by Dutra and colleagues have found that there is no significant association of smoking and prognosis of direct restoration either in retention, marginal discoloration, color matching, integrity, and sensitivity after 6 and 12 months follow-up.[86]

SUMMARY

The summary of systemic factors and likely prosthodontic complications with reasons is outlined in **Table 1**. The oral cavity is considered the gateway to the body. Systemic factors of a patient have a profound impact on the oral health and possibly the outcome of dental treatments. This review explored the relationship between systemic factors and prosthodontic treatment outcomes. Success or failure of prosthodontic treatment is dependent on identifying the risk factors stemming from the systemic conditions and formulating a plan for the patient from the oral health care provider. Customizing a patient-specific recall regimen and home care instruction based on the patient's medical condition is imminent for a successful outcome.

CLINICS CARE POINTS

- It's essential to assess the medical history of all systemic diseases related to metabolic, cardiovascular, autoimmune, and bone disorders.
- These conditions can significantly impact the healing and overall treatment outcomes.

DISCLOSURE

None.

REFERENCES

1. Gade DJ, Mahule DA, Trivedi DV, et al. Prosthodontic management of patients with systemic disorders. Eur J Mol Clin Med 2021;8(3):1439–51.
2. Le Bars P, Kouadio AA, N'goran JK, et al. Relationship between removable prosthesis and some systemics disorders. J Indian Prosthodont Soc 2015;15(4):292.
3. Ioannidis G, Paschalidis T, Petridis HP, et al. The influence of age on tooth supported fixed prosthetic restoration longevity. A systematic review. J Dent 2010; 38(3):173–81.
4. Ioannidou E. The Sex and Gender Intersection in Chronic Periodontitis. Front Public Health 2017;5:189.
5. Hintao J, Teanpaisan R, Chongsuvivatwong V, et al. Root surface and coronal caries in adults with type 2 diabetes mellitus. Community Dent Oral Epidemiol 2007;35(4):302–9.
6. Hintao J, Teanpaisan R, Chongsuvivatwong V, et al. Root surface and coronal caries in adults with type 2 diabetes mellitus. Prim Dent Care 2008;4:152.
7. Weinstein M, Schuchman J, Lieberman J, et al. Age and denture experience as determinants in patient denture satisfaction. J Prosthet Dent 1988;59(3):327–9.
8. Zarb GA. Oral motor patterns and their relation to oral prostheses. J Prosthet Dent 1982;47(5):472–8.
9. De Backer H, Van Maele G, De Moor N, et al. The influence of gender and age on fixed prosthetic restoration longevity: an up to 18- to 20-year follow-up in an undergraduate clinic. Int J Prosthodont (IJP) 2007;20(6):579–86.
10. van de Sande FH, Collares K, Correa MB, et al. Restoration Survival: Revisiting Patients' Risk Factors Through a Systematic Literature Review. Oper Dent 2016; 41(S7):S7–26.
11. van de Sande FH, Opdam NJ, Rodolpho PADR, et al. Patient risk factors' influence on survival of posterior composites. J Dent Res 2013;92(7 Suppl):78s–83s.
12. Critchlow SB, Ellis JS. Prognostic indicators for conventional complete denture therapy: a review of the literature. J Dent 2010;38(1):2–9.
13. Fenlon MR, Sherriff M, Douglas Walter J. An investigation of factors influencing patients' use of new complete dentures using structural equation modelling techniques. Community Dent Oral Epidemiol 2000;28(2):133–40.
14. Diehl RL, Foerster U, Sposetti VJ, et al. Factors associated with successful denture therapy. J Prosthodont 1996;5(2):84–90.
15. Allen PF, McMillan AS. A review of the functional and psychosocial outcomes of edentulousness treated with complete replacement dentures. J Can Dent Assoc 2003;69(10):662.
16. Palmqvist S, Swartz B. Artificial crowns and fixed partial dentures 18 to 23 years after placement. Int J Prosthodont (IJP) 1993;6(3):279–85.
17. Schulz P, Johansson A, Arvidson K. A retrospective study of Mirage ceramic inlays over up to 9 years. Int J Prosthodont (IJP) 2003;16(5):510–4.
18. van Dijken JW, Hasselrot L. A prospective 15-year evaluation of extensive dentin-enamel-bonded pressed ceramic coverages. Dent Mater 2010;26(9): 929–39.
19. Gruythuysen RJ, Kreulen CM, Tobi H, et al. 15-year evaluation of Class II amalgam restorations. Community Dent Oral Epidemiol 1996;24(3):207–10.

20. Koc D, Dogan A, Bek B. Bite force and influential factors on bite force measurements: a literature review. Eur J Dermatol 2010;4(2):223–32.
21. Powter G, Cleaton-Jones P. Quantitative assessment of some factors governing complete denture success. J Dent Assoc S Afr 1980;35(1):5–8.
22. Müller S, Eickholz P, Reitmeir P, et al. Long-term tooth loss in periodontally compromised but treated patients according to the type of prosthodontic treatment. A retrospective study. J Oral Rehabil 2013;40(5):358–67.
23. Kim H-K, Kim YG, Cho JH, et al. The effect of periodontal and prosthodontic therapy on glycemic control in patients with diabetes. The Journal of Advanced Prosthodontics 2019;11(5):247–52.
24. Bala S, Kumari R. Assessment of effect of periodontal and prosthodontic therapy on glycemic control in patients with diabetes. J Pharm BioAllied Sci 2021; 13(Suppl 2):S1561.
25. Ambikathanaya U, Swamy KR, Gujjari AK, et al. Effect of Acrylic Removable Partial Denture in Caries Prevalence Among Diabetic and Non-Diabetic Patients. J Pharm BioAllied Sci 2022;14(Suppl 1):S917.
26. Bayram YE, Eskan MA. Mastication inefficiency due to diminished or lack of occlusal support is associated with increased blood glucose levels in patients with type 2 diabetes. PLoS One 2023;18(4):e0284319.
27. Bianchi CM, Bianchi HA, Tadano T, et al. Factors related to oral candidiasis in elderly users and non-users of removable dental prostheses. Rev Inst Med Trop Sao Paulo 2016;58:17.
28. Azogui-Lévy S, Dray-Spira R. Sociodemographic factors associated with the dental health of persons with diabetes in France. Spec Care Dentist 2012; 32(4):142–9.
29. Dragomir LP, Nicolae FM, Gheorghe DN, et al. The Influence of Fixed Dental Prostheses on the Expression of Inflammatory Markers and Periodontal Status—Narrative Review. Medicina 2023;59(5):941.
30. Elsalhin AA, Afaf. Clinical evaluation of fixed-fixed bridge design and cantilever bridge design in diabetic patient. Int J Sci Res 2022;11(12):436–9.
31. Chien WC, Fu E, Chung CH, et al. Type 2 Diabetes mellitus and periodontitis: bidirectional association in population-based 15-year retrospective cohorts. J Clin Endocrinol Metab 2023;108(11):e1289–97.
32. Rahman B. Prosthodontic concerns in a diabetic patient. Int J Health Sci Res 2013;3(10):117–20.
33. Stavreva N. Most common systemic disorders: implications and considerations for prosthodontic treatment. KNOWLEDGE-International Journal 2021;47(4): 543–8.
34. Stavreva N, Cana A, Jakupi JA. Considerations of oral manifestations and prosthodontic management of patients with diabetes mellitus. IOSR J Dent Med Sci 2019;18:21–3.
35. Detert J, Pischon N, Burmester GR, et al. The association between rheumatoid arthritis and periodontal disease. Arthritis Res Ther 2010;12(5):218.
36. Canalis E, Giustina A. Glucocorticoid-induced osteoporosis: summary of a workshop. J Clin Endocrinol Metab 2001;86(12):5681–5.
37. Saccucci M, Di Carlo G, Bossù M, et al. Autoimmune Diseases and Their Manifestations on Oral Cavity: Diagnosis and Clinical Management. J Immunol Res 2018;2018:6061825.
38. Daneshparvar H, Esfahanizadeh N, Vafadoost R. Dental Implants in Sjögren Syndrome. Eur J Transl Myol 2020;30(2):8811.

39. Mosaddad SA, Abdollahi Namanloo R, Ghodsi R, et al. Oral rehabilitation with dental implants in patients with systemic sclerosis: A systematic review. Immun Inflamm Dis 2023;11(3):e812.

40. Raviv E, Harel-Raviv M, Shatz P, et al. Implant-supported overdenture rehabilitation and progressive systemic sclerosis. Int J Prosthodont (IJP) 1996;9(5):440–4.

41. al-Hashimi I. The management of Sjögren's syndrome in dental practice. J Am Dent Assoc 2001;132(10):1409–17, quiz 1460-1.

42. Rossie K, Guggenheimer J. Oral candidiasis: clinical manifestations, diagnosis, and treatment. Pract Periodontics Aesthet Dent 1997;9(6):635–41, quiz 642.

43. Sinclair GF, Frost PM, Walter JD. New design for an artificial saliva reservoir for the mandibular complete denture. J Prosthet Dent 1996;75(3):276–80.

44. Mendoza AR, Tomlinson MJ. The split denture: a new technique for artificial saliva reservoirs in mandibular dentures. Aust Dent J 2003;48(3):190–4.

45. NIH Consensus conference. Optimal calcium intake. NIH Consensus Development Panel on Optimal Calcium Intake. JAMA 1994;272(24):1942–8.

46. Periodontology, A.A. Glossary of periodontal terms. Chicago: American Academy of Periodontology; 1992.

47. Wright NC, Looker AC, Saag KG, et al. The recent prevalence of osteoporosis and low bone mass in the United States based on bone mineral density at the femoral neck or lumbar spine. J Bone Miner Res 2014;29(11):2520–6.

48. Cimões R, Pinho RCM, Gurgel BCdV, et al. Impact of tooth loss due to periodontal disease on the prognosis of rehabilitation. Braz Oral Res 2021;35(Supp 2):e101.

49. Martínez-Maestre M, González-Cejudo C, Machuca G, et al. Periodontitis and osteoporosis: a systematic review. Climacteric 2010;13(6):523–9.

50. Genco RJ, Borgnakke WS. Risk factors for periodontal disease. Periodontol 2000 2013;62(1):59–94.

51. Wactawski-Wende J, Grossi SG, Trevisan M, et al. The role of osteopenia in oral bone loss and periodontal disease. J Periodontol 1996;67(10 Suppl):1076–84.

52. Weyant RJ, Pearlstein ME, Churak AP, et al. The association between osteopenia and periodontal attachment loss in older women. J Periodontol 1999;70(9):982–91.

53. Dixon D, Hildebolt CF, Miley DD, et al. Calcium and vitamin D use among adults in periodontal disease maintenance programmes. Br Dent J 2009;206(12):627–31 ; discussion 617.

54. Brincat SD, Borg M, Camilleri G, et al. The role of cytokines in postmenopausal osteoporosis. Minerva Ginecol 2014;66(4):391–407.

55. Verron E, Bouler JM. Is bisphosphonate therapy compromised by the emergence of adverse bone disorders? Drug Discov Today 2014;19(3):312–9.

56. Rodan GA, Fleisch HA. Bisphosphonates: mechanisms of action. J Clin Invest 1996;97(12):2692–6.

57. Faienza MF, Chiarito M, D'amato G, et al. Monoclonal antibodies for treating osteoporosis. Expert Opin Biol Ther 2018;18(2):149–57.

58. Metwally T, Burke A, Tsai JY, et al. Fibrous Dysplasia and Medication-Related Osteonecrosis of the Jaw. J Oral Maxillofac Surg 2016;74(10):1983–99.

59. Ruggiero SL, Dodson TB, Fantasia J, et al. American Association of Oral and Maxillofacial Surgeons position paper on medication-related osteonecrosis of the jaw–2014 update. J Oral Maxillofac Surg 2014;72(10):1938–56.

60. Borm JM, Moser S, Locher M, et al. [Risk assessment in patients undergoing osseous antiresorptive therapy in dentistry. An update]. Schweiz Monatsschr Zahnmed 2013;123(11):985–1001, 955.

61. da Silva Maganhoto A, Garcia Margute T, Quirino Mota da Silva T, et al. Considerations about bisphosphonate therapy and patients using dental prosthesis: a literature review. Brazilian Journal of Case Reports 2021;1(3):103–15.

62. Wang X, Hu J, Jiang Q. Tooth Loss-Associated Mechanisms That Negatively Affect Cognitive Function: A Systematic Review of Animal Experiments Based on Occlusal Support Loss and Cognitive Impairment. Front Neurosci 2022;16:811335.

63. Sun X, Lu Y, Pang Q, et al. Tooth loss impairs cognitive function in SAMP8 mice via the NLRP3/Caspase-1 pathway. Oral Dis 2024;30(4):2746–55.

64. Marchini L, Ettinger R, Caprio T, et al. Oral health care for patients with Alzheimer's disease: An update. Spec Care Dentist 2019;39(3):262–73.

65. Campos CH, Ribeiro GR, Costa JLR, et al. Correlation of cognitive and masticatory function in Alzheimer's disease. Clin Oral Investig 2017;21(2):573–8.

66. Campos CH, Ribeiro GR, Rodrigues Garcia RCM. Mastication and oral health-related quality of life in removable denture wearers with Alzheimer disease. J Prosthet Dent 2018;119(5):764–8.

67. Campos CH, Ribeiro GR, Stella F, et al. Mandibular movements and bite force in Alzheimer's disease before and after new denture insertion. J Oral Rehabil 2017;44(3):178–86.

68. Minagi Y, Ono T, Hori K, et al. Relationships between dysphagia and tongue pressure during swallowing in Parkinson's disease patients. J Oral Rehabil 2018;45(6):459–66.

69. Ribeiro GR, Campos CH, Garcia R. Removable prosthesis hygiene in elders with Parkinson's disease. Spec Care Dentist 2017;37(6):277–81.

70. Ribeiro GR, Campos CH, Garcia RC. Oral Health in Elders with Parkinson's Disease. Braz Dent J 2016;27(3):340–4.

71. Ribeiro GR, Campos CH, Rodrigues Garcia RCM. Influence of a removable prosthesis on oral health-related quality of life and mastication in elders with Parkinson disease. J Prosthet Dent 2017;118(5):637–42.

72. Ribeiro GR, Campos CH, Rodrigues Garcia RCM. Parkinson's disease impairs masticatory function. Clin Oral Investig 2017;21(4):1149–56.

73. Beech N, Robinson S, Porceddu S, et al. Dental management of patients irradiated for head and neck cancer. Aust Dent J 2014;59(1):20–8.

74. Marx RE. Osteoradionecrosis: a new concept of its pathophysiology. J Oral Maxillofac Surg 1983;41(5):283–8.

75. Marx RE, Johnson RP. Studies in the radiobiology of osteoradionecrosis and their clinical significance. Oral Surg Oral Med Oral Pathol 1987;64(4):379–90.

76. Vissink A, Burlage FR, Spijkervet FKL, et al. Prevention and treatment of the consequences of head and neck radiotherapy. Crit Rev Oral Biol Med 2003;14(3):213–25.

77. Vissink A, Jansma J, Spijkervet FKL, et al. Oral sequelae of head and neck radiotherapy. Crit Rev Oral Biol Med 2003;14(3):199–212.

78. Jham BC, Reis PM, Miranda EL, et al. Oral health status of 207 head and neck cancer patients before, during and after radiotherapy. Clin Oral Invest 2008;12:19–24.

79. Porter S, Fedele S, Habbab K. Xerostomia in head and neck malignancy. Oral Oncol 2010;46(6):460–3.

80. Tanaka A, Kellesarian SV, Arany S. Xerostomia and patients' satisfaction with removable denture performance: systematic review. Quintessence Int 2021; 52(1):46–55.

81. Turner M, Jahangiri L, Ship JA. Hyposalivation, xerostomia and the complete denture: a systematic review. J Am Dent Assoc 2008;139(2):146–50.

82. Gupta S, Bogra P, Sharma D, et al. Impact of radiotherapy and shielding on the efficacy of the self-etch adhesive technique. J Conserv Dent: J Comput Dynam 2022;25(4):444.

83. Soares C, Roscoe MG, Castro CG, et al. Effect of gamma irradiation and restorative material on the biomechanical behaviour of root filled premolars. Int Endod J 2011;44(11):1047–54.

84. Başer Can ED, Barut G, Işık V, et al. Push-out bond strength of fiber posts to irradiated and non-irradiated intraradicular dentin. Clin Oral Invest 2022;26(12): 7057–69.

85. De Moor RJ, Stassen IG, van 't Veldt Y, et al. Two-year clinical performance of glass ionomer and resin composite restorations in xerostomic head-and neck-irradiated cancer patients. Clin Oral Invest 2011;15:31–8.

86. de Carvalho LD, Gondo R, Lopes GC. One-year clinical evaluation of resin composite restorations of noncarious cervical lesions in smokers. J Adhes Dent 2015;17(5):405–11.

87. Singh H, Sharma S, Singh S, et al. Problems faced by complete denture-wearing elderly people living in jammu district. J Clin Diagn Res 2014;8(12):Zc25–7.

88. Ogunrinde TJ, Dosumu OO. The influence of demographic factors and medical conditions on patients complaints with complete dentures. Ann Ib Postgrad Med 2012;10(2):16–21.

89. Ramasamy J, Sivapathasundharam B. A study on oral mucosal changes among tobacco users. J Oral Maxillofac Pathol 2021;25(3):470–7.

90. Arendorf TM, Walker DM. Tobacco smoking and denture wearing as local aetiological factors in median rhomboid glossitis. Int J Oral Surg 1984;13(5):411–5.

91. Sreebny LM. Recognition and treatment of salivary induced conditions. Int Dent J 1989;39(3):197–204.

92. Carr L, Lucas VS, Becker PJ. Diseases, medication, and postinsertion visits in complete denture wearers. J Prosthet Dent 1993;70(3):257–60.

93. Andrade KM, Alfenas BFM, Rodrigues Garcia RCM. Influence of removable prostheses on mastication in elderly subjects with rheumatoid arthritis. J Oral Rehabil 2018;45(4):295–300.

94. Laurell L, Hugoson A, Håkansson J, et al. General oral status in adults with rheumatoid arthritis. Community Dent Oral Epidemiol 1989;17(5):230–3.

95. Kalladka M, Quek S, Heir G, et al. Temporomandibular joint osteoarthritis: diagnosis and long-term conservative management: a topic review. J Indian Prosthodont Soc 2014;14(1):6–15.

96. Tan CXW, Brand HS, Kalender B, et al. Dental and periodontal disease in patients with inflammatory bowel disease. Clin Oral Invest 2021;25(9):5273–80.

97. Bandela V, Munagapati B, Karnati RKR, et al. Osteoporosis: Its Prosthodontic Considerations - A Review. J Clin Diagn Res 2015;9(12):Ze01–4.

98. Akintoye SO, Boyce AM, Collins MT. Dental perspectives in fibrous dysplasia and McCune-Albright syndrome. Oral Surg Oral Med Oral Pathol Oral Radiol 2013;116(3):e149–55.

99. Smith BJ, Eveson JW. Paget's disease of bone with particular reference to dentistry. J Oral Pathol 1981;10(4):233–47.

100. Pinto A, Glick M. Management of patients with thyroid disease: oral health considerations. J Am Dent Assoc 2002;133(7):849–58.
101. Loevy HT, Aduss H, Rosenthal IM. Tooth eruption and craniofacial development in congenital hypothyroidism: report of case. J Am Dent Assoc 1987;115(3):429–31.
102. Bhat V, Bhat VS, Vadakkan J, et al. Prosthodontic Management of Congenital Hypothyroidism with Anodontia: A Case Report. Int J Clin Pediatr Dent 2021; 14(4):586–9.
103. Little JW. Thyroid disorders. Part I: hyperthyroidism. Oral Surg Oral Med Oral Pathol Oral Radiol Endod 2006;101(3):276–84.
104. Haralur SB. Clinical strategies for complete denture rehabilitation in a patient with Parkinson disease and reduced neuromuscular control. Case Rep Dent 2015;2015:352878.

Medications Affecting Outcomes and Prognosis of Dental Treatment: Part 1

Davis C. Thomas, BDS, DDS, MSD, MSc Med, MSc[a],*,
Saurabh K. Shah, BDS, PGDMLS[b], Jitendra Chawla, BDS, MDS[c],
Linda Sangalli, DDS, MS, PhD[d]

KEYWORDS

- Implant prognosis • Implant osseointegration • Implant failure
- SSRIs and dental treatment • Bisphosphonates and implants
- Proton pump inhibitors and implant failure
- Parkinson's disease and dental prognosis • Alzheimer's and dental prognosis

KEY POINTS

- Succinct knowledge about the effect of medications on prognosis and outcomes in dentistry is essential for the clinician.
- Clinicians need to carefully evaluate the effect of the current and past medications on their potential effects on the proposed treatment plan.
- Certain drug classes including, but not limited to, proton pump inhibitors, serotonin medications, have a significant impact on prognosis of dental treatment.

INTRODUCTION

This article gives valuable insights into the effect of selected groups of medications on the dental treatment outcome and prognosis. Medications affect surgical procedures, wound healing, periodontal health, salivation, and dental implants osseointegration and survival, among others. The review highlights the importance of taking these factors into consideration while managing and formulating treatment options for patients suffering from systemic diseases, and their impact on prognosis of dental treatment. The following are classes of drugs and their interactions discussed in this article:

[a] Department of Diagnostic Sciences, Center for Temporomandibular Disorders and Orofacial Pain, Rutgers School of Dental Medicine, Newark, NJ, USA; [b] Private Practice, Mumbai, India; [c] Department of Dentistry, All India Institute of Medical Sciences, Mangalagiri. Dist, Guntur, Andhra Pradesh, India; [d] College of Dental Medicine - Illinois, Midwestern University, 555 31st Street, Downers Grove, IL, USA
* Corresponding author. Department of Diagnostic Sciences, Rutgers School of Dental Medicine, 110 Bergen Street, Newark NJ 07103.
E-mail address: davisct1@gmail.com

Dent Clin N Am 68 (2024) 767–783
https://doi.org/10.1016/j.cden.2024.07.006
0011-8532/24/© 2024 Elsevier Inc. All rights reserved, including those for text and data mining, AI training, and similar technologies.

dental.theclinics.com

1. Drugs used in neurodegenerative diseases (Parkinson's and Alzheimer's):
   - Dopamine agonist therapy
   - Anticholinergic therapy
2. Drugs that affect the respiratory system
   - Beta-agonists, bronchodilators
   - Steroids and anticholinergic drugs
3. Drugs used in mood disorders
   - Serotonin-specific reuptake inhibitors (SSRIs)
   - Serotonin/norepinephrine reuptake inhibitors (SNRIs)
   - Heterocyclics/tricyclic antidepressants (TCAs)
4. Drugs that affect the endocrine system
   - Insulin, glucagon, and oral hypoglycemic drugs
   - Parathyroid drugs
5. Drugs that affect the gastrointestinal tract
   - Histamine (H2) antagonists
   - Proton pump inhibitors (PPIs)
   - Antacids and ulcer protective agents
6. Drugs used in osteoporosis
   - Bisphosphonates
   - Selective estrogen receptor modulators (SERMs)
   - Estrogens replacement therapies (ERTs)

MEDICATIONS FOR NEURODEGENERATIVE DISEASES

The most common neurodegenerative diseases are Parkinson's and Alzheimer's diseases.

Parkinson's Disease

Parkinson's disease (PD) has an estimated prevalence of 1% to 4% among adults aged older than 60 years, and its incidence increases with aging.[1]

Although the exact pathophysiology in not fully understood, PD is characterized by the accumulation of Lewy bodies and a loss of dopamine-containing neurons in the substantia nigra.[1,2] There are several oral side-effects of medications used for the management of PD. In addition, the motor effects of PD affect daily oral hygiene care[3–7] and contribute to problems in the patient's ability to insert and remove the prosthesis.[8–10] One of the most frequent oral side-effects of antiparkinsonism drugs is dry mouth.[11–15] Dry mouth is a side-effect of amantadine, used in patients with PD.[16] This may result in a higher caries index[11,14,17,18] compared to age-matched and sex-matched controls without xerostomia.[18] Dry mouth has also been related to higher dental plaque formation and increased bleeding on probing,[19] with negative consequences for postoperative periodontal maintenance with fixed prosthesis. Consequently, patients with PD have more dental caries and periodontal diseases, conceivably due to oral dysbiosis associated with their condition.[20,21] Notably, the literature revealed that patients with PD under treatment with levodopa/carbidopa exhibited significantly different oral microbiota compared to patients with PD not taking such medications.[22,23] The use of anticholinergic drugs does not seem to influence the prognosis of dental implants.[24–28]

It is advisable to refrain from the use of epinephrine when patients with PD are managed with levodopa and certain monoamine oxidase (MAO) inhibitors, as epinephrine could interfere with such drugs and result in a rise in blood pressure.[8] Other studies advise to reduce the use of epinephrine.[8] Moreover, dental procedures should be scheduled in the morning, possibly at least 1 hour before taking levodopa.

Long-term use of levodopa may result in the development of dyskinesias (ie, levodopa-induced dyskinesia) in about 30% to 80% of the cases.[29-32] As a result, patients develop erratic jaw opening and closing movements, lip protrusion, tongue movements, muscle twitching, and tooth clenching and grinding.[29,33] It is conceivable that these patients have jaw fatigue and possible failure of restoration.[33]

The literature presents contradictory findings on the effects of dopaminergic medications on bruxism,[34] some supporting a decrease,[35-37] while some others failing to reveal any effects.[38-41]

Alzheimer's Disease

Alzheimer's disease (AD) affects approximately 40 million people globally.[42]

The presence of periodontal disease compromised oral hygiene, higher risk of dental caries, and higher number of teeth loss were correlated to the likelihood of presenting with AD compared to healthy controls.[42-48] There is a lack of evidence relating AD-medications to periodontal disease. Cholinesterase inhibitors may reduce salivary flow,[49] conceivably resulting in higher caries index.[46] Yet, other studies contradict this.[50,51] Increased salivation may interfere with those dental procedures that require a dry working field.[51] Moreover, another study has suggested impairment in the retention of removable prostheses due to the change in saliva consistency.[52] A change in the salivary total protein content has also been documented elsewhere.[49]

The most common medications utilized for the treatment of these neurodegenerative conditions are presented in **Table 1**.

MEDICATIONS FOR RESPIRATORY CONDITIONS

The most common respiratory conditions are asthma and chronic obstructive pulmonary disease. Asthma is a chronic inflammation of the airways characterized by increased mucus production and hyperreactivity of the tracheobronchial tree.[53] Its prevalence has significantly increased nowadays, with estimates of more than 300 million people worldwide.[53-55] The therapeutic approaches for respiratory conditions are based on 2 main categories of drugs, that is, bronchodilators and anti-inflammatory drugs. Most of the adverse oral effects are observed particularly due to the route of administration of inhalation or nebulization.[53]

A significantly higher prevalence of dental caries has been reported by the majority of the studies among patients with asthma of various age groups treated with β-agonists and glucocorticoids.[56-66] This has been particularly observed with chronic use, inhaler formulation, use of bronchodilators, high frequency of dosing times, and combination therapy.[58,67-69] The increased predilection to dental caries is attributed to a decreased salivary flow, buffering capacity, and pH, which in turn lowers the protective mechanism of the saliva (ie, decreased salivary peroxidase, salivary amylase, lysozyme, and immunoglobulin A) and favors a higher cariogenic bacteria concentration (ie, *Streptococcus mutans* and *Lactobacillus acidophilus*).[53,59-61,67,68,70-74] Moreover, a higher plaque index has also been reported among children and adolescents with asthma compared to age-matched controls.[75] Furthermore, antiasthmatic medications are frequently utilized before going to sleep with no other oral hygiene procedures performed after the administration, with further negative consequences on tooth structure and salivary composition.[53,76] Hence, prescription of fluoride supplements to patients with asthma is advised, especially for those under treatment with beta adrenergic agonists.

Patients with asthma under treatment with beta-agonists, anticholinergic drugs, and/or oral and inhaled corticosteroids exhibited significantly higher occurrence of

Table 1
Common medications utilized for the treatment of these neurodegenerative conditions

Condition	Class of Drug	Name of Drugs	Mechanism of Action	Side Effects that May Affect Dental Treatment Prognosis and Outcomes
Neurodegenerative Conditions				
Parkinson disease	Dopamine replacement therapy	Carbidopa and levodopa	Metabolic precursor of dopamine, which crosses the BBB	Nausea, confusion, and anxiety
		Tolcapone and entacapone	Plasma COMT inhibitors used to prolong the half-life of levodopa	Liver dysfunction and dyskinesia
		Selegiline (deprenyl) and rasagiline	Inhibitor of MAO, the enzyme that metabolizes dopamine in the CNS	Dry mouth, headache, difficulty swallowing, and nausea
		Amantadine	Antiviral drug, which enhances synthesis, release, and reuptake of dopamine from nigral neurons	Nausea, suicidal ideation, and dry mouth
	Dopamine agonist therapy	Bromocriptine and pergolide	Ergotamine derivatives used to stimulate postsynaptic dopamine receptors and restore the imbalance of dopamine	Nausea
		Pramipexole, ropinirole, and rotigotine	Nonergotamine derivatives used to stimulate postsynaptic dopamine receptors and restore the imbalance of dopamine	Dry mouth and nausea
	Anticholinergic therapy	Trihexyphenidyl, benztropine, and biperiden	Muscarinic antagonists used to reduce the activity of the uninhibited cholinergic neurons in the basal ganglia	Dry mouth
AD	Cholinesterase inhibitors	Donepezil, galantamine, rivastigmine, and tacrine	Inhibition of the breakdown activity of acetylcholinesterase enzyme in the synaptic cleft	Nausea, muscle cramps, myalgia, sialorrhea, salivary dysfunction, and xerostomia
	NMDA receptor antagonists	Memantine	Noncompetitive antagonist at the NMDA glutamate receptor	Nausea, hypertension, and dry mouth
	Amyloid-beta monoclonal antibodies	Aducanumab and lecanemab	Monoclonal antibodies against amyloid beta in the brain	Nausea

Abbreviations: BBB, blood–brain barrier; CNS, central nervous system; COMT, catechol-o-methyltransferase; MAO, monoamine oxidase. NMDA, N-methyl-ᴅ–aspartate.

periodontitis[77] and gingival bleeding compared to controls.[61] A decreased salivary flow and reduction of protective salivary mechanisms seem to be responsible for worsening of periodontal health (ie, plaque index, gingival index, clinical attachment loss, probing depth, periodontal index status, calculus index, and gingival bleeding) with the use of antiasthmatic drugs.[53,78–81] In addition, patients with asthma tend to be mouth breathers, which further worsens oral mucosa dehydration.[53,74,81] The immunosuppressive action of corticosteroids is also suggested to influence the response of the periodontal tissue by hampering the host response, thus predisposing to clinical expression of gingivitis.[79,82] In particular, in patients treated with inhaled corticosteroids, maintaining a good gingival health has also been suggested to reduce the frequency of respiratory attacks.[79,83] Patients under treatment with topical steroids and other medications that induce dryness of the oral mucosa as side effect are particularly vulnerable to oral candidiasis, with a prevalence ranging from 0% to 77%.[53,84] Regular dental checkups, use of topic antifungals, modalities, and medications that increase salivary flow are also recommended.[53,84,85]

Antiasthmatic medications may contribute to the development of dental erosion due to a decreased salivary protection against oral acids,[61,86–89] a reduction of the oral pH below 5.5, and the relaxation of smooth muscles (ie, lower esophageal sphincter) with potential gastric reflux as a result.[53] Interestingly, a cross-sectional study revealed a significant association between adolescents with asthma not under treatment with any medication and the number of teeth affected by molar incisor hypomineralization.[90] Prevention strategies include rinsing the mouth with neutral sodium fluoride or sodium bicarbonate after inhalers use, and restrain from brushing their teeth soon after the exposure to the acids.[53,88]

MEDICATIONS USED IN MOOD DISORDERS

SSRIs are currently classified primarily as antidepressants. There is mounting evidence in the literature of a positive association between failure of osseointegrated implants and the use of SSRIs.[91–97] Although the exact mechanism of how SSRIs cause implant failure is not fully understood, it has been proposed that these drugs increase osteoclastic activity and reduce bone apposition.[91,97] Conversely, a few articles have proposed a lack of association between SSRI usage and implant failure.[98] The mode of action of SSRIs involves the 5-HT1B receptor on osteoblasts, leading to bone loss, while binding to the 5-HT1C receptor in the brain promotes bone formation. SSRIs may contribute to dysregulation of this process, thereby causing increased risk of implant loss.[99]

Antidepressants have been shown to induce xerostomia.[100] TCAs tend to have a higher impact causing xerostomia, due to their antimuscarinic effects. With regards to inducing xerostomia, SSRIs and SNRIs have been proposed to have less potential.[101] The prevalence of periapical abscesses were thought to be higher with concomitant use of SSRIs compared to controls.[102] Patients on TCAs, SNRIs, and SSRIs are considered to be at higher risk of implant loss compared to controls.[103–105]

DRUGS THAT AFFECT THE ENDOCRINE SYSTEM

Type 1 diabetes mellitus (DM) has negative effects on bone microarchitecture, mineralization, and bone microhardness. Insulin, when used to regulate the blood sugar level, minimizes these effects on bone.[106,107] When type 1 DM is controlled with insulin, there was an observed positive effect on the bone implant contact (BIC), bone mineral content, and implant removal torque values. Similar conclusive effect has not been shown in type 2 DM.[107] There is evidence of higher incidence of periodontal disease and tooth-loss with type 1 and type 2 DM.[108,109] Sodium glucose cotransporter 2 inhibitors such as canagliflozin (oral hypoglycemic drug) have been shown to have potential adverse effects on bone healing, increased fracture risk, and reduced bone mineral density.[110–112]

Metformin, an oral hypoglycemic drug, improves osseointegration and has osteogenic effect on peri-implant tissues. The drug was shown in in vitro studies to help in proliferation and differentiation of stem cells in the periodontal ligament.[113,114] In animal studies, metformin used in conjunction with insulin yielded superior results with regards to periodontal tissue response to orthodontic forces.[115]

The use of synthetic parathyroid hormone for osteoporosis lacks extensive literature regarding dental treatment outcomes. However, animal studies have shown favorable results, including outcomes of periodontal therapy, increased BIC and apposition, enhanced implant retention, and greater orthodontic stability.[116,117] Further studies need to be done in this regard.

DRUGS THAT AFFECT THE GASTROINTESTINAL TRACT

H2 antagonists are effective in the management of peptic ulcer and hyperacidity but have been surpassed by proton-pump inhibitors, which are relatively safer and more efficient.[118] Due to the cholinergic activity of H2 receptor antagonists such as cimetidine, ranitidine, and nizatidine, there is an increase in parotid (salivary) secretions, which could potentially alleviate burning mouth symptoms in patients with dry mouth.[119,120] H2-blockers have negative interactions with various medications such as antibiotics, antifungals, oral iron, and fluoride, a consideration clinicians should bear in mind when prescribing these drugs in a dental setting.[121]

The basis of using PPIs in peptic ulcer disease is their ability to irreversibly inhibit proton pumps in acid-secreting parietal cells of the stomach.[122] Concomitantly, these drugs may lead to xerostomia and secondary burning mouth symptoms, due to their action on salivary glands.[121,123]

PPIs are known to reduce the absorption of calcium, leading to decreased bone mineral density. This reduction can hinder the bone's ability to integrate with the implant, increasing the risk of implant failure.[124] The literature consistently supports that PPI use is associated with an increased risk of dental implant failure, particularly prior to loading. Clinicians need to carefully consider this risk when planning and managing dental implant treatments for patients on PPIs.[124,125]

It is interesting to note that PPIs have been proposed to have the potential for protective effects on periodontal tissues, due to their possible inhibitive effects on osteoclasts.[126,127] The same literature seemingly suggests that PPIs may be prescribed for short-term use in patients with higher periodontitis risk. However, the available evidence supporting this is not as robust and requires further research.[127] Isolated animal studies have referred to the increased rate of orthodontic tooth movement with PPIs, possibly due to their tendency to affect bone metabolism.[128] The mechanism of this phenomenon is not fully understood.

Antacids are drugs that act by neutralizing the gastric acid by raising the pH, in both stomach and in oral cavity. These drugs have known to counteract gastric acid induced enamel loss by forming acid-resistant coating over the teeth.[129] There is lack of robust evidence as to the other possible effects of antacids on teeth or supporting structures.

Mucosal protective agents, such as sucralfate, have been experimented with as a supplement to analgesics for managing recurrent aphthous stomatitis, oral ulcers, and as a topical analgesic for oral wounds and oral mucositis. However, there are conflicting reports in the literature regarding its effectiveness for these conditions.[130–133] In vitro studies have demonstrated the protective effects of sucralfate against dental erosion.[134]

Bismuth compounds are used for the management of duodenal ulcers associated with *Helicobacter pylori* infections in combination with PPI, imidazoles, and tetracyclines.[135] Bismuth compounds tend to have a tendency to discolor oral mucosa specifically when administered orally via chewable tablets.[136] Patients taking bismuth compounds and undergoing cosmetic periodontal procedures such as gingival depigmentation treatments should be advised about the potential recurrence or discoloration.

DRUGS USED IN OSTEOPOROSIS

Bisphosphonates are employed to alleviate bone pain, lower hypercalcemia in patients with cancer, and manage skeletal issues in individuals with multiple myeloma and other malignancies as well as Paget's disease of the bone.[137] Jaw osteonecrosis (ONJ) is the most common dentistry-related side effect associated with bisphosphonates use. Bisphosphonates-related ONJ is more common in patients with cancer as compared to patients with osteoporosis.[138,139] This discrepancy may be related to higher frequency and varied route of administration of bisphosphonates. Most ONJ cases reportedly occur upon surgical dental procedures, but spontaneous initiation has also been reported.[137,140,141] The clinical manifestation of osteoradionecrosis comprises an intraoral wound that fails to heal, characterized by exposed necrotic bone. It may also entail tooth loosening, the presence of infected sequestra, and, in severe instances, pathologic fractures of the bone.[138] Bisphosphonates reduce the resorption of the infected bone by reducing the activity of osteoclasts.[142] Endodontic and restorative procedures are generally considered safe in patients undergoing bisphosphonates therapy. Surgical interventions should be planned and executed with abundance of caution.[143,144]

A variety of effects of bisphosphonates on orthodontic treatment have been reported. These include, but are not limited to, reduced clinical outcomes leading to longer treatment durations, root resorption, and bone changes.[145] Interestingly, bisphosphonates use is proposed to be associated with only a slightly elevated risk of possible reduced implant success rate.[146–148] The same literature also mentioned specific bisphosphonates drug (risedronate) and other systemic and surgical risk factors associated with such implant failure. When patients with implants that have integrated successfully undergo bisphosphonates therapy, implant failure may occur, clinically presenting as a sequestrum that remains attached to the implant.[149] In a strange way, local application of bisphosphonates has been shown to improve and favor osseointegration of dental implants.[150,151] Further, there is some evidence of bisphosphonates improving the efficacy of scaling and root planning in periodontitis cases.[152]

ERTs and other classes that act with similar results have been popularized recently. Robust literature regarding the effects of these classes of drugs on dental treatment prognosis is lacking. Earlier studies on the effect of ERTs on dental treatment prognosis have proposed a positive/beneficial effect of these drugs on dental implants.[153–155] However, there are more recent apparently conflicting reports of varied effects of hormone replacement therapies (HRTs) on dental treatment prognosis. Some studies including systematic reviews have concluded little or no effect of HRTs on periodontal or dental implant treatments.[156] Meanwhile other more recent publications have referred to relatively good beneficial periodontal results with HRTs.[157]

A newer class of drugs called SERMs, such as raloxifene, is increasingly being used in the field. There are recent isolated reports of this class of medications purportedly predisposing to osteonecrosis of jaws.[158,159] The clinician should carefully consider the possible effects of these drugs on the prognosis of surgical dental therapies. Interestingly, animal studies indicate the protective nature of the same class of drugs on the periodontium and peri-implant tissues.[160–165]

SUMMARY

Systemic conditions, and medications used in the management of these conditions affect the prognosis and outcome of dental treatments. The medications that affect dental treatment prognosis in the respiratory, neurodegenerative, mood disorders, and GI categories may do so, by affecting quantity and quality of saliva. In addition, PPIs and SSRIs adversely affect bone healing and implant osseointegration. Some of these drugs also may affect patients' physical and psychological response to treatment procedures and results.

CLINICS CARE POINTS

- During the dental treatment planning phase, it is essential to thoroughly assess and consider the medications regularly taken by the patient, as these can impact the outcome of dental procedures.
- It is crucial for clinicians to stay updated with current research on how these medications can influence the outcomes and prognosis of dental treatments, enabling them to anticipate and manage potential complications effectively.
- It is important to inform patients about the possible impact that their medications may have on dental treatment prognosis.
- Clinicians should carefully evaluate the balance between the risks and benefits of treatment in relation to the impact of these medications.

DISCLOSURE

D.C. Thomas, S.K. Shah, J. Chawla, L. Sangalli declare no conflict of interest. Funding statement: None. Statement of institutional review board approval or waiver: Institutional review and approval were not necessary for this article.

REFERENCES

1. Verhoeff MC, Eilenboom D, Koutris M, et al. Parkinson's disease and oral health: A systematic review. Arch Oral Biol 2023;151:105712.
2. Verhoeff MC, Lobbezoo F, Wetselaar P, et al. Parkinson's disease, temporomandibular disorders and bruxism: A pilot study. J Oral Rehabil 2018;45(11):854–63.
3. Vanbellingen T, Kersten B, Bellion M, et al. Impaired finger dexterity in Parkinson's disease is associated with praxis function. Brain Cognit 2011;77:48–52.
4. Chaudhuri KR, Healy DG, Schapira AHV. Non-motor symptoms of Parkinson's disease: diagnosis and management. Lancet Neurol 2006;5:235–45.
5. van Stiphout MAE, Marinus J, van Hilten JJ, et al. Oral health of Parkinson's Disease patients: a case-control study. Parkinsons Dis 2018;2018:9315285.
6. Kaur T, Uppoor A, Naik D. Parkinson's disease and periodontitis - the missing link? A review. Gerodontology 2016;33(4):434–8.

7. Anastassiadou V, Katsarou Z, Naka O, et al. Evaluating dental status and prosthetic need in relation to medical findings in Greek patients suffering from idiopathic Parkinson's disease. Eur J Prosthodont Restor Dent 2002;10(2):63–8.
8. Bollero P, Franco R, Cecchetti F, et al. Oral health and implant therapy in Parkinson's patients: review. Oral Implantol (Rome) 2017;10:105–11.
9. Nakayama Y, Wwashio M, Mori M. Oral health conditions in patients with Parkinson's disease. J Epidemiol 2004;14:143–50.
10. Fiske J, Hyland K. Parkinson's disease and oral care. Dent Update 2000;27: 58–65.
11. Kakkar M, Caetano de Souza VE, Barmak AB, et al. Potential association of anticholinergic medication intake and caries experience in young adults with xerostomia. J Dent Sci 2023;18:1693–8.
12. Stenbäck J, Tilisanoja A, Syrjälä AM, et al. High anticholinergic burden and hyposalivation and xerostomia in the elderly. Acta Odontol Scand 2023;81:436–42.
13. Tiisanoja A, Syrjala AM, Komulainen K, et al. Anticholinergic burden and dry mouth among Finnish, community-dwelling older adults. Gerodontology 2018; 35:3–10.
14. Arany S, Kopycka-Kedzierawski DT, Caprio TV, et al. Anticholinergic medication: Related dry mouth and effects on the salivary glands. Oral Surg Oral Med Oral Pathol Oral Radiol 2021;132:662–70.
15. Barbe AG. Medication-induced xerostomia and hyposalivation in the elderly: culprits, complications, and management. Drugs Aging 2018;35:877–85.
16. Chang C, Rramphul K. Amantadine. In: StatPearls [Internet]. Treasure Island (FL): StatPearls Publishing; 2023 Jan. Available at: https://wwwncbinlmnihgov/books/NBK499953/.
17. Kakkar M, Barmak AB, Arany S. Anticholinergic medication and dental caries status in middle-aged xerostomia patients-a retrospective study. J Dent Sci 2022;17(3):1206–11.
18. Cheah HL, Gray M, Aboelmagd S, et al. Anticholinergic medication and caries status predict xerostomia under 65. Dent J 2023;11:87.
19. Mizutani S, Ekuni D, Tomofuji T, et al. Relationship between xerostomia and gingival condition in young adults. J Periodontal Res 2015;50:74–9.
20. Fleury V, Zekeridou A, Lazarevic V, et al. Oral dysbiosis and inflammation in Parkinson's Disease. J Parkinsons Dis 2021;11:619–31.
21. Hanaoka A, Kashihara K. Increased frequencies of caries, periodontal disease and tooth loss in patients with Parkinson's disease. J Clin Neurosci 2009;16: 1279–82.
22. Rozas NS, Tribble GD, Jeter CB. Oral factors that impact the oral microbiota in Parkinson's disease. Microorganisms 2021;9(8):1616.
23. Bardow A, Nyvad B, Nauntofte B. Relationships between medication intake, complaints of dry mouth, salivary flow rate and composition, and the rate of tooth demineralization in situ. Arch Oral Biol 2001;46:413–23.
24. Packer M, Nikitin V, Coward T, et al. The potential benefits of dental implants on the oral health quality of life of people with Parkinson's disease. Gerodontol 2009;26:11–8.
25. Chu FC, Deng FL, Siu AS, et al. Implant-tissue supported, magnet-retained mandibular overdenture for an edentulous patient with Parkinson's disease: a clinical report. J Prosthet Dent 2004;91:219–22.
26. Schimmel M, Srinivasan M, McKenna G, et al. Effect of advanced age and/or systemic medical conditions on dental implant survival: A systematic review and meta-analysis. Clin Oral Implants Res 2018;29(Suppl 16):311–30.

27. Heckmann SM, Heckmann JG, Weber HP. Clinical outcomes of three Parkinson's disease patients treated with mandibular implant overdentures. Clin Oral Impl Res 2000;11:566–71.

28. Bera RN, Tripathi R, Bhattacharjee B, et al. Implant survival in patients with neuropsychiatric, neurocognitive, and neurodegenerative disorders: A meta-analysis. Natl J Maxillofac Surg 2021;12:162–70.

29. Tee TY, Khoo CS, Norlinah MI. Prominent oromandibular dystonia as levodopa-induced dyskinesia in idiopathic Parkinson's Disease. Mov Disord Clin Pract 2019;6(4):330–1.

30. Fabbrini G, Brotchie JM, Grandas F, et al. Levodopa-induced dyskinesias. Mov Disord 2007;22(10):1379–89.

31. Davie CA. A review of Parkinson's disease. Br Med Bull 2008;86:109–27.

32. Zesiewicz TA, Sullivan KL, Hauser RA. Levodopa-induced dyskinesia in Parkinson's disease: epidemiology, etiology, and treatment. Curr Neurol Neurosci Rep 2007;7(4):302–10.

33. Bakke M, Henriksen T, Biernat HB, et al. Interdisciplinary recognizing and managing of drug-induced tardive oromandibular dystonia: two case reports. Clin Case Rep 2018;6(11):2150–5.

34. Magee KR. Bruxism related to levodopa therapy. J Am Med Assoc 1970;214(1):147.

35. Harris M, Nora L, Tanner CM. Neuroleptic malignant syndrome responsive to carbidopa/levodopa: support for a dopaminergic pathogenesis. Clin Neuropharmacol 1987;10(2):186–9.

36. Lobbezoo F, Soucy JP, Hartman NG, et al. Effects of the D2 receptor agonist bromocriptine on sleep bruxism: report of two single-patient clinical trials. J Dent Res 1997;76(9):1610–4.

37. Lobbezoo F, Lavigne GJ, Tanguay R, et al. The effect of the catecholamine precursor L-dopa on sleep bruxism: a controlled clinical trial. Mov Disord 1997;12(1):73–8.

38. Lavigne GJ, Soucy JP, Lobbezoo F, et al. Double-blind, crossover, placebo-controlled trial of bromocriptine in patients with sleep bruxism. Clin Neuropharmacol 2001;24(3):145–9.

39. Winocur E, Gavish A, Voikovitch M, et al. Drugs and bruxism: a critical review. J Orofac Pain 2003;17(2):99–111.

40. Cahlin BJ, Hedner J, Dahlström L. A randomised, open-label, crossover study of the dopamine agonist, pramipexole, in patients with sleep bruxism. J Sleep Res 2017;26(1):64–72.

41. Verhoeff MC, Koutris M, van Selms MKA, et al. Is dopaminergic medication dose associated with self-reported bruxism in Parkinson's disease? A cross-sectional, questionnaire-based study. Clin Oral Invest 2021;25(5):2545–53.

42. Matsushita K, Yamada-Furukawa M, Kurosawa M, et al. Periodontal disease and periodontal disease-related bacteria involved in the pathogenesis of Alzheimer's Disease. J Inflamm Res 2020;13:275–83.

43. Fang WL, Jiang MJ, Gu BB, et al. Tooth loss as a risk factor for dementia: systematic review and meta-analysis of 21 observational studies. BMC Psychiatr 2018;18:345.

44. Chen CK, Wu YT, Chang YC. Association between chronic periodontitis and the risk of Alzheimer's disease: a retrospective, population-based, matched-cohort study. Alzheimer's Res Ther 2017;9(1):56.

45. Chalmers J, Carter K, Spencer AJG. Caries incidence and increments in community-living older adults with and without dementia. Gerodontology 2002;19:80–94.

46. Gao SS, Chen KJ, Duangthip D, et al. The oral health status of chinese elderly people with and without dementia: a cross-sectional study. Int J Environ Res Publ Health 2020;17(6):1913.

47. Ellefsen B, Holm-Pedersen P, Morse DE, et al. Caries prevalence in older persons with and without dementia. J Am Geriatr Soc 2008;56:59–67.

48. Foley NC, Affoo RH, Siqueira WL, et al. A systematic review examining the oral health status of persons with dementia. JDR Clin Trans Res. 2017;2(4):330–42.

49. Zalewska A, Klimiuk A, Zięba S, et al. Salivary gland dysfunction and salivary redox imbalance in patients with Alzheimer's disease. Sci Rep 2021;11:23904.

50. Khosravani N, Birkhed D, Ekström J. The cholinesterase inhibitor physostigmine for the local treatment of dry mouth: a randomized study. Eur J Oral Sci 2009; 117(3):209–17.

51. Ahmed SE, Begum R, Kumar AS, et al. Drug therapy in cognitive disorders and its effects on oral health. Cureus 2022;13(7):e27194.

52. Friedlander AH, Norman DC, Mahler ME, et al. Alzheimer's disease: psychopathology, medical management and dental implications. J Am Dent Assoc 2006; 137:1240–51.

53. Pacheco-Quito EM, Jaramillo J, Sarmiento-Ordoñez J, et al. Drugs prescribed for asthma and their adverse effects on dental health. Dent J 2023;11(5):113.

54. Dharmage SC, Perret JL, Custovic A. Epidemiology of asthma in children and adults. Front Pediatr 2019;7:246.

55. Stern J, Pier J, Litonjua AA. Asthma epidemiology and risk factors. Semin Immunopathol 2020;42:5–15.

56. Chumpitaz-Cerrate V, Bellido-Meza JA, Chávez-Rimache L, et al. Impact of inhaler use on dental caries in asthma pediatrics patients: A case-control study. Arch Argent Pediatr 2020;118(1):38–46.

57. Samec T, Amaechi BT, Jan J. Influence of childhood asthma on dental caries: A longitudinal study. Clin Exp Dent Res 2021;7(6):957–67.

58. Jan BM, Khayat MA, Bushnag AI, et al. The association between long-term corticosteroids use and dental caries: a systematic review. Cureus 2023;15(9): e44600.

59. Ersin NK, Gulen F, Eronat N, et al. Oral and dental manifestations of young asthmatics related to medication, severity and duration of condition. Pediatr Int 2006;48(6):549–54.

60. Mazzoleni S, Stellini E, Cavaleri E, et al. Dental caries in children with asthma undergoing treatment with short-acting beta2-agonists. Eur J Paediatr Dent 2008;9(3):132–8.

61. Bairappan S, Puranik MP, Sowmya KR. Impact of asthma and its medication on salivary characteristics and oral health in adolescents: A cross-sectional comparative study. Spec Care Dent 2020;40(3):227–37.

62. Boskabady M, Nematollahi H, Boskabady MH. Effect of inhaled medication and inhalation technique on dental caries in asthmatic patients. Iran Red Crescent Med J 2012;14:816–21.

63. Arafa A, Aldahlawi S, Fathi A. Assessment of the oral health status of asthmatic children. Eur J Dermatol 2017;11.

64. Wu F, Liu J. Asthma medication increases dental caries among children in taiwan: an analysis using the national health insurance research database. J Dent Sci 2019;14:413–8.

65. Rezende G, dos Santos NML, Stein C, et al. Asthma and oral changes in children: associated factors in a community of Southern Brazil. Int J Paediatr Dent 2019;29:456–63.

66. Hassanpour K, Tehrani H, Goudarzian M, et al. Comparison of the frequency of dental caries in asthmatic children under treatment with inhaled corticosteroids and healthy children in Sabzevar in 2017–2018. Electron J Gen Med. 2019;16:em119.

67. Alaki SM, Ashiry EA, Bakry NS, et al. The effects of asthma and asthma medication on dental caries and salivary characteristics in children. Oral Health Prev Dent 2013;11(2):113–20.

68. Gani F, Caminati M, Bellavia F, et al. Oral health in asthmatic patients: a review: asthma and its therapy may impact on oral health. Clin Mol Allergy 2020;18:22.

69. Shashikiran ND, Reddy VVS, Krishnam Raju P. Effect of antiasthmatic medication on dental disease: dental caries and periodontal disease. J Indian Soc Pedod Prev Dent 2007;25:65–8.

70. Brigic A, Kobaslija S, Zukanovic A. Cariogenic potential of inhaled antiasthmatic drugs. Med Arch 2015;69:247–50.

71. Brigic A, Kobaslija S, Zukanovic A. Antiasthmatic inhaled medications as favoring factors for increased concentration of Streptococcus mutans. Mater Soc Med 2015;27:237.

72. Botelho MPJ, Maciel SM, Cerci Neto A, et al. Cariogenic microorganisms and oral conditions in asthmatic children. Caries Res 2011;45:386–92.

73. Doğan M, Şahiner ÜM, Ataç AS, et al. Oral health status of asthmatic children using inhaled corticosteroids. Turk J Pediatr 2021;63:77–85.

74. Stensson M, Wendt LK, Koch G, et al. Oral health in young adults with long-term, controlled asthma. Acta Odontol Scand 2011;69:158–64.

75. Moreira LV, Galvao EL, Mourão PS, et al. Association between asthma and oral conditions in children and adolescents: a systematic review with meta-analysis. Clin Oral Invest 2023;27(1):45–67.

76. Maupomé G, Shulman JD, Medina-Soils CE, et al. Is There a relationship between asthma and dental caries?: a critical review of the literature. J Am Dent Assoc 2010;141:1061–74.

77. Khassawneh B, Alhabashneh R, Ibrahim F. The association between bronchial asthma and periodontitis: a case-control study in jordan. J Asthma 2019;56:404–10.

78. Yaghobee S, Paknejad M, Khorsand A. Association between asthma and periodontal disease. Front Dent (J Dent Tehran Univ Med Sci) 2018;5:47–51.

79. Moraschini V, de Albuquerque Calasans-Maja J, Calasans-Maia MD. Association between asthma and periodontal disease: a systematic review and meta-analysis. J Periodontol 2017;89:440–55.

80. Rivera R, Andriankaja OM, Perez CM, et al. Relationship between periodontal disease and asthma among overweight/obese adults. J Clin Periodontol 2016;43:566–71.

81. Mappangara S, Basir I, Oktawati S, et al. Periodontal disease associated with corticosteroidin asthma patients-a systematic review. Int J Appl Pharm 2019;11:68–70.

82. Trombelli L, Farina R. A review of factors influencing the incidence and severity of plaque-induced gingivitis. Minerva Stomatol 2013;62:207–34.

83. Santos NC, Jamelli S, Costa L, et al. Assessing caries, dental plaque and salvary flow in asthamtic adolescents using inhaled corticosteroids. Allergol Immunopathol 2012;40:220–4.

84. GÜMRÜ B, Akkitap MP. Oral candidiasis as a local adverse effect of inhaled corticosteroids: what the dental practitioner should know. Black Sea J Health Sci. 2021;5:107–15.

85. Cuenca-León K, Pachieco-Quito EM, Granda-Granda Y, et al. Phytotherapy: a solution to decrease antifungal resistance in the dental field. Biomolecules 2022;12:789.

86. Manuel ST, Kundabaka M, Shetty N, et al. Asthma and dental erosion. Kathmandu Univ Med J 2008;6:370–4.

87. Gupta M, Pandit IK, Srivastava N, et al. Dental erosion in children. J Oral Health Community Dent 2009;3:56–61.

88. Lussi A, Jaeggi T. Dental erosion in children. Monogr Oral Sci 2006;20:140–51.

89. Dugmore CR, Rock WP. A multifactorial analysis of factors associated with dental erosion. Br Dent J 2004;196:283–6.

90. Flexeder C, Kabary Hassan L, Standl M, et al. Is There an association between asthma and dental caries and molar incisor hypomineralisation? Caries Res 2020;54(1):87–95.

91. Wu X, Al-Abedalla K, Rastikerdar E, et al. Selective serotonin reuptake inhibitors and the risk of osseointegrated implant failure: a cohort study. J Dent Res 2014; 93:1054–61.

92. Altay MA, Sindel A, Özalp Ö, et al. Does the intake of selective serotonin reuptake inhibitors negatively affect dental implant osseointegration? a retrospective study. J Oral Implantol 2018;44:260–5.

93. Kotsailidi EA, Gagnon C, Johnson L, et al. Association of selective serotonin reuptake inhibitor use with marginal bone level changes around osseointegrated dental implants: a retrospective study. J Periodontol 2023;94:1008–17.

94. Shariff JA, Gurpegui Abud D, Bhave MB, et al. Selective serotonin reuptake inhibitors and dental implant failure: a systematic review and meta-analysis. J Oral Implantol 2023;49:436–43.

95. Jung RE, Al-Nawas B, Araujo M, et al. Group 1 ITI Consensus Report: The influence of implant length and design and medications on clinical and patient-reported outcomes. Clin Oral Implants Res 2018;29(Suppl 16):69–77.

96. Ball J, Darby I. Mental health and periodontal and peri-implant diseases. Periodontol 2000 2022;90:106–24.

97. Deepa MK, Dhillon K, Jadhav P, et al. Prognostic implication of selective serotonin reuptake inhibitors in osseointegration of dental implants: a 5-year retrospective study. J Contemp Dent Pract 2018;19:842–6.

98. Chrcanovic BR, Kisch J, Albrektsson T, et al. Is the intake of selective serotonin reuptake inhibitors associated with an increased risk of dental implant failure? Int J Oral Maxillofac Surg 2017;46:782–8.

99. Wadhwa R, Kumar M, Talegaonkar S, et al. Serotonin reuptake inhibitors and bone health: A review of clinical studies and plausible mechanisms. Osteoporos Sarcopenia 2017;3:75–81.

100. Hunter KD, Wilson WS. The effects of antidepressant drugs on salivary flow and content of sodium and potassium ions in human parotid saliva. Arch Oral Biol 1995;40:983–9.

101. Johnsson M, Winder M, Zawia H, et al. In vivo studies of effects of antidepressants on parotid salivary secretion in the rat. Arch Oral Biol 2016;67:54–60.

102. Rotstein I, Katz J. Acute periapical abscesses in patients using selective serotonin reuptake inhibitors. Spec Care Dent 2024;44:143–7.

103. Hakam AE, Vila G, Duarte PM, et al. Effects of different antidepressant classes on dental implant failure: A retrospective clinical study. J Periodontol 2021;92: 196–204.

104. Apostu D, Lucaciu O, Lucaciu GD, et al. Systemic drugs that influence titanium implant osseointegration. Drug Metab Rev 2017;49:92–104.

105. Nicolaev N, Romanos GE, Malmstrom H, et al. Commonly used systemic drugs interfering with bone remodeling: a case report and literature review. Quintessence Int 2021;52:880–6.

106. Limirio PHJO, Soares PBF, Venâncio JF, et al. Type I diabetes mellitus and insulin therapy on bone microarchitecture, composition and mechanical properties. Curr Diabetes Rev 2022;18. e301121198427.

107. Tan SJ, Baharin B, Mohd N, et al. Effect of anti-diabetic medications on dental implants: a scoping review of animal studies and their relevance to humans. Pharmaceuticals 2022;15:1518.

108. Saleh W, Xue W, Katz J. Diabetes mellitus and periapical abscess: a cross-sectional study. J Endod 2020;46:1605–9.

109. Kaur G, Holtfreter B, Rathmann W, et al. Association between type 1 and type 2 diabetes with periodontal disease and tooth loss. J Clin Periodontol 2009;36: 765–74.

110. Blevins TC, Farooki A. Bone effects of canagliflozin, a sodium glucose co-transporter 2 inhibitor, in patients with type 2 diabetes mellitus. Postgrad Med 2017;129:159–68.

111. Jackson K, Moseley KF. Diabetes and bone fragility: SGLT2 inhibitor use in the context of renal and cardiovascular benefits. Curr Osteoporos Rep 2020;18: 439–48.

112. Alba M, Xie J, Fung A, et al. The effects of canagliflozin, a sodium glucose co-transporter 2 inhibitor, on mineral metabolism and bone in patients with type 2 diabetes mellitus. Curr Med Res Opin 2016;32:1375–85.

113. Patel V, Sadiq MS, Najeeb S, et al. Effects of metformin on the bioactivity and osseointegration of dental implants: A systematic review. J Taibah Univ Med Sci 2022;18:196–206.

114. Zhang R, Liang Q, Kang W, et al. Metformin facilitates the proliferation, migration, and osteogenic differentiation of periodontal ligament stem cells in vitro. Cell Biol Int 2020;44:70–9.

115. Mena Laura EE, Cestari TM, Almeida R, et al. Metformin as an add-on to insulin improves periodontal response during orthodontic tooth movement in type 1 diabetic rats. J Periodontol 2019;90:920–31.

116. Aggarwal P, Zavras A. Parathyroid hormone and its effects on dental tissues. Oral Dis 2012;18:48–54.

117. Javed F, Al Amri MD, Kellesarian SV, et al. Efficacy of parathyroid hormone supplementation on the osseointegration of implants: a systematic review. Clin Oral Invest 2016;20:649–58.

118. Mejia A, Kraft WK. Acid peptic diseases: pharmacological approach to treatment. Expert Rev Clin Pharmacol 2009;2:295–314.

119. Boros I, Keszler P, Szombath D, et al. H2-receptor-blokkolók (cimetidin és ranitidin) hatása patkányok gl. parotisának szekréciójára és a nyál szénsavanhidráz-aktivitására [The effect of H2-receptor blockers (cimetidine and ranitidin) on parotid gland secretion and salivary carbonic anhydrase activity in the rat]. Fogorv Sz 1993;86:265–73.

120. Kikuchi T, Hirano K, Genda T, et al. A study of the effects of saliva stimulation by nizatidine on dry mouth symptoms of primary biliary cirrhosis. World J Hepatol 2013;5:90–6.

121. Karthik R, Karthik KS, David C, et al. Oral adverse effects of gastrointestinal drugs and considerations for dental management in patients with gastrointestinal disorders. J Pharm BioAllied Sci 2012;4(Suppl 2):S239–41.

122. Stedman CA, Barciay ML. Review article: comparison of the pharmacokinetics, acid suppression and efficacy of proton pump inhibitors. Aliment Pharmacol Ther 2000;14:963–78.

123. Krajewski MP Jr, Mo Q, Lu CH, et al. Medication use among patients reporting xerostomia of an academic dental clinic. J Pharm Technol 2022;38:264–71.

124. Altay MA, Sindel A, Özalp Ö, et al. Proton pump inhibitor intake negatively affects the osseointegration of dental implants: a retrospective study. J Korean Assoc Oral Maxillofac Surg 2019;45:135–40.

125. Vinnakota DN, Kamatham R. Effect of proton pump inhibitors on dental implants: A systematic review and meta-analysis. J Indian Prosthodont Soc 2020;20: 228–36.

126. Chawla BK, Cohen RE, Stellrecht EM, et al. The influence of proton pump inhibitors on tissue attachment around teeth and dental implants: A scoping review. Clin Exp Dent Res 2022;8:1045–58.

127. Costa-Rodrigues J, Reis S, Teixeira S, et al. Dose-dependent inhibitory effects of proton pump inhibitors on human osteoclastic and osteoblastic cell activity. FEBS J 2013;280:5052–64.

128. Makrygiannakis MA, Kaklamanos EG, Athanasiou AE. Does common prescription medication affect the rate of orthodontic tooth movement? A systematic review. Eur J Orthod 2018;40:649–59.

129. Turssi CP, Vianna LM, Hara AT, et al. Counteractive effect of antacid suspensions on intrinsic dental erosion. Eur J Oral Sci 2012;120:349–52.

130. Rattan J, Schneider M, Arber N, et al. Sucralfate suspension as a treatment of recurrent aphthous stomatitis. J Intern Med 1994;236:341–3.

131. Loprinzi CL, Ghosh C, Camoriano J, et al. Phase III controlled evaluation of sucralfate to alleviate stomatitis in patients receiving fluorouracil-based chemotherapy. J Clin Oncol 1997;15:1235–8.

132. Singh NV, Gabriele GA, Wilkinson MH. Sucralfate as an adjunct to analgesia to improve oral intake in children with infectious oral ulcers: a randomized, double-blind, placebo-controlled trial. Ann Emerg Med 2021;78:331–9.

133. Suparakchinda C, Rawangban W. Effectiveness of Sucralfate comparing to normal saline as an oral rinse in pain reduction and wound healing promotion in oral surgery. Laryngoscope Investig Otolaryngol 2023;8:1226–32.

134. Turssi CP, Amaral FLB, França FMG, et al. Effect of sucralfate against hydrochloric acid-induced dental erosion. Clin Oral Invest 2019;23:2365–70.

135. Vanderah TW. Katzung's basic & clinical pharmacology. McGraw-Hill; 2024.

136. Dekker W, Dal Monte PR, Bianchi Porro G, et al. An international multi-clinic study comparing the therapeutic efficacy of colloidal bismuth subcitrate coated tablets with chewing tablets in the treatment of duodenal ulceration. Scand J Gastroenterol 1986;122:46–50.

137. American Dental Association Council on Scientific Affairs. Dental management of patients receiving oral bisphosphonate therapy: expert panel recommendations. J Am Dent Assoc 2006;137:1144–50.

138. Sedghizadeh PP, Sun S, Jones AC, et al. Bisphosphonates in dentistry: Historical perspectives, adverse effects, and novel applications. Bone 2021;147:115933.

139. Khan AA, Morrison A, Hanley DA, et al. Diagnosis and management of osteonecrosis of the jaw: a systematic review and international consensus. J Bone Miner Res 2015;30:3–23.

140. Kawahara M, Kuroshima S, Sawase T. Clinical considerations for medication-related osteonecrosis of the jaw: a comprehensive literature review. Int. J. Implant Dent. 2021;7:47.

141. Nicolatou-Galitis O, Schiodt M, Mendes RA, et al. Medication-related osteonecrosis of the jaw: definition and best practice for prevention, diagnosis, and treatment. Oral Surg Oral Med Oral Pathol Oral Radiol 2019;127:117–35.

142. Katsarelis H, Shah NP, Dhariwal DK, et al. Infection and medication-related osteonecrosis of the jaw. J Dent Res 2015;94:534–9.

143. Zamparini F, Pelliccioni GA, Spinelli A, et al. Root canal treatment of compromised teeth as alternative treatment for patients receiving bisphosphonates: 60-month results of a prospective clinical study. Int Endod J 2021;54:156–71.

144. AlRahabi MK, Ghabbani HM. Clinical impact of bisphosphonates in root canal therapy. Saudi Med J 2019;39:232–8.

145. Zymperdikas VF, Yavropoulou MP, Kaklamanos EG, et al. Effects of systematic bisphosphonate use in patients under orthodontic treatment: a systematic review. Eur J Orthod 2020;42:60–71.

146. Fiorillo L, Cicciu M, Tözüm TF, et al. Impact of bisphosphonate drugs on dental implant healing and peri-implant hard and soft tissues: a systematic review. BMC Oral Health 2022;22:291.

147. Mendes V, Dos Santos GO, Calasans-Maia MD, et al. Impact of bisphosphonate therapy on dental implant outcomes: An overview of systematic review evidence. Int J Oral Maxillofac Surg 2019;48:373–81.

148. de-Freitas NR, Lima LB, de-Moura MB, et al. Bisphosphonate treatment and dental implants: A systematic review. Med Oral Patol Oral Cir Bucal 2016;21:e644–51.

149. Pogrel MA, Ruggiero SL. Previously successful dental implants can fail when patients commence anti-resorptive therapy-a case series. Int J Oral Maxillofac Surg 2018;47:220–2.

150. Guimarães MB, Antes TH, Dolacio MB, et al. Does local delivery of bisphosphonates influence the osseointegration of titanium implants? A systematic review. Int J Oral Maxillofac Surg 2017;46:1429–36.

151. Najeeb S, Siddiqui F, Khurshid Z, et al. Effect of bisphosphonates on root resorption after tooth replantation - a systematic review. Dent Traumatol 2017;33:77–83.

152. Wang Y, He F. Meta-analysis of the efficacy of alendronate-assisted cleansing and root planing in the treatment of periodontitis. Panminerva Med 2024;66:90–2.

153. Qi MC, Zhou XQ, Hu J, et al. Oestrogen replacement therapy promotes bone healing around dental implants in osteoporotic rats. Int J Oral Maxillofac Surg 2004;33:279–85.

154. Nociti FH Jr, Sallum AW, Sallum EA, et al. Effect of estrogen replacement and calcitonin therapies on bone around titanium implants placed in ovariectomized rats: a histometric study. Int J Oral Maxillofac Implants 2002;17:786–92.

155. Duarte PM, Cesar-Neto JB, Sallum AW, et al. Effect of estrogen and calcitonin therapies on bone density in a lateral area adjacent to implants placed in the tibiae of ovariectomized rats. J Periodontol 2023;74:1618–24.
156. Chaves JDP, Figueredo TFM, Warnavin SVSC, et al. Sex hormone replacement therapy in periodontology-A systematic review. Oral Dis 2020;26:270–84.
157. Man Y, Zhang C, Cheng C, et al. Hormone replacement therapy and periodontitis progression in postmenopausal women: A prospective cohort study. J Periodontal Res 2024. https://doi.org/10.1111/jre.13258.
158. Bindakhil M, Shanti RM, Mupparapu M. Raloxifene-induced osteonecrosis of the jaw (MRONJ) with no exposure to bisphosphonates: clinical and radiographic findings. Quintessence Int 2021;52:258–63.
159. Chiu WY, Chien JY, Yang WS, et al. The risk of osteonecrosis of the jaws in Taiwanese osteoporotic patients treated with oral alendronate or raloxifene. J Clin Endocrinol Metab 2014;99:2729–35.
160. Gomes-Filho JE, Wawama M, Dornelles RC, et al. Effect of raloxifene on periapical lesions in ovariectomized rats. J Endod 2015;41:671–5.
161. Ramalho-Ferreira G, Faverani LP, Prado FB, et al. Raloxifene enhances peri-implant bone healing in osteoporotic rats. Int J Oral Maxillofac Surg 2015;44:798–805.
162. Ichimaru R, Tominari T, Yoshinouchi S, et al. Raloxifene reduces the risk of local alveolar bone destruction in a mouse model of periodontitis combined with systemic postmenopausal osteoporosis. Arch Oral Biol 2018;85:98–103.
163. Heo HA, Park S, Jeon YS, et al. Effect of raloxifene administration on bone response around implant in the maxilla of osteoporotic rats. Implant Dent 2019;28:272–8.
164. Azami N, Chen PJ, Mehta S, et al. Raloxifene administration enhances retention in an orthodontic relapse model. Eur J Orthod 2020;42:371–7.
165. Park S, Heo HA, Min JS, et al. Effect of raloxifene on bone formation around implants in the osteoporotic rat maxilla: histomorphometric and microcomputed tomographic analysis. Int J Oral Maxillofac Implants 2020;35:249–456.

Medications Affecting Treatment Outcomes in Dentistry: Part 2

Gayathri Subramanian, PhD, DMD[a],*,
Davis C. Thomas, BDS, DDS, MSD, MSc Med, MSc[a],
Dipti Bhatnagar, BDS, MDS[b], Samuel Y.P. Quek, DMD, MPH[a]

KEYWORDS

- Medications • Dental treatment outcomes • Critical appraisal
- Pharmacoepidemiologic studies • Causation • Association • Risk factors

KEY POINTS

- The literature is rife with studies describing the impact of medications on dental treatment outcomes.
- An incremental process of critical appraisal of the literature is essential for the clinician/practitioner to comprehend the true implications of such studies.
- Using key examples, this article outlines:
  ○ The concepts of association and causation.
  ○ The hierarchy of the evidence pyramid.
  ○ Critical appraisal of literature.
- The practitioner is encouraged to actively and critically appraise the literature and comprehend the difference between association and causation, refrain from premature risk attribution, recognize study weaknesses or biases, and ascertain study validity.

INTRODUCTION

Chronic diseases being so prevalent, it is not unusual for dental patients to present for elective, and sometimes, emergent dental care while taking multiple medications to manage medical comorbidities. Although the focus is naturally on the impact of these health conditions, it is essential to recognize that these medications may impact the patient's ability to tolerate the proposed dental treatment and the prognosis or the treatment outcome.

[a] Department of Diagnostic Sciences, Rutgers School of Dental Medicine, 110 Bergen Street, Newark, NJ 07103, USA; [b] Department of Oral Medicine and Radiology, Rayat Bahra Dental College and Hospitals, Sahibzada Ajit Singh Nagar, Punjab 140301, India
* Corresponding author.
E-mail address: subramga@sdm.rutgers.edu

Dent Clin N Am 68 (2024) 785–797
https://doi.org/10.1016/j.cden.2024.07.005
0011-8532/24/© 2024 Elsevier Inc. All rights reserved, including those for text and data mining, AI training, and similar technologies.

dental.theclinics.com

The patient's ability to tolerate the proposed treatment is influenced by the underlying health conditions and the medications prescribed. Broad considerations include their collective impact on the risk of bleeding, infection susceptibility, healing, drug interactions/toxicity, and pharmacokinetics, and the ability to compromise the patient's capacity to withstand the proposed treatment.

However, a medication may impact the treatment outcome, likely driven by its effects on the integrity of the oral mucosa, dental, and periodontal tissues. Such an effect may either be a direct extension of the mechanism of action of the medication or a side effect, or idiosyncratic in nature. In some instances, such an impact is readily apparent. In such a case, it is straightforward to attribute the impact to the medication in question, factor in such a consequence into treatment considerations, and help plan the patient's treatment, setting treatment expectations accordingly. In other instances, such an impact is subtle and becomes apparent only when viewing and analyzing treatment outcome data at an epidemiologic level. Nevertheless, it is critical to recognize the latter to provide optimal treatment recommendations for the patient, and to anticipate adverse outcomes.

This article provides insight into both types of such instances and reviews the current knowns and unknowns in the context of selected classes of medications that illustrate these nuances best. These include antiresorptive medications, drugs used in the management of HIV disease, immunosuppressive medications, and cancer medications, in addition to cardiovascular drugs, and nonsteroidal anti-inflammatory drugs (NSAIDs).

The article also underscores the need for a keen awareness of current scientific literature and its critical appraisal to comprehend its importance and to recognize the clinical implications.

PARADIGM 1. WHEN A MEDICATION'S ADVERSE EFFECTS ON DENTAL OUTCOMES ARE DIRECT AND READILY APPARENT

In this section, a few medications with an established impact on either the patient's ability to withstand the planned treatment or on dental treatment outcomes are reviewed. It should be noted that although the relationship between the medication and adverse dental treatment outcomes is established as one with increased adverse outcomes, the frequency of the adverse outcome may still be a small fraction of those exposed to the medication.

Antiresorptive Medications

This discussion pertains to antiresorptive medications, such as bisphosphonates and denosumab, and does not include discussion of osteoanabolic medications, such as teriparatide or abaloparatide. As a class of medications, antiresorptives directly impact dental treatment outcomes by imparting a risk for medication-related osteonecrosis of the jaw (MRONJ) through its effects on bone remodeling.

Bisphosphonates become bound to the mineralized bone matrix, to the calcium in calcium hydroxyapatite, particularly in surfaces undergoing active bone remodeling. When endocytosed by incoming osteoclasts, they interfere with osteoclast survival. The early nonnitrogen-containing etidronate, clodronate, and tiludronate get incorporated into nonhydrolyzable ATP analogues. The nitrogen-containing bisphosphonates interfere with the mevalonate pathway, and ultimately result in osteoclast apoptosis.[1] Denosumab is a monoclonal antibody directed against receptor activator of nuclear factor-KappaB ligand (RANKL), a molecule critical for osteoclast activation, function, and survival.[2]

Because bone-remodeling involves the close and reciprocal interactions of osteo-clasts and osteoblasts, antiresorptive medications plausibly compromise bone remodeling and healing in the postdental extraction socket. There are additional aber-rations in host-microbe immune interactions that seem to predispose the jawbone to developing osteonecrosis, in contrast to other bones in the body. The summary pre-sented so far is at best an oversimplification of the pathogenesis of MRONJ but suf-fices for this discussion.[3]

Antiresorptive medications can precipitate MRONJ either spontaneously or second-ary to invasive dental procedures performed in the context of endodontic or peri-odontal disease. In patients with cancer receiving antiresorptive therapy, an invasive procedure, such as a dental extraction, can impart a 33-fold increase in the risk for MRONJ.[4] Bone remodeling is key in dental implant osseointegration and its ongoing survival; as an extension, it is conceivable that the adverse effects should impact the success of dental implant–based therapy. However, MRONJ is a rare complication.

The risk for MRONJ is determined by the potency and half-life of the medication, the route, duration and frequency of administration, compounded by the risk of an inva-sive dental procedure[5] performed in the context of dental disease. Accordingly, oral bisphosphonates carry the least risk for MRONJ (nearly a 1 in 10,000), whereas intra-venously administered zoledronate and pamidronate carry a much higher risk (1–18 in 100). Denosumab is believed to carry a risk similar to that[6] of intravenous bisphosphonates.[7]

The risk of implant failure is less well understood and seems to be less frequent than MRONJ occurrence; however, in the absence of a personalized risk assess-ment to estimate an individual's risk for an adverse outcome, it is best that caution is exercised during treatment decisions.[8–10] Implant-related MRONJ reported in literature predominantly has occurred as late events presenting greater than 12 months following implant surgery, often occurring at sites of implant placed before the initiation of antiresorptive therapy.[3,5,6,11] Given the absence of rigorous studies quantifying the risk for implant-related MRONJ and identifying specific risk factors, at this time, a detailed informed consent process that acknowledges the MRONJ risk and regular recall assessments are essential elements of appropriate patient care.[3]

Osteoanabolic Agents

Osteoanabolic agents, such as teriparatide, abaloparatide (parathyroid hormone frag-ments), and romozosumab (antisclerostin antibody), originally introduced for reducing fracture risk and managing refractory osteoporosis, increase bone mineral density by stimulating osteogenesis.[12–14] Their use as first line in patients with very high fracture risk is now rising.[15] In addition, preoperative teriparatide is being considered for oste-oporotic, elderly (65 years or older) patients undergoing spinal orthopedic surgery, for 2 to 6 months, and at least 8 months when used postoperatively. It will be interesting to watch this evolving field closely to understand implications osteoanabolic therapy could hold for oral surgical procedures that involve bone grafts.[16,17]

The other evolving area of scientific literature is in the potential for osteoanabolic therapy to facilitate management of MRONJ.[18,19]

Cytotoxic Medications and Immune Suppressants

Cytotoxic medications potently impact rapidly dividing cells; these include white and red blood cells, epithelial cells, and the lining of the gastrointestinal tract. The most common indication of use is as part of cancer chemotherapy. Apart from being an easy illustration of medications that profoundly impact the ability of the patient to tolerate the planned procedure, because of the risk of infection, bleeding and mucositis, and so forth, discussing these medications does not add much relevance because concurrent elective dental treatment is unlikely to be planned at the time of active cancer chemotherapy.

In contrast, those cytotoxic medications that are taken in conjunction with such diseases as rheumatoid arthritis, such as methotrexate and azathioprine, require careful consideration along the lines explained later in Paradigm 2. Low-impact studies have raised concerns of increased frequency of adverse dental treatment outcomes, especially when the bioavailability of methotrexate is abruptly increased because of reduced renal clearance or breakdown, something to bear in mind with concomitant treatment with NSAIDs or selected antibiotics, such as trimethoprim/sulfamethoxazole; however, adverse dental treatment outcomes in absence of such overt toxicity has not been consistently documented.[20,21] There are sporadic reports of an increased risk for osteonecrosis of the jaw with concomitant antiresorptive therapy; however, pharmacoepidemiologic evidence for the same, as elaborated under Paradigm 2, is lacking.[22]

Immune suppressants, such as prednisone, impact the patient's ability to tolerate the planned dental procedure because of compromised resistance to bacterial infection and to tolerate the stress associated with invasive dental procedures, and long-term dental outcomes because of its ability to undermine bone health, secondarily leading to osteoporotic changes. Sporadic reports in literature have documented a similar increased risk for osteonecrosis of the jaw with concomitant prednisone therapy. However, similar to the scenario with methotrexate, the exact frequency of such adverse effects, and specific risk factors have not been determined and require pharmacoepidemiologic validation, again, as elaborated in Paradigm 2.

Cardiovascular Medications

Diuretics are commonly used in the management of hypertension. These drugs induce xerostomia/dry mouth and alter the composition of the saliva.[23] Thiazides have been reported to be the most robust in inducing xerostomia.[24] Because hyposalivation results in change of salivary composition (buffering capacity, pH, immunoproteins) with increased viscosity it can also lead to rapid fall of pH contributing in the development of dental caries.[25] Also, less saliva results in immunoprotein deficiencies, which hereby affects oral flora and increase in incidence of cariogenic microorganisms. Saliva is essential for retention and stability in removable prosthesis. Decreased salivation can lead to dislodgement of the prosthesis during function.[26] Implants may be a better option in the appropriate type of patients within the cohort of xerostomia. However, maintaining hygiene could be cause of concern in these patients.

Dry mouth may reduce the survival rate and life of various restorations.[27,28] Cardiovascular drugs, such as angiotensin-converting enzyme inhibitors and angiotensin II receptor blockers, also induce xerostomia, which also has effect on gingival tissues because decreased salivation leads to accumulation of dental plaque.[29]

Antiplatelet drugs/anticoagulants have been given to prevent and treat thromboembolism in patients suffering from cardiac diseases. Adequate hemostasis is essential for the success of dental procedures. These drugs have an increased risk of prolonged oral bleeding following oral surgical procedures.[30,31] A clinician attempting to perform optimal impression procedures (including such adjuncts as cord packing) may find it more difficult to make the finer details especially around crown margins if there is concomitant gingival bleeding.

Nonsteroidal Anti-inflammatory Drugs

NSAIDs have been the mainstay of medications used for pain control in dentistry. Because most dental pains are of inflammatory origin, this class has been widely used for dental/postoperative pain management. However, the impact of NSAIDs on tissue healing in surgical cases seems to be evolving in recent literature.[32] Several studies and reviews have proposed a negative impact of NSAIDs on postoperative periodontal procedure healing and on implant healing.[33–35] A recent systematic review with meta-analysis of animal studies showed that acetyl salicylic acid may act to inhibit orthodontic tooth movement.[36] The same study found that acetaminophen and celecoxib do not inhibit orthodontic tooth movement. Ibuprofen may have a role in masking endodontic diagnosis.[37] Both diclofenac and parecoxib were shown not to affect osseointegration in animal surgical implant model.[38]

PARADIGM 2. WHEN A MEDICATION'S ADVERSE IMPACT ON DENTAL OUTCOMES IS NOT READILY APPARENT FROM ITS MECHANISM OF ACTION

Attributing adverse dental outcomes in such instances is much more difficult. It first needs to be established beyond doubt that the medication does undermine dental outcomes, and that, even if an association with an adverse outcome existed, such a risk resulted from the medication and not, for example, the underlying disease or another confounding factor.

Large pharmacoepidemiologic studies are necessary to validate such associations.[39] Currently, literature is rife with much smaller studies, mostly retrospective cohorts. In contrast, especially when the occurrence is rare, large cohorts need to be studied in a systematic, and unbiased manner, to detect a true association of increased risk for an adverse outcome.

For example, if we were to hypothetically attribute an increased risk for implant failure to a drug A, then, the occurrence of implant failures must be demonstrated as more frequently encountered in the group of individuals exposed to drug A, when compared with the baseline frequency of implant failures normally encountered. An adequate minimum sample size of a representative study population, studied in an unbiased manner are key in being able to detect a true association of increased risk of implant failure. Increased relative risk for an adverse event in an exposed cohort would imply a meaningful association.

Assuming a success rate of 95% for dental implants, to detect a two-fold increase in failure as a result of exposure to drug A (power of 80% and α of 0.05), a sample size of 590 individuals receiving implant-based treatment and exposed to drug A will need to be compared with 590 unexposed control subjects (https://riskcalc.org/samplesize/). Furthermore, the study population should be derived in an unbiased manner to obtain generalizable results. Any smaller population, or derived in a biased manner (eg, single office study) would render the results unusable because the results may not be generalizable. For rarer events, the required minimum sample size will need to be even larger.

Until such rigorous, systematic assessments are performed, it should be recognized that such high-quality evidence does not exist and the current literature is inadequate to draw any conclusion on the presence or absence of such an increased risk for adverse outcomes.

HIV Medications

It is harder to discern the impact of the disease from its treatment in case of HIV disease and its management given the multiple comorbidities that may accompany the disease and the polypharmacy that is usually used to manage the disease in those instances where antiretroviral treatment is warranted. Like most other instances, these medications seem be well-tolerated, and well-managed HIV disease does not seem to be associated with increased adverse dental outcomes.[40]

Antihypertensive Medications

Hypertension and therapy with antihypertensives are thought to not affect implant survival.[9,41] This class of medications is currently depicted in the dental literature as increasing the survival rate of implants.[42,43] Other studies have shown comparable implant success between patients taking antihypertensives and those who are not taking them.[44] Nonselective β-blocker drugs, such as propranolol, were shown to not affect new bone formation in peri-implant defects.[45] Improved remodeling of bone and increased osseointegration were shown in initial studies of patients taking renin-angiotensin system inhibitors.[46] Initial studies on calcium channel blockers show a tendency toward higher tooth loss rate with these drugs.[47] Furthermore, these drugs may induce gingival enlargement, necessitating further procedures associated with restorative dentistry.

DISCUSSION

The examples provided in this article share a common factor: much remains unknown about the impact of medications on dental treatment outcomes. Validating a given medication's anticipated impact on treatment outcomes depend on the paradigm under which it may fall. A biologic, mechanistic basis may be apparent in Paradigm A. In such a case, a continuity of evidence may exist from a preclinical model (cell-culture to preclinical animal model) through case series or cohort studies demonstrating a risk relationship for an adverse outcome, eventually validated through pharmacoepidemiologic outcome studies generating clinical practice guidelines, the apex synthesis of systematic review/meta-analyses of such epidemiologic studies.

In Paradigm B, this sequence of scientific data validating a medication's impact on treatment outcome may be altered in that a search for a biologic basis or mechanism that drives the adverse outcome may only ensue once a link has unambiguously been established through pharmacoepidemiologic studies and triggers the quest for understanding the biologic basis behind such an impact.

Thus, recognizing the paradigm a given medication's anticipated impact on a treatment outcome may fall under, can cue in the practitioner as to the scientific process that may come into play in validating such a role.

Several factors come sequentially into play in comprehending the impact any given medication may have on a treatment outcome. These include a clear understanding of the following elements (each of which is elaborated next): the concepts of risk factor association and causation of an outcome; and the pyramid of evidence.

CRITICAL APPRAISAL OF LITERATURE
Association and Causation

Although elucidating the mechanistic basis for biologic events, the key differences between association and causation must also be understood. Risk factors may simply amplify the odds of an outcome, rather than cause an adverse outcome. However, the possibility that epidemiologic associations are causal are strengthened when Bradford Hill criteria are fulfilled. These include strength of association (magnitude and statistical significance), consistency (reproducibility), specificity (preferential choice of outcome as opposed to other outcomes), temporality (precedence of exposure to event), biologic gradient (dose response), biologic plausibility (mechanistic relationship based on known biologic potential), coherence (corroborative natural history and biology with causal implications), experimental manipulation of outcome (causal factor withdrawal mitigating impact on outcome), and analogy (precedence in similar outcome).[48,49]

There are two additional factors that are essential to understanding the true impact of a given medication on treatment outcome. One is a clear understanding of the hierarchy of the evidence pyramid, to clearly grasp the import of the scientific literature. An understanding of a serial and incremental integration of the rungs of the evidence pyramid allows the reader to recognize the value of sentinel events, such as case reports, case series, and case-control studies, while at the same time avoid an exaggerated or premature risk assessment and attribution. Similar considerations are relevant to interpretation of preclinical studies that explore preliminary or mechanistic basis for biologic events. Each of these elements is elaborated further.

The Pyramid of Evidence

The fundamental tenet of evidence-based medicine has been that not all evidence is equal, that a hierarchy of evidence exists. The traditional hierarchy of evidence places at the apex systematic and meta-analytic studies, followed by the randomized controlled trials, cohort and case-control studies, case series, reports, opinions and preclinical studies placed toward the base, respectively.[50] Although this is broadly true, a data-synthetic systematic review or meta-analytic study of observational studies may have a lot less rigor and credibility than that of well-designed randomized clinical trials. Thus, clinical practice guidelines incorporated the assessment of the GRADE approach (Grading of Recommendations Assessment, Development and Evaluation) as best practice, while assessing the strength of recommendation.[51] Another improvisation was the modified evidence pyramid, which recognizes systematic reviews and meta-analyses as the lens through which any body of evidence may be appraised.[52]

Critical Appraisal of Scientific Literature

A process of critical appraisal of scientific literature is essential to verify the validity of the claims made in scientific publications. Today, this is broadly viewed as an essential skill a clinician needs to possess and exercise while analyzing such scientific articles, and ultimately, to practice evidence-based medicine.[53–55]

Specifically, scientific literature needs to be evaluated for internal and external validity. Internal validity reflects the rigor with which the study addressed the questions it was meant to address. The reliability and accuracy of study results is undermined by bias and confounding; this can undermine a study's internal validity, as can poor study design, execution, or data analysis and interpretation.[56] Thus, random or systematic errors can be unknowingly introduced into the study design. Thus, regardless of the rung occupied by a given study design in the hierarchy of evidence, any study may irreparably be compromised by such factors. Thus, study-specific methodologic limitations may significantly compromise the validity of even the much-respected randomized clinical trial study design. The clinician should closely appraise the given literature for such internal validity. Similarly, how applicable/generalizable the given study results are to a real-life clinical situation, or external validity, may be compromised by narrow eligibility criteria or other patient/disease characteristics.

Thus, the clinician must learn and cultivate critical appraisal skills to ascertain the validity of individual works of scientific literature, incorporating this as an essential element of an evidence-based practice.

Applying the Key Concepts Identified to Analyze the Medications Described in this Manuscript

It is important to revisit the body of evidence described in this article based on the previous discussion.

Since the original case series drawing attention to the entity of bisphosphonate-related osteonecrosis of the jaw,[57,58] a large body of evidence has contributed toward knowledge of this adverse effect of an expanding class of medications that include antiresorptive therapy. The spectrum of recent scientific literature spans across primary research, that is, basic, clinical, and epidemiologic research, and systematic and meta-analytic studies.[59–61] Apex organizations, such as the American Association of Oral and Maxillofacial Surgeons, or task forces, such as International Task Force on Osteonecrosis of the Jaw, have synthesized the body of literature to provide position papers, which serve as the equivalent of clinical practice guidelines, that have periodically been updated, incorporating critical appraisal of the evolving basic and clinical knowledge.[3,62–65] Thus, the data on the development of MRONJ are abundant and robust.

Other medications that have been reported to amplify this risk include methotrexate and corticosteroids as described previously, and antiangiogenic medications and other targeted therapeutics, such as bevacizumab, sunitinib, everolimus, osimertinib, and so forth, although these data are preliminary and lack quantification and pharmacoepidemiologic validation.[3,66–69]

In contrast to MRONJ, the body of knowledge pertaining to increased risk for implant failure following antiresorptive therapy, while consistent and established, is less robust and is still emerging.[3,70]

Nevertheless, the data consistently implicate a causative role of antiresorptive medications in the development of jaw osteonecrosis and in implant failure, although the overall pathogenesis is likely multifactorial.

When it comes to the impact of antihypertensives and their impact on dental treatment outcomes, it should be noted that the context for any such compromise in dental outcomes as a result of xerostomia is in the setting of objective xerostomia impacting the survival or oral restorations and/or the cariogenic risk, rather than subjective xerostomia. Overt, objective, xerostomia is more evident in such diseases/conditions as Sjögren syndrome, and post–head and neck radiation, all medical conditions rather than medication-induced and hence, beyond the scope of this discussion. Alternately, in the context of periodontal outcomes, gingival hyperplasia in relation to calcium channel blockers in particular, there seems to be a consistent increased risk for gingival hyperplasia principally in the context of compromised oral hygiene.[71] Institution of appropriate periodontal care, and switching medications, as medically advised, seem to be adequate interventions. Hence, the current body of literature is inadequate to directly draw conclusions regarding the specific impact of antihypertensive medications and dental treatment outcomes.

Antiplatelet medications and anticoagulants have a direct impact on bleeding and coagulation parameters. Although it is conceivable that an increased tendency for gingival hemorrhage can undermine the ability to record accurate dental impressions, there is a paucity of literature that assesses the ability or the lack thereof of local hemostatic agents currently in clinical use to circumvent this situation in the context of such medication use. The predominant literature focuses on bleeding tendency or challenges to achieving hemostasis primarily in the context of oral and periodontal surgery rather than prosthodontic procedures. Hence it is not possible to provide any recommendations or draw conclusions based on literature currently available.

Similarly, the literature is too preliminary to gain any clinical insight regarding the impact of medications, such as β-blockers, on bone remodeling and thereby their impact on treatment outcomes pertaining to implant-based rehabilitation. At this time, clinicians are cautioned against drawing any conclusive inferences and encouraged to await higher quality evidence.

SUMMARY

With a plethora of medical comorbidities and their pharmacologic management, dentists need to factor in the adverse impact medications may have on dental treatment outcomes. Save for a few well-established interactions of systemic medications and adverse treatment outcomes, the evidence implicating most medications is weak. Systematic efforts are required to design and conduct pharmacoepidemiologic studies that can interrogate and validate such associations. Only such rigorously conducted studies will generate reliable evidence that can inform clinical practice guidelines. Until then, practitioners need to carefully appraise and interpret the available evidence to best manage their patients.

A combination of a clear understanding of the hierarchy of the evidence pyramid and a critical appraisal of a given literature implicating a given medication to an altered treatment outcome, is vital in accurately gauging the reliability, accuracy, and the applicability of the scientific literature in guiding an evidence-based practice.

CLINICS CARE POINTS

- During treatment planning discussions, it is essential for the practitioner to factor in the impact of medications a patient may be taking on any of the proposed treatment outcomes.

- Accurate prognostication and assessment of the risks and benefits for a planned treatment should include such clinical considerations.

- Among the medications reviewed in this article, such an impact has been validated for antiresorptive medications, with an increased risk for MRONJ, and less well-established adverse impact on the success of implant-based treatments.

- The literature is still evolving for other medications reviewed here and warrants more stringent validation from pharmacoepidemiologic studies.

- In the absence of clinical practice guidelines that integrate and appraise the body of evidence, the practitioner should factor in the level of evidence, and engage in active critical appraisal of the literature before incorporating study findings into practice.

DISCLOSURE

The authors report no conflict of interests. Author contributions are as follows: G. Subramanian: Concept, manuscript first draft, discussion. D.C. Thomas: Cardiovascular drugs (diuretics, antiplatelets and anticoagulants, antihypertensives). D. Bhatnagar: NSAIDs. S.Y. P. Quek: Concept, manuscript review/edits.

REFERENCES

1. Drake MT, Clarke BL, Khosla S. Bisphosphonates: mechanism of action and role in clinical practice. Mayo Clin Proc 2008;83(9):1032–45.
2. Pageau SC. Denosumab. mAbs 2009;1(3):210–5.

3. Ruggiero SL, Dodson TB, Aghaloo T, et al. American Association of Oral and Maxillofacial Surgeons' Position Paper on Medication-Related Osteonecrosis of the Jaws-2022 Update. J Oral Maxillofac Surg 2022;80(5):920–43.

4. Vahtsevanos K, Kyrgidis A, Verrou E, et al. Longitudinal cohort study of risk factors in cancer patients of bisphosphonate-related osteonecrosis of the jaw. J Clin Oncol 2009;27(32):5356–62.

5. Gelazius R, Poskevicius L, Sakavicius D, et al. Dental implant placement in patients on bisphosphonate therapy: a systematic review. J Oral Maxillofac Res 2018;9(3):e2.

6. Giovannacci I, Meleti M, Manfredi M, et al. Medication-related osteonecrosis of the jaw around dental implants: implant surgery-triggered or implant presence-triggered osteonecrosis? J Craniofac Surg 2016;27(3):697–701.

7. O'Carrigan B, Wong MHF, Willson ML, et al. Bisphosphonates and other bone agents for breast cancer. Cochrane Database Syst Rev 2017;(10):CD003474.

8. Jung J, Ryu JI, Shim GJ, et al. Effect of agents affecting bone homeostasis on short- and long-term implant failure. Clin Oral Implants Res 2023;34(Suppl 26): 143–68.

9. D'Ambrosio F, Amato A, Chiacchio A, et al. Do systemic diseases and medications influence dental implant osseointegration and dental implant health? An umbrella review. Dent J 2023;11(6):146.

10. Chappuis V, Avila-Ortiz G, Araujo MG, et al. Medication-related dental implant failure: systematic review and meta-analysis. Clin Oral Implants Res 2018; 29(Suppl 16):55–68.

11. Kwon TG, Lee CO, Park JW, et al. Osteonecrosis associated with dental implants in patients undergoing bisphosphonate treatment. Clin Oral Implants Res 2014; 25(5):632–40.

12. Kostenuik PJ, Binkley N, Anderson PA. Advances in osteoporosis therapy: focus on osteoanabolic agents, secondary fracture prevention, and perioperative bone health. Curr Osteoporos Rep 2023;21(4):386–400.

13. Kendler DL, Marin F, Zerbini CAF, et al. Effects of teriparatide and risedronate on new fractures in post-menopausal women with severe osteoporosis (VERO): a multicentre, double-blind, double-dummy, randomised controlled trial. Lancet 2018;391(10117):230–40.

14. Russow G, Jahn D, Appelt J, et al. Anabolic therapies in osteoporosis and bone regeneration. Int J Mol Sci 2018;20(1).

15. Cosman F. The evolving role of anabolic therapy in the treatment of osteoporosis. Curr Opin Rheumatol 2019;31(4):376–80.

16. Zandi M, Dehghan A, Gheysari F, et al. Evaluation of teriparatide effect on healing of autografted mandibular defects in rats. J Cranio-Maxillo-Fac Surg 2019;47(1): 120–6.

17. Pelled G, Lieber R, Avalos P, et al. Teriparatide (recombinant parathyroid hormone 1-34) enhances bone allograft integration in a clinically relevant pig model of segmental mandibulectomy. J Tissue Eng Regen Med 2020;14(8):1037–49.

18. Beth-Tasdogan NH, Mayer B, Hussein H, et al. Interventions for managing medication-related osteonecrosis of the jaw. Cochrane Database Syst Rev 2022;7(7):CD012432.

19. Sim IW, Borromeo GL, Tsao C, et al. Teriparatide promotes bone healing in medication-related osteonecrosis of the jaw: a placebo-controlled, randomized trial. J Clin Oncol 2020;38(26):2971–80.

20. Deeming GM, Collingwood J, Pemberton MN. Methotrexate and oral ulceration. Br Dent J 2005;198(2):83–5.

21. Schelzel G, Palicherla A, Tauseef A, et al. Low-dose methotrexate toxicity leading to pancytopenia: leucovorin as a rescue treatment. SAVE Proc 2024;37(2): 339–43.

22. Mathai PC, Andrade NN, Aggarwal N, et al. Low-dose methotrexate in rheumatoid arthritis: a potential risk factor for bisphosphonate-induced osteonecrosis of the jaw. Oral Maxillofac Surg 2018;22(2):235–40.

23. Prasanthi B, Kannan N, Patil R. Effect of diuretics on salivary flow, composition and oral health status: a clinico-biochemical study. Ann Med Health Sci Res 2014;4(4):549–53.

24. Wolff A, Joshi RK, Ekstrom J, et al. A guide to medications inducing salivary gland dysfunction, xerostomia, and subjective sialorrhea: a systematic review sponsored by the World Workshop on Oral Medicine VI. Drugs R 2017; 17(1):1–28.

25. Tschoppe P, Wolgin M, Pischon N, et al. Etiologic factors of hyposalivation and consequences for oral health. Quintessence Int 2010;41(4):321–33.

26. Turner M, Jahangiri L, Ship JA. Hyposalivation, xerostomia and the complete denture: a systematic review. J Am Dent Assoc 2008;139(2):146–50.

27. Leinonen J, Vahanikkila H, Raninen E, et al. The survival time of restorations is shortened in patients with dry mouth. J Dent 2021;113:103794.

28. Hahnel S, Schwarz S, Zeman F, et al. Prevalence of xerostomia and hyposalivation and their association with quality of life in elderly patients in dependence on dental status and prosthetic rehabilitation: a pilot study. J Dent 2014;42(6): 664–70.

29. Mizutani S, Ekuni D, Tomofuji T, et al. Relationship between xerostomia and gingival condition in young adults. J Periodontal Res 2015;50(1):74–9.

30. Mingarro-de-Leon A, Chaveli-Lopez B, Gavalda-Esteve C. Dental management of patients receiving anticoagulant and/or antiplatelet treatment. J Clin Exp Dent 2014;6(2):e155–61.

31. Thean D, Alberghini M. Anticoagulant therapy and its impact on dental patients: a review. Aust Dent J 2016;61(2):149–56.

32. Apostu D, Lucaciu O, Lucaciu GD, et al. Systemic drugs that influence titanium implant osseointegration. Drug Metab Rev 2017;49(1):92–104.

33. Corbella S, Morandi P, Alberti A, et al. The effect of the use of proton pump inhibitors, serotonin uptake inhibitors, antihypertensive, and anti-inflammatory drugs on clinical outcomes of functional dental implants: a retrospective study. Clin Oral Implants Res 2022;33(8):834–43.

34. Etikala A, Tattan M, Askar H, et al. Effects of NSAIDs on periodontal and dental implant therapy. Compend Contin Educ Dent 2019;40(2):e1–9.

35. Winnett B, Tenenbaum HC, Ganss B, et al. Perioperative use of non-steroidal anti-inflammatory drugs might impair dental implant osseointegration. Clin Oral Implants Res 2016;27(2):e1–7.

36. Fang J, Li Y, Zhang K, et al. Escaping the adverse impacts of NSAIDs on tooth movement during orthodontics: current evidence based on a meta-analysis. Medicine (Baltim) 2016;95(16):e3256.

37. Read JK, McClanahan SB, Khan AA, et al. Effect of ibuprofen on masking endodontic diagnosis. J Endod 2014;40(8):1058–62.

38. Cai WX, Ma L, Zheng LW, et al. Influence of non-steroidal anti-inflammatory drugs (NSAIDs) on osseointegration of dental implants in rabbit calvaria. Clin Oral Implants Res 2015;26(4):478–83.

39. Strom BL, Kimmel SE, Hennessy S. Pharmacoepidemiology. Hoboken, United Kingdom. Incorporated: John Wiley & Sons; 2012.

40. Sivakumar I, Arunachalam S, Choudhary S, et al. Does HIV infection affect the survival of dental implants? A systematic review and meta-analysis. J Prosthet Dent 2021;125(6):862–9.

41. Tonini KR, Hadad H, Egas LS, et al. Successful osseointegrated implants in hypertensive patients: retrospective clinical study. Int J Oral Maxillofac Implants 2022;37(3):501–7.

42. Seki K, Hasuike A, Iwano Y, et al. Influence of antihypertensive medications on the clinical parameters of anodized dental implants: a retrospective cohort study. Int. J. Implant Dent. 2020;6(1):32.

43. Wu X, Al-Abedalla K, Eimar H, et al. Antihypertensive medications and the survival rate of osseointegrated dental implants: a cohort study. Clin Implant Dent Relat Res 2016;18(6):1171–82.

44. Mishra SK, Sonnahalli NK, Chowdhary R. Do antihypertensive medications have an effect on dental implants? A systematic review. Oral Maxillofac Surg 2024; 28(2):459–68.

45. Gunes N, Gul M, Dundar S, et al. Effects of systemic propranolol application on the new bone formation in periimplant guided bone regeneration. J Oral Maxillofac Res 2021;12(3):e2.

46. Saravi B, Vollmer A, Lang G, et al. Impact of renin-angiotensin system inhibitors and beta-blockers on dental implant stability. Int. J. Implant Dent. 2021;7(1):31.

47. Fardal O, Lygre H. Management of periodontal disease in patients using calcium channel blockers: gingival overgrowth, prescribed medications, treatment responses and added treatment costs. J Clin Periodontol 2015;42(7):640–6.

48. Hill AB. The environment and disease: association or causation? Proc R Soc Med 1965;58(5):295–300.

49. Hill AB. The environment and disease: association or causation? 1965. J R Soc Med 2015;108(1):32–7.

50. Greenhalgh T. How to read a paper: the basics of evidence-based medicine and healthcare. 6th edition. Hoboken, NJ: Wiley-Blackwell; 2019.

51. Guyatt GH, Oxman AD, Vist GE, et al. GRADE: an emerging consensus on rating quality of evidence and strength of recommendations. BMJ 2008;336(7650): 924–6.

52. Murad MH, Asi N, Alsawas M, et al. New evidence pyramid. Evid Based Med 2016;21(4):125–7.

53. Sackett DL, Rosenberg WM, Gray JA, et al. Evidence based medicine: what it is and what it isn't. BMJ 1996;312(7023):71–2.

54. du Prel JB, Röhrig B, Blettner M. Critical appraisal of scientific articles: part 1 of a series on evaluation of scientific publications. Dtsch Arztebl Int 2009;106(7): 100–5.

55. Röhrig B, du Prel JB, Blettner M. Study design in medical research: part 2 of a series on the evaluation of scientific publications. Dtsch Arztebl Int 2009; 106(11):184–9.

56. Grimes DA, Schulz KF. Bias and causal associations in observational research. Lancet 2002;359(9302):248–52.

57. Marx RE. Pamidronate (Aredia) and zoledronate (Zometa) induced avascular necrosis of the jaws: a growing epidemic. J Oral Maxillofac Surg 2003;61(9): 1115–7.

58. Ruggiero SL, Mehrotra B, Rosenberg TJ, et al. Osteonecrosis of the jaws associated with the use of bisphosphonates: a review of 63 cases. J Oral Maxillofac Surg 2004;62(5):527–34.

59. Zhang C, Shen G, Li H, et al. Incidence rate of osteonecrosis of jaw after cancer treated with bisphosphonates and denosumab: a systematic review and meta-analysis. Spec Care Dentist 2024;44(2):530–41.

60. Everts-Graber J, Lehmann D, Burkard JP, et al. Risk of osteonecrosis of the jaw under denosumab compared to bisphosphonates in patients with osteoporosis. J Bone Miner Res 2022;37(2):340–8.

61. Tetradis S, Allen MR, Ruggiero SL. Pathophysiology of medication-related osteonecrosis of the jaw: a minireview. JBMR Plus 2023;7(8):e10785.

62. Ruggiero SL, Dodson TB, Assael LA, et al. American Association of Oral and Maxillofacial Surgeons position paper on bisphosphonate-related osteonecrosis of the jaws: 2009 update. J Oral Maxillofac Surg 2009;67(5 Suppl):2–12.

63. Ruggiero SL, Dodson TB, Fantasia J, et al. American Association of Oral and Maxillofacial Surgeons position paper on medication-related osteonecrosis of the jaw: 2014 update. J Oral Maxillofac Surg 2014;72(10):1938–56.

64. Advisory Task Force on Bisphosphonate-Related Osteonecrosis of the Jaws AAoO, Maxillofacial S. American Association of Oral and Maxillofacial Surgeons position paper on bisphosphonate-related osteonecrosis of the jaws. J Oral Maxillofac Surg 2007;65(3):369–76.

65. Khan AA, Morrison A, Hanley DA, et al. Diagnosis and management of osteonecrosis of the jaw: a systematic review and international consensus. J Bone Miner Res 2015;30(1):3–23.

66. Fusco V, Santini D, Armento G, et al. Osteonecrosis of jaw beyond antiresorptive (bone-targeted) agents: new horizons in oncology. Expert Opin Drug Saf 2016;15(7):925–35.

67. Nicolatou-Galitis O, Kouri M, Papadopoulou E, et al. Osteonecrosis of the jaw related to non-antiresorptive medications: a systematic review. Support Care Cancer 2019;27(2):383–94.

68. King R, Tanna N, Patel V. Medication-related osteonecrosis of the jaw unrelated to bisphosphonates and denosumab-a review. Oral Surg Oral Med Oral Pathol Oral Radiol 2019;127(4):289–99.

69. Sacco R, Shah S, Leeson R, et al. Osteonecrosis and osteomyelitis of the jaw associated with tumour necrosis factor-alpha (TNF-alpha) inhibitors: a systematic review. Br J Oral Maxillofac Surg 2020;58(1):25–33.

70. Al-Nawas B, Lambert F, Andersen SWM, et al. Group 3 ITI Consensus Report: materials and antiresorptive drug-associated outcomes in implant dentistry. Clin Oral Implants Res 2023;34(Suppl 26):169–76.

71. Khairnar S, Bhate K, S NS, et al. Comparative evaluation of low-level laser therapy and ultrasound heat therapy in reducing temporomandibular joint disorder pain. J Dent Anesth Pain Med 2019;19(5):289–94.

Systemic Factors Affecting Healing in Dentistry

Mahnaz Fatahzadeh, DMD, MSD[a], Anjali Ravi, BDS[b],*,
Prisly Thomas, BDS, MDS[c], Vincent B. Ziccardi, DDS, MD[d]

KEYWORDS

- Wound • Healing • Cancer • Inflammation • Re-epithelization • Bone healing
- Oral mucosa

KEY POINTS

- Oral Wound healing, is a dynamic process consisting of precisely sequences and continuous stages. It occurs in a dynamic environment with variations in temperature, moisture, and a rich oral microbiome.
- Oral wound healing is significantly influenced by systemic factors such as but not limited to age, sex, stress, diet, medical conditions (diabetes), and behaviors (drinking alcohol and smoking) by various mechanisms.
- Diabetes disrupts the healing of oral mucosal wounds through various mechanisms including inflammation, growth factor imbalances, and changes in saliva composition.
- Smoking impedes the healing of oral wounds in numerous ways, eventually causing complications and prolonging healing time.
- Challenges posed by chemotherapy may exacerbate the healing process for cancer patients.

INTRODUCTION

Dentistry is primarily considered a surgical discipline with a variety of soft and hard tissue procedures, the success of which relies on the innate ability of the body to repair itself. Exodontia, one of the most commonly performed oral surgical procedures, also follows an uncomplicated process of healing in most cases.[1,2] Wound healing is

Funding statement: There was no funding for this article.
[a] Division of Oral Medicine, Department of Diagnostic Sciences, Rutgers School of Dental Medicine, 110 Bergen Street, Newark, NJ 07103, USA; [b] University of Pittsburgh School of Dental Medicine, 341 Darragh Street, Unit 313, Pittsburgh, PA 15213, USA; [c] Diplomate American Board of Orofacial Pain, Believers Church Medical College Hospital, St. Thomas Nagar Kuttapuzha, Thiruvalla Kerala-689103, India; [d] Department of Oral and Maxillofacial Surgery, Rutgers School of Dental Medicine, Room B854, 110 Bergen Street, Newark, NJ 07103, USA
* Corresponding author. DMD Candidate, Class of 2026, University of Pittsburgh School of Dental Medicine, 341 Darragh Street, Unit 313, Pittsburgh, PA 15213.
E-mail address: aanjali1296@gmail.com

Dent Clin N Am 68 (2024) 799–812
https://doi.org/10.1016/j.cden.2024.05.008
0011-8532/24/© 2024 Elsevier Inc. All rights reserved, including those for text and data mining, AI training, and similar technologies.

dental.theclinics.com

considered a dynamic biological process composed of 4 precisely sequenced and continuous stages including hemostasis, inflammation, proliferation, and remodeling, which ultimately restores the structure and function of the damaged or lost tissues.[3–7] Wound healing is the body's innate defense mechanism, prioritizing rapid recovery and restoration. The oral environment is considerably dynamic, with variations in temperatures, moisture, and the diversity of the oral microbiome.[8] The success of wound healing in the oral cavity is influenced by local factors, systemic factors, and a possible interplay between them.[8] Local factors such as early clot dissolution, improper surgical techniques, infection, and presence of foreign bodies directly impact the site of injury.[1,5] In contrast, systemic factors refer to the patient's overall state of health or disease that influences the propensity for healing.[5] Examples of systemic factors include aging, malnutrition, immunosuppression, metastatic cancer, medications, diabetes mellitus, and smoking.[1,3,4] As our current knowledge and perception of wound healing advances, the relevance of systemic factors on the same is becoming more apparent.

DEFINITION

A wound is described as a disturbance in the normal anatomic structures and their proper functioning.[9,10] The term healing is derived from the word, "haelen," which denotes wholeness. It also refers to a systematic series of steps in order to achieve a state of completeness or cohesion.[11] This process consists of a series of complex cellular and biochemical steps to ensure the restoration of normal anatomy and function of the injured tissues.[9,12] Regeneration restores tissue structurally and functionally, while repair relies on fibrous scar tissue for tissue integrity.[9,13]

CLASSIFICATION OF WOUND HEALING

Wound healing is divided into 3 types namely primary, secondary, and tertiary wound healing.[9,14] In healing by primary intention, the tissues are approximated by sutures. It is characterized by clean healing with minimal tissue loss and scar formation.[9,14–16] Wounds that heal by secondary intention present with extensive loss of tissue and a large defect that is allowed to granulate and heal on its own.[9,14–16] The wound is unable to be sutured and healing may be delayed for several weeks depending on the size, depth, and location of the wound. Inherent in this process is the formation of a scar and increased amount of granulation tissue.[9,14,17] Formation of eschar within the wound bed can lead to further delays in healing and subsequent scar formation. Intentional delay in closing a wound is healing by tertiary intention. This is utilized when resolution of inflammation or infection prior to closing the wound to clear microorganisms, debris, or edema is anticipated. When healing by secondary intention is interrupted, healing by tertiary intention ensues.[9,17,18]

PROCESS OF WOUND HEALING

A variety of cell types contribute to this highly regulated progression of events and perform various functions depending on the specific phase of healing. The 4 phases of wound healing include hemostasis, inflammatory, proliferative, and remodeling.[5] Wound healing begins with hemostasis characterized by vascular contraction together with formation and stabilization of a platelet plug.[5] During inflammatory phase, the release of proinflammatory cytokines and growth factors from the clot and the wound promotes migration of neutrophils, macrophages, and lymphocytes to the injured site.[4,5,7,19] The proliferative phase involves the activation of keratinocytes, fibroblasts, and endothelial cells, together with angiogenesis, collagen synthesis, and formation of a provisional scaffold (glycosaminoglycans, proteoglycan) for tissue regeneration and re-epithelialization.[4,5,20] Finally, during the remodeling phase, wound contracts and assumes nearly normal architecture and vascular density.[5,7,19] When repair involves osseous tissues such as the one encountered in an extraction socket, osteoprogenitor and mesenchymal cells produce osteoid, which develops into woven bone. Upon remodeling by osteoblasts and osteoclasts, this tissue becomes mature lamellar bone.[1,20] Although wound healing is a routine intrinsic process, a variety of local and systemic factors could modify or disrupt it.[1,3–6,21]

WOUND HEALING IN THE ORAL CAVITY VERSUS SKIN

The skin and gingiva are thought to be structurally and functionally homogenous tissues and exhibit identical wound-healing patterns. Each is distinguished by the presence of keratinized epithelium with underlying connective tissue, which serves as a defense against microorganisms and other contaminants.[22] Cutaneous and gingival tissues share macroscopic healing stages—hemostasis, inflammation, proliferation, and collagen remodeling—but exhibit distinct responses at the molecular level.[23] Oral wounds heal considerably faster than skin wounds, demonstrating quick re-epithelialization and remodeling that results in minimal scarring despite the presence

Table 1 Wound healing process in various areas of the oral cavity	
Hard palate[8,27]	a. Healthy underlying bone is critical for wound healing b. Complications: • Significant scarring or communication to the antrum and nasal cavity • Decreased maxillary transverse width, in the case of patients in active phase of growth
Socket healing[8,23]	Part of the healing process after tooth extraction Approximate sequence following extraction: • Clot formation • Re-epithelialization commences after 24 h • Granulation tissue replaces the clot after a week • Bone completely fills the extraction site in 8 wk Bone remodeling reduces alveolar width and height over the course of 6 mo caused by bone remodeling
Dental pulp[8,28]	• Maintenance of odontoblastic layer and apical blood supply is crucial • When intact, odontoblasts and Hoehl's cells promote reactionary tubular/atubular dentin formation • Pulpal stem/progenitor cells can differentiate into cells that make osteodentin or reparative dentin
Implant–tissue interface[8]	• Healing of the soft tissue over the cover screw occurs without extensive granulation tissue • At the implant-osteotomy interface post placement—blood clots form within implant grooves—immune cell infiltration occurs—granulation tissue vascularized by endothelial cells—created by fibroblast granulation tissue matures into osteoblasts—formation of bone reaches their peak in 3 mo
Areas affected by burn[8,27]	• Burns to the face or oral cavity cause compromised wound healing and noticeable scarring • These burns continue to affect deeper structures for 48–72 h due to vascular and inflammatory reactions

of oral microorganisms and saliva.[8,23,24] Growth factors and cytokines found in saliva, as well as the critical function of fibroblasts, may be responsible for this efficiency. Presence of proteins such as lactoferrin, lysozyme, and epidermal growth factors (EGFs) in saliva also contribute to antimicrobial and anti-inflammatory properties of oral biofluid.[25,26] Specifics of the wound healing process in various areas of the oral cavity is elaborated in **Table 1**.

SYSTEMIC FACTORS AFFECTING HEALING IN THE ORAL CAVITY
Age

Aging affects every phase of the healing process. Older adults tend to heal wounds slower than younger adults, even after accounting for factors such as medication use and concomitant health conditions.[29] The contributing mechanisms include increased platelet aggregation, elevation of mediators of inflammation, impaired function of macrophages and lymphocytes, reduction in growth factors, and delay in re-epithelialization. Aging also adversely affects angiogenesis, collagen formation, and wound strength.[5,7] The concentration of histatins, a group of salivary antimicrobial peptides (AMPs), reduces with aging. Histatin-1 and Histatin-2 play a crucial role in oral wound healing by facilitating tissue re-epithelialization and angiogenesis.[30–32] Age-related alterations in immune and nonimmune cells within the oral mucosa also hinder the wound healing process.[30]

Sex

Reduction in inflammation is associated with enhanced wound healing and generally forms the foundation for faster mucosal healing as compared to dermal.[33,34] Studies reveal that sex hormones affect the healing of both oral mucosal and dermal wounds, but they may do so in distinct ways, potentially promoting opposing outcomes in the healing process.[29,35] Oral mucosal wound healing in women has been found to be slower compared to men.[29] It is postulated that increased levels of testosterone (known for its potent anti-inflammatory properties) in saliva and mucosal fluids may serve as a potential factor in enhanced mucosal wound healing in men.[29,35] In contrast, it has been shown that estrogen deficiency-induced osteoporosis in rats could lead to reduction of cancellous bone volume and disruption of contact between the bone and implant. This results in impaired healing of bone around dental implants.[36] It has been reported that both age and gender play significant roles in mucosal wound healing, with women of older age, particularly at risk for delayed healing following oral or mucosal surgery or injury.[29]

Stress

The negative influence of stress on wound healing primarily occurs through the involvement of the hypothalamic-pituitary-adrenal and sympathetic-adrenal medullary systems.[5,37,38] These systems control the release of certain hormones and other biological molecules such as cortisol, adrenocorticotrophic hormones, prolactin, epinephrine, and norepinephrine. Stress increases cortisol levels and reduces proinflammatory cytokines, which are critical for wound healing. It also decreases the expression of interleukin (IL)-1α and IL-8, essential for the initial phase of inflammatory cascade in healing.[5,37,38] Furthermore, cortisol affects the function of immune cells.[5,39] These anti-inflammatory actions of cortisol delay the normal immune response at the wound site and prolong wound healing under psychological stress.[5,37] Besides the direct effects of stress-induced anxiety and depression on the endocrine and immune systems, individuals under stress may be prone to adopting unhealthy habits, including irregular sleep patterns, malnutrition, reduced physical activity, and a higher likelihood of substance abuse (alcohol, cigarettes, and other drugs). These various factors could collectively undermine the healing process.[5]

Nutrition

The impact of nutritional state on optimal healing of wounds created by trauma or surgical intervention has long been recognized.[40] This is particularly relevant to patients with cancer who frequently undergo surgical procedures, receive therapeutic regimens with deleterious effects on tissues, suffer from disease or treatment-related stress, and are often malnourished due to inability to eat or tolerate food.[1,5,6,41,42] An elevation of up to 40% in basal energy consumption caused by disease and stress has been reported in patients with advanced disease states.[6] Metabolic demands of patients with cancer could also be magnified by expanding local tumor burden and/or progressive metastatic disease.[6] In addition, nutritional depletion and the onset of catabolic state in severely ill individuals have a profound and detrimental impact on cellular and humoral immunity, capacity for tissue repair, susceptibility to wound infection, and thereby potentially affecting the disease outcome.[6,43,44] Therefore, the evaluation of nutritional status is an essential component of therapeutic planning for these patients in order to minimize complications and optimize healing.[6] Adequate and timely correction of nutritional deficiencies in this patient population is necessary to improve tolerance of therapeutic interventions, support proper wound healing, and reduce disease-related morbidity and mortality.[5,6,41] In some patients, nutritional

Table 2	
Nutritional substances and their role in healing process	
Protein	a. Essential role in wound healing (angiogenesis, fibroblastic proliferation, collagen formation, proteoglycan production, and wound remodeling)[1,5]
Glucose	a. Generation of cellular ATP and energy for neovascularization and tissue repair during the healing process[5,43]
	b. Prevents breakdown of proteins for energy production during gluconeogenesis[42]
Arginine	a. Supports collagen synthesis (precursor to proline, a component of collagen), vascular proliferation, and wound contraction[19,40]
Glutamine	a. Major source of metabolic energy for rapidly dividing cells[5,19]
	b. Critical contribution to early inflammatory phase of wound healing[5,45]
Lipids	a. Provide energy and critical building blocks for tissue regeneration[5,43]
Vitamin C	a. An important cofactor for collagen synthesis (hydroxylation of proline and lysine residues involved in collagen polymerization, cross-linking, stability, and extracellular secretion)[6,40]
	b. Promotes angiogenesis and fibroblastic proliferation[5]
	c. Contributes to wound tensile strength[6]
Vitamin A	a. Recruitment of macrophages into wounds[6]
	b. Fibroblastic proliferation, collagen synthesis, and cross-linking[40]
	c. Epithelialization and wound closure[6]
Magnesium	a. Cofactor for many enzymes involved in protein and collagen production[45]
Copper	a. Optimal cross-linking of collagen[43]
Zinc	a. DNA and RNA synthesis, protein production, and cellular proliferation[6,40]
Iron	a. Support for collagen synthesis (required for hydroxylation of proline and lysine)[5,19]

support and exogenous supplementation of appropriate substrates may be started preoperatively to build up resources in anticipation of diminished dietary intake and increased metabolic needs associated with disease and planned therapeutic interventions.[6] The energy demands and nutritional needs of patients with cancer are complex and intended to support wound repair, attenuate tissue catabolism, and promote recovery. Dietary requirements of these patients include proteins, carbohydrates, lipids, amino acids, vitamins, minerals, and hematinic including iron, folate, and vitamin B12 required for the formation of blood cells.[1,6,41,42,45] **Table 2** provides a summary of the role of various elements of composite nutrition in the healing process.

Ischemic Conditions

Sufficient oxygen is crucial for producing adenosine triphosphate (ATP), vital in the energy-intensive wound healing process. Optimal oxygen levels are necessary to

Table 3	
The influence of diabetes on the re-epithelization of oral wounds	
Slower oral mucosal healing in diabetes[49,51,52]	• Both type 1 and type 2 diabetes models exhibit slower oral mucosal wound healing • Delayed healing is attributed to the direct impact of elevated glucose levels and indirect effects • Increased inflammation together with elevated advanced glycation end-product (AGE) and reactive oxygen species hinder the migration of oral and skin keratinocytes
Inflammatory and growth factor imbalance[49,52]	• Increased levels of tumor necrosis factor (TNF) and IL-1β and reduced levels of growth factors such as fibroblast growth factor 2 (FGF-2) and transforming growth factor -β (TGF-β) in oral wounds of diabetics. This combination negatively affects keratinocyte migration and the overall healing process
Role of saliva[49,53]	• Diabetes alters saliva composition (reduced EGF levels). This negatively impacting re-epithelialization • Diabetics have lower levels of AMPs such as histatins. This hinders keratinocyte migration and the body's defense against microbes
MMPs and delayed healing[49,54]	• High MMP-9 levels are associated with reduced keratinocyte migration in high-glucose conditions • Elevated MMP-2 and MMP-9 levels in the saliva from patients with diabetes may further impair re-epithelialization
Inflammation and neutrophils[49,50]	• Diabetes extends the inflammatory phase of oral wound healing, characterized by increased neutrophils • TNF inhibitors enhance re-epithelialization in diabetic wounds, emphasizing the problematic role of elevated TNF levels
Bacterial challenges[5,49]	• Bacterial colonization exacerbates inflammation, delaying the healing process
Direct effects of bacteria[49,55]	• Bacteria directly influence keratinocytes by causing apoptosis, impairing cell migration, and inhibiting cell proliferation • *Porphyromonas gingivalis* and *Fusobacterium nucleatum* infiltrate oral keratinocytes, disrupting the re-epithelialization process

prevent infections and facilitate wound contraction, promote angiogenesis, support the regrowth of skin cells (re-epithelialization) and the subsequent synthesis of collagen.[46] Insufficient oxygen levels lead to compromised wound healing.[47] Ischemia, a condition associated with chronic wounds that resist healing, can occur due to problems like inadequate arterial blood flow, high venous pressure, and pressure-related injuries.[48]

Diabetes

Diabetes disrupts the healing of oral mucosal wounds through various mechanisms including inflammation, growth factor imbalances, changes in saliva composition, increased levels of matrix metalloproteinases (MMPs), and alteration in macrophage phenotypes. Dysregulation of MMPs can lead to prolonged inflammation and delayed wound healing. Additionally, bacterial colonization can further delay the healing process in the oral cavity.[49–52] The mechanisms by which diabetes influences the re-epithelization of oral wounds is summarized in **Table 3**. Diabetes also significantly impacts bone healing in the oral cavity. It disrupts the coordinated activity of osteoclasts, osteoblasts, and mesenchymal stem cells, impairing bone formation. High glucose levels in diabetes increase osteoclast numbers, inhibit fibroblast and osteoblast expansion, and hinder progenitor cell proliferation and osteogenic differentiation. This results in reduced osteoid matrix production and cellularity in diabetic bone healing. Diabetes also suppresses the expression of critical transcription factors responsible for osteoblast formation.[56,57] Furthermore, diabetes can activate inflammatory pathways and reduce the expression of growth factors necessary for osteogenesis.

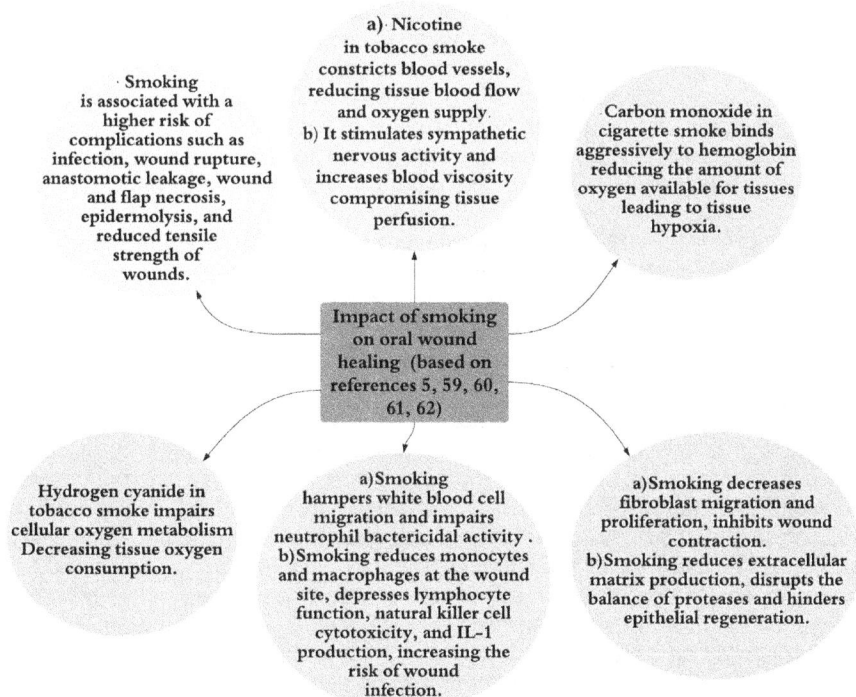

Fig. 1. Key concepts regarding detrimental impact of smoking on oral healing.

Prolonged inflammation due to diabetes negatively affects bone formation by blocking the expression of bone matrix proteins. Additionally, diabetes interferes with proper immune functions, increasing the risk of infectious complications during bone healing.[49,58] Patients with diabetes should be optimized medically prior to any elective surgical procedures.

Smoking

Smoking has a multitude of detrimental effects on oral wound healing, leading to various complications and delayed recovery. The key concepts regarding detrimental impact of smoking on oral wound healing are illustrated in **Fig. 1**.[5,59–62]

Alcohol

Alcohol consumption is known to significantly hinder wound healing and increase the risk of infections.[5,63] Acute alcohol exposure tends to suppress the release of proinflammatory cytokines leading to decreased neutrophil recruitment and impaired phagocytic function, all of which promote the risk of infection postinjury.[64] Acute alcohol exposure can also disrupt various aspects of the healing process including re-epithelialization, angiogenesis, collagen production, and wound closure.[5,65] Notably, wound angiogenesis is significantly reduced after even a single episode of alcohol consumption. This results in increased wound hypoxia and oxidative stresses. Chronic alcohol exposure also impairs wound healing and host resistance to infections, but the underlying mechanisms require further investigation.[5,66]

Hereditary Conditions

Wound healing is a complex process also influenced by genetic factors. Genetic defects can result in various clinical conditions including immune system disorders, hemoglobin synthesis disorders, vasculopathies, connective tissue diseases, and progeroid syndromes, which are hereditary conditions causing premature physiologic aging.[67,68] Certain genetic conditions, like Down's syndrome and Ataxia-telangiectasia, can also lead to abnormal wound healing.[67,69,70] Furthermore, immune system disorders like leukocyte adhesion deficiencies and transporter associated with antigen processing deficiency syndrome are recognized as risk factors for impaired wound healing because they play a specific role in the inflammatory phase of the healing process.[67,68,71,72] The literature indicates that Ehlers-Danlos and Marfan syndromes are associated with impaired wound healing.[73] However, there is limited evidence to suggest that these inherited conditions impact the healing process in the oral cavity.[8] Wound healing in the mouth poses challenges for individuals with osteogenesis imperfecta or epidermolysis bullosa.[8]

Metastatic Cancer

Metastasis is a hallmark of malignancy and accounts for the majority of cancer deaths.[74] It refers to the spread of malignant cells to distant locations and formation of secondary tumors at the new sites. Metastasis to the cutaneous site of injury including surgical incisions is a well-recognized but rare phenomenon.[75,76] In general, metastasis to the oral cavity is uncommon with mandible and gingiva being the most commonly reported osseous and soft tissue targets, respectively.[77] In a 1993 study, authors reported 55 cases of metastasis to postextraction sites, the majority of which were nonhealing sockets and contained a soft tissue mass. They surmised that, in some cases, cancer was likely present at the site prior to the tooth removal while in others metastasis could have developed after the tooth extraction; they postulated that tooth extraction might promote metastatic spread.[77] Metastasis is a complex process, which requires cells to successfully detach from the primary tumor, penetrate tissues, intravasate blood or lymphatics, extravasate, take hold, and generate secondary growths at the new sites.[74] Only a small number of cells separated from the original tumor actually survive immune surveillance and the harsh microenvironment to ultimately develop metastatic neoplasia.[74] Some investigators propose that cells capable of metastasizing have unique properties different from the original tumor and are able to use the natural wound healing processes to their advantage and form cancerous growths in remote locations.[74] The consideration of "wound healing gone wrong" is not a new notion.[78] In 1858, Rudolph Virchow proposed a role for irritation and its resulting inflammation in the generation of neoplastic growth (irritation theory).[74,79] In 1980, Harold Dvorak who stated tumors are "wounds that do not heal" revisited this idea.[74,80] A 2020 study found that the expression of L1 cell adhesion molecule (L1CAM) on cells disseminated from colorectal cancer is necessary for successful metastasis to distant sites but not for the initiation of primary tumors.[78] Interestingly, normal wound repair also requires expression of L1CAM by epithelial cells separated from each other during tissue injury. They postulated that both normal and metastatic cells separated from their neighbors share the same marker of wound healing, which would allow them to, respectively, make new tissues for the closure of epithelial breach or colonize new sites and form secondary neoplasms.[78] As described earlier, natural wound healing is a well-coordinated and tightly controlled pathway with built-in positive and negative feedback mechanisms, the goal of which is to replace lost tissue mass and prevent excess regeneration.[74] It is also possible that in the context of a malignancy, chronic signaling emanated from tumor cells drive or override respective positive and/or negative feedback loops and lead to a state of pathologic inflammation.[3,5,74] This unchecked viscous cycle could not only impede progression to the final remodeling phase and postpone completion of wound healing but also support propagation of metastasis and cancer progression.[5,74] Understanding details of how wound healing and metastasis processes intersect may provide therapeutic opportunities to prevent the spread of malignancies.[74]

Chemotherapy for Cancer

In addition to malignant disease itself, factors such as chemotherapy, poor nutrition, and smoking could also compromise healing in patients afflicted with cancer.[6] Advanced chemotherapeutics, alone or as part of complex multimodal approaches can help reduce preoperative disease burden, eliminate postsurgical residual disease and improve cancer survival.[6] However, collateral tissue injury and impaired healing of wounds irrespective of their origin (caused by the primary disease, created by cancer surgery, or induced by chemo/radiation) remain significant concerns.[6] Available chemotherapy protocols utilize different classes of drugs such as alkylating agents (cyclophosphamide, chlorambucil, thiopeta, mechlorethamine, and cisplatin), antimetabolites (methotrexate, 5-fluorouracil, 6-mercaptopurine, and azathioprine), plant alkaloids (vincristine and vinblastine), antitumor antibiotics (bleomycin, doxorubicin, actinomycin D, and mitomycin C), and angiogenesis inhibitors (bevacizumab) in various combinations with each class having a unique anticancer mode of action.[6] Investigations in both animals and humans indicate that severity of healing complications varies with the specific class and number of drugs administered as well as dose, frequency, duration, and timing of chemotherapy.[6] In general, standard chemotherapeutic agents primarily target particular aspects of replication cycle in the rapidly dividing cells such as those found in bone marrow, hair follicles, gastrointestinal tract, or healing wounds.[6] These drugs could also negatively impact other cell types such as macrophages and fibroblasts that are critically involved in wound repair.[6] The overall effect of these agents on regeneration of lost tissue is a consequence of delayed cellular migration into the wound, reduced angiogenesis, decreased formation of early scaffold, impaired fibroblastic proliferation, attenuation of collagen synthesis, and prevention of wound contraction.[5,6,81] In addition, chemotherapy could impair proliferation of cells in bone marrow and induce neutropenia, anemia, and thrombocytopenia. These could, respectively, interfere with the inflammatory phase of healing cascade and render wounds susceptible to infection, diminish oxygen perfusion of tissues and promote local bleeding all of which are detrimental to optimal wound repair.[5] From a clinical stand point, timing of surgery and specific drug used in chemotherapy are important considerations for healing when planning surgical interventions or discussing potential complications with patients with cancer.[6]

SUMMARY

Wound healing in the oral cavity is a complex process influenced by a wide array of systemic factors. These include age, sex, stress, nutrition, underlying health status such as diabetes or hereditary conditions, and behavioral factors such as smoking and alcohol consumption all of which can significantly impact the body's ability to heal after oral procedures. In patients with cancer, challenges posed by chemotherapy could further complicate the healing process. Recognizing the intricate interplay between these systemic factors and the phases of wound healing is critical for providing effective and tailored care to dental patients. By understanding and addressing these systemic influences, dental professionals can minimize complications, optimize healing outcomes, and ultimately improve the overall well-being of individuals undergoing dental treatment.

CLINICS CARE POINTS

- Understanding the impact of various systemic factors on healing in the oral cavity is paramount for minimizing complications and optimizing outcomes while delivering dental care.
- Patients with diabetes should be optimized medically prior to any elective oral surgical procedures.
- Alcohol consumption is known to hinder wound healing and increase the risk of infections.
- Dental treatment failure can be attributed to persistent smoking habits particularly during the critical preoperative and postoperative healing periods.
- Understanding details of how wound healing and metastasis processes intersect may provide therapeutic opportunities to prevent the spread of malignancies.

ACKNOWLEDGMENTS

Stephen F Modica, MLS, Librarian for Information and Education Services, George F. Smith Library of the Health Sciences, Rutgers Biomedical and Health Sciences, Newark, NJ, USA.

DISCLOSURE

M. Fatahzadeh, A. Ravi, P. Thomas, and V.B. Ziccardi declare no conflict of interest. Statement of institutional review board approval or waiver: Institutional review and approval were not necessary for this article.

REFERENCES

1. Henry CJ, Stassen LFA. The non-healing extraction socket: a diagnostic dilemma - case report and discussion. J Ir Dent Assoc 2016;62(4):215–20.
2. Huebsch RF, Coleman RD, Frandsen AM, et al. The healing process following molar extraction. I. Normal male rats (long-evans strain). Oral Surg Oral Med Oral Pathol 1952;5(8):864–76.
3. Calis H, Sengul S, Guler Y, et al. Non-healing wounds: Can it take different diagnosis? Int Wound J 2020;17(2):443–8.
4. Deptuła M, Zieliński J, Wardowska A, et al. Wound healing complications in oncological patients: perspectives for cellular therapy. Postepy Dermatol Alergol 2019; 36(2):139–46.
5. Guo S, Dipietro LA. Factors affecting wound healing. J Dent Res 2010;89(3): 219–29.
6. Payne WG, Naidu DK, Wheeler CK, et al. Wound healing in patients with cancer. Eplasty 2008;8:e9.
7. Gosain A, DiPietro LA. Aging and wound healing. World J Surg 2004;28(3):321–6.
8. Politis C, Schoenaers J, Jacobs R, et al. Wound Healing Problems in the Mouth. Front Physiol 2016;7:507.
9. Chhabra S, Chhabra N, Kaur A, et al. Wound Healing Concepts in Clinical Practice of OMFS. J Maxillofac Oral Surg 2017;16(4):403–23.
10. Robson MC, Steed DL, Franz MG. Wound healing: biologic features and approaches to maximize healing trajectories. Curr Probl Surg 2001;38(2):72–140.
11. Firth K, Smith K, Sakallaris BR, et al. Healing, a Concept Analysis. Glob Adv Health Med 2015;4(6):44–50.
12. Wilkinson HN, Hardman MJ. Wound healing: cellular mechanisms and pathological outcomes. Open Biol 2020;10(9):200223.
13. Miloro M, Ghali GE, Larsen PE, et al. Peterson's principles of oral and maxillofacial surgery. Cham, Switzerland: Springer International Publishing; 2022.
14. Azmat CE, Council M. Wound closure techniques. StatPearls. Treasure Island (FL): StatPearls Publishing LLC; 2024.
15. Ozgok Kangal MK, Regan JP. Wound healing. StatPearls. Treasure Island (FL): StatPearls Publishing LLC; 2024.
16. Gantwerker EA, Hom DB. Skin: histology and physiology of wound healing. Facial Plast Surg Clin North Am 2011;19(3):441–53.
17. Kumar V, Abbas AK, Aster JC. Robbins and cotran pathologic basis of disease, professional edition E-book. Philadelphia, PA: Elsevier Health Sciences; 2014.
18. Healing by Intention. Adv Skin Wound Care 2017;246–7.
19. Campos AC, Groth AK, Branco AB. Assessment and nutritional aspects of wound healing. Curr Opin Clin Nutr Metab Care 2008;11(3):281–8.
20. Devlin H, Sloan P. Early bone healing events in the human extraction socket. Int J Oral Maxillofac Surg 2002;31(6):641–5.
21. Pollack SV. The wound healing process. Clin Dermatol 1984;2(3):8–16.
22. Nikoloudaki G, Creber K, Hamilton DW. Wound healing and fibrosis: a contrasting role for periostin in skin and the oral mucosa. Am J Physiol, Cell Physiol 2020; 318(6):C1065–77.
23. Cho YD, Kim KH, Lee YM, et al. Periodontal Wound Healing and Tissue Regeneration: A Narrative Review. Pharmaceuticals (Basel) 2021;14(5).
24. Iglesias-Bartolome R, Uchiyama A, Molinolo AA, et al. Transcriptional signature primes human oral mucosa for rapid wound healing. Sci Transl Med 2018; 10(451).

25. Katsani KR, Sakellari D. Saliva proteomics updates in biomedicine. J Biol Res (Thessalon) 2019;26:17.
26. Ahangar P, Mills SJ, Smith LE, et al. Human gingival fibroblast secretome accelerates wound healing through anti-inflammatory and pro-angiogenic mechanisms. NPJ Regen Med 2020;5(1):24.
27. Glim JE, van Egmond M, Niessen FB, et al. Detrimental dermal wound healing: what can we learn from the oral mucosa? Wound Repair Regen 2013;21(5): 648–60.
28. Dimitrova-Nakov S, Baudry A, Harichane Y, et al. Pulp stem cells: implication in reparative dentin formation. J Endod 2014;40(4 Suppl):S13–8.
29. Engeland CG, Bosch JA, Cacioppo JT, et al. Mucosal wound healing: the roles of age and sex. Arch Surg 2006;141(12):1193–7 ; discussion 98.
30. Villalobos V, Garrido M, Reyes A, et al. Aging envisage imbalance of the periodontium: A keystone in oral disease and systemic health. Front Immunol 2022; 13:1044334.
31. Cabras T, Pisano E, Boi R, et al. Age-dependent modifications of the human salivary secretory protein complex. J Proteome Res 2009;8(8):4126–34.
32. Oudhoff MJ, Kroeze KL, Nazmi K, et al. Structure-activity analysis of histatin, a potent wound healing peptide from human saliva: cyclization of histatin potentiates molar activity 1,000-fold. Faseb j 2009;23(11):3928–35.
33. Dovi JV, Szpaderska AM, DiPietro LA. Neutrophil function in the healing wound: adding insult to injury? Thromb Haemost 2004;92(2):275–80.
34. Szpaderska AM, Zuckerman JD, DiPietro LA. Differential injury responses in oral mucosal and cutaneous wounds. J Dent Res 2003;82(8):621–6.
35. Engeland CG, Sabzehei B, Marucha PT. Sex hormones and mucosal wound healing. Brain Behav Immun 2009;23(5):629–35.
36. Qi MC, Zhou XQ, Hu J, et al. Oestrogen replacement therapy promotes bone healing around dental implants in osteoporotic rats. Int J Oral Maxillofac Surg 2004;33(3):279–85.
37. Godbout JP, Glaser R. Stress-induced immune dysregulation: implications for wound healing, infectious disease and cancer. J Neuroimmune Pharmacol 2006;1(4):421–7.
38. Boyapati L, Wang HL. The role of stress in periodontal disease and wound healing. Periodontol 2000 2007;44:195–210.
39. Sternberg EM. Neural regulation of innate immunity: a coordinated nonspecific host response to pathogens. Nat Rev Immunol 2006;6(4):318–28.
40. Kavalukas SL, Barbul A. Nutrition and wound healing: an update. Plast Reconstr Surg 2011;127(Suppl 1):38s–43s.
41. Lach K, Peterson SJ. Nutrition Support for Critically Ill Patients With Cancer. Nutr Clin Pract 2017;32(5):578–86.
42. Ondrey FG, Hom DB. Effects of nutrition on wound healing. Otolaryngol Head Neck Surg 1994;110(6):557–9.
43. Posthauer ME, Dorner B, Collins N. Nutrition: a critical component of wound healing. Adv Skin Wound Care 2010;23(12):560–72, quiz 73-4.
44. de Launoit Y, Kiss R, Paridaens R, et al. Effect of estradiol -17- beta (E2) on cell proliferation in the uterus and the MXT mammary tumor borne by intact, ovariectomized and/or hypophysectomized mice. In Vivo 1987;1(3):173–9.
45. Arnold M, Barbul A. Nutrition and wound healing. Plast Reconstr Surg 2006;117(7 Suppl):42s–58s.
46. Yip WL. Influence of oxygen on wound healing. Int Wound J 2015;12(6):620–4.

47. Raunaq Shah FD, Nirmal S, Domah J. Surgical wound healing in the oral cavity: a review. Dent Update 2020;47(2).

48. Non-healing wounds. American College of Surgeons Division of Education Page 2 of 36 Blended Surgical Education and Training for Life. Available at: https://www.facs.org/media/buthal55/nonhealing_wounds.pdf.

49. Ko KI, Sculean A, Graves DT. Diabetic wound healing in soft and hard oral tissues. Transl Res 2021;236:72–86.

50. Wang Y, Graves DT. Keratinocyte function in normal and diabetic wounds and modulation by FOXO1. J Diabetes Res 2020;2020:3714704.

51. Kim JH, Ruegger PR, Lebig EG, et al. High levels of oxidative stress create a microenvironment that significantly decreases the diversity of the microbiota in diabetic chronic wounds and promotes biofilm formation. Front Cell Infect Microbiol 2020;10:259.

52. Brizeno LA, Assreuy AM, Alves AP, et al. Delayed healing of oral mucosa in a diabetic rat model: Implication of TNF-α, IL-1β and FGF-2. Life Sci 2016;155:36–47.

53. Cabras T, Pisano E, Mastinu A, et al. Alterations of the salivary secretory peptidome profile in children affected by type 1 diabetes. Mol Cell Proteomics 2010; 9(10):2099–108.

54. Kuehl MN, Rodriguez H, Burkhardt BR, et al. Tumor necrosis factor-α, matrix-metalloproteinases 8 and 9 levels in the saliva are associated with increased hemoglobin A1c in type 1 diabetes subjects. PLoS One 2015;10(4):e0125320.

55. Bhattacharya R, Xu F, Dong G, et al. Effect of bacteria on the wound healing behavior of oral epithelial cells. PLoS One 2014;9(2):e89475.

56. Kim HS, Park JW, Yeo SI, et al. Effects of high glucose on cellular activity of periodontal ligament cells in vitro. Diabetes Res Clin Pract 2006;74(1):41–7.

57. Liu R, Bal HS, Desta T, et al. Diabetes enhances periodontal bone loss through enhanced resorption and diminished bone formation. J Dent Res 2006;85(6): 510–4.

58. Ko KI, Syverson AL, Kralik RM, et al. Diabetes-Induced NF-κB Dysregulation in Skeletal Stem Cells Prevents Resolution of Inflammation. Diabetes 2019;68(11): 2095–106.

59. Chan LK, Withey S, Butler PE. Smoking and wound healing problems in reduction mammaplasty: is the introduction of urine nicotine testing justified? Ann Plast Surg 2006;56(2):111–5.

60. Ahn C, Mulligan P, Salcido RS. Smoking-the bane of wound healing: biomedical interventions and social influences. Adv Skin Wound Care 2008;21(5):227–36, quiz 37-8.

61. Sørensen LT, Jørgensen S, Petersen LJ, et al. Acute effects of nicotine and smoking on blood flow, tissue oxygen, and aerobe metabolism of the skin and subcutis. J Surg Res 2009;152(2):224–30.

62. McMaster SK, Paul-Clark MJ, Walters M, et al. Cigarette smoke inhibits macrophage sensing of Gram-negative bacteria and lipopolysaccharide: relative roles of nicotine and oxidant stress. Br J Pharmacol 2008;153(3):536–43.

63. Szabo G, Mandrekar P. A recent perspective on alcohol, immunity, and host defense. Alcohol Clin Exp Res 2009;33(2):220–32.

64. Greiffenstein P, Molina PE. Alcohol-induced alterations on host defense after traumatic injury. J Trauma 2008;64(1):230–40.

65. Radek KA, Matthies AM, Burns AL, et al. Acute ethanol exposure impairs angiogenesis and the proliferative phase of wound healing. Am J Physiol Heart Circ Physiol 2005;289(3):H1084–90.

66. Radek KA, Kovacs EJ, Gallo RL, et al. Acute ethanol exposure disrupts VEGF receptor cell signaling in endothelial cells. Am J Physiol Heart Circ Physiol 2008; 295(1):H174–84.

67. Avishai E, Yeghiazaryan K, Golubnitschaja O. Impaired wound healing: facts and hypotheses for multi-professional considerations in predictive, preventive and personalised medicine. EPMA J 2017;8(1):23–33.

68. Elsharkawi-Welt K, Hepp J, Scharffetter-Kochanek K. [Genetic causes of impaired wound healing. Rare differential diagnosis of the non-healing wound]. Hautarzt 2008;59(11):893–903.

69. Mik G, Gholve PA, Scher DM, et al. Down syndrome: orthopedic issues. Curr Opin Pediatr 2008;20(1):30–6.

70. Götz A, Eckert F, Landthaler M. Ataxia-telangiectasia (Louis-Bar syndrome) associated with ulcerating necrobiosis lipoidica. J Am Acad Dermatol 1994;31(1): 124–6.

71. Roos D, Law SK. Hematologically important mutations: leukocyte adhesion deficiency. Blood Cells Mol Dis 2001;27(6):1000–4.

72. Gadola SD, Moins-Teisserenc HT, Trowsdale J, et al. TAP deficiency syndrome. Clin Exp Immunol 2000;121(2):173–8.

73. Trudgian J, Trotman S. Ehlers-Danlos syndrome and wound healing: injury in a collagen disorder. Br J Nurs 2011;20(6):S10–2. S14 Passim.

74. Deyell M, Garris CS, Laughney AM. Cancer metastasis as a non-healing wound. Br J Cancer 2021;124(9):1491–502.

75. Boaz RJ, Vig T, Manojkumar R, et al. Incision site metastasis: Adding insult to injury. J Cancer Res Ther 2017;13(6):1068–9.

76. Otsuka I. Cutaneous metastasis after surgery, injury, lymphadenopathy, and peritonitis: possible mechanisms. Int J Mol Sci 2019;20(13).

77. Hirshberg A, Leibovich P, Horowitz I, et al. Metastatic tumors to postextraction sites. J Oral Maxillofac Surg 1993;51(12):1334–7.

78. Ganesh K, Basnet H, Kaygusuz Y, et al. L1CAM defines the regenerative origin of metastasis-initiating cells in colorectal cancer. Nat Cancer 2020;1(1):28–45.

79. Byun JS, Gardner K. Wounds that will not heal: pervasive cellular reprogramming in cancer. Am J Pathol 2013;182(4):1055–64.

80. Dvorak HF. Tumors: wounds that do not heal-redux. Cancer Immunol Res 2015; 3(1):1–11.

81. Franz MG, Steed DL, Robson MC. Optimizing healing of the acute wound by minimizing complications. Curr Probl Surg 2007;44(11):691–763.

Systemic Factors Affecting Prognosis and Outcome of Endodontic Therapy

Carla Y. Falcon, DMD, MDS[a],*, Varsha Agnihotri, DMD, MBS[b,1],
Amrita Gogia, BDS, MDS[c,2],
Anu Priya Guruswamy Pandian, BDS, MDS[d,3]

KEYWORDS

- Systemic diseases • Endodontic treatment • Endodontic treatment outcome
- Apical periodontitis • Healing of periapical tissues • Endodontic prognosis

KEY POINTS

- The prognosis of endodontic therapy is most commonly evaluated by the presence and/or size of a radiographic periapical lesion.
- An increased prevalence of apical periodontitis is associated with several systemic disease conditions and systemic factors including diabetes, irritable bowel disease, osteoporosis, renal disease, inherited coagulation disorders, and smoking.
- Few studies have established a causal relationship between systemic conditions/systemic factors and endodontic outcomes. Further studies are needed.
- Despite optimal endodontic therapy, the biological mechanisms involved in the process of periapical healing, namely, the host immune system and genetic polymorphism play a major role in determining the outcome of endodontic treatment.

INTRODUCTION

Apical periodontitis (AP) is a chronic inflammatory disease affecting almost half of the adult population globally.[1] Infections of endodontic origin elicit an immune or inflammatory response in the periapical tissues leading to AP.[2,3] Root canal treatment (RCT) is performed to prevent or treat AP and restore the functionality of the tooth.[4]

---

[a] Diplomate, American Board of Endodontics, Department of Endodontics, Rutgers School of Dental Medicine, 110 Bergen Street, D883, Newark, NJ 07103, USA; [b] Tend Rockefeller Center, 12 West 48th Street, 4th Floor, New York, NY 10029, USA; [c] Department of Dental Sciences, Medanta - The Medicity, Sector 38, Gurugram, Haryana 1220011, India; [d] Durga Dental, Chennai 600054, Tamil Nadu
[1] Present address: 1399 Park Avenue, Apartment 10B, New York, NY 10029.
[2] Present address: 46, Ashoka Road, New Delhi 110001, India.
[3] Present address: 6121 Glade Avenue, Apartment B218, Woodland Hills, Los Angeles, CA 91367.
* Corresponding author.
E-mail address: falconcy@sdm.rutgers.edu

Dent Clin N Am 68 (2024) 813–826
https://doi.org/10.1016/j.cden.2024.05.009
0011-8532/24/© 2024 Elsevier Inc. All rights are reserved, including those for text and data mining, AI training, and similar technologies.

dental.theclinics.com

Healing of periapical tissues following endodontic treatment is influenced by various local and systemic factors (**Fig. 1**)[5–7] involving a series of inflammatory responses and dynamic balance between host immune reaction and infection.[8] The biological mechanisms of periapical healing can be altered by the overall health condition of a patient including systemic diseases and genetic polymorphism.[4]

Endodontic medicine has evolved over the last few decades investigating the potential interrelationship between endodontic infections and systemic diseases.[4,9–11] Understanding the interrelationship of systemic diseases and endodontic infections may assist clinicians in optimizing endodontic treatment outcomes and further research is needed.

Systemic Conditions Influencing the Outcome of Endodontic Treatment

Diabetes mellitus

Diabetes mellitus (DM) is the third most common chronic disease amongst dental patients[12,13] and is a prognostic factor affecting the success of root canal therapy.[10,12,14–16] Diabetic patients are more susceptible to pulpal and periapical infections[17] due to impaired collateral circulation, and decreased oxygen diffusion in the capillaries.[13] The incidence of flare-up post endodontic treatment in diabetics is 2-fold higher when compared to non-diabetics.[2,13,18]

DM negatively affects the healing of periapical tissues following endodontic procedures (**Fig. 2**)[10,14,19] leading to the persistence of AP and endodontic treatment failure.[19–21] Long-term diabetic patients have a higher frequency of AP than short-term diabetics.[14,18,22] Type-2 diabetic patients have a polymorphism of certain specific genes, which may affect the healing of AP.[4,23]

Hyperglycemia, a hallmark of DM, is associated with delayed healing,[24] and a lower success of RCT in diabetic patients.[25] Uncontrolled diabetes can delay healing[4] and lead to the progression and increased size of periapical pathology, following RCT.[10,26,27] Proper glycemic control is vital for a good endodontic treatment outcome.[28] Additionally, the presence of pre-operative AP in diabetic patients also significantly decreased the success of RCT compared to non-diabetics.[9,29–31] DM is a risk factor for extraction of tooth following non-surgical endodontic therapy.[4,20,30]

Hypertension

Inconsistent bone mineralization in hypertensive patients can be attributed to elevated levels of parathyroid hormones and abnormal vitamin D metabolism.[32] Heightened

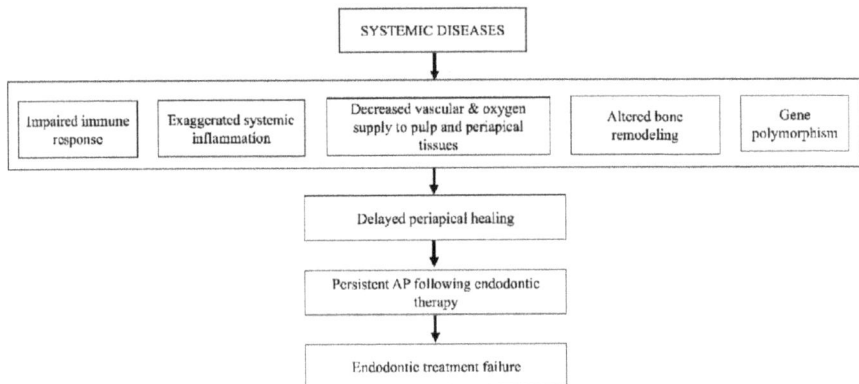

Fig. 1. Summary of mechanisms by which systemic diseases may influence prognosis of endodontic therapy.

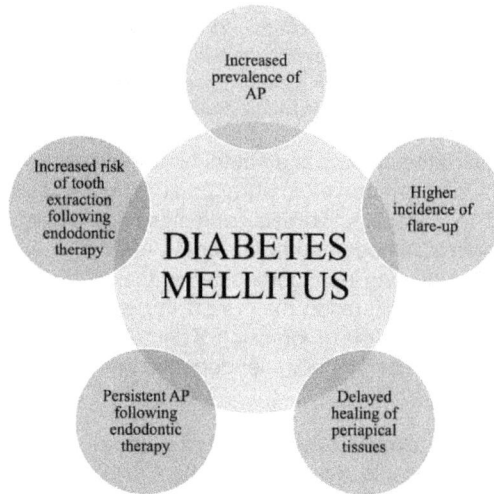

The figure shows "DIABETES MELLITUS" in the center surrounded by six circles:
- Increased prevalence of AP
- Increased risk of tooth extraction following endodontic therapy
- Higher incidence of flare-up
- Persistent AP following endodontic therapy
- Delayed healing of periapical tissues

Fig. 2. Influence of diabetes mellitus on endodontic infections.

periapical bone destruction is attributed to angiotensin II-induced osteoclast differentiation and an increased number of mature osteoclasts.[33] Genetic variations are common to both hypertension and AP.[4,34] Hypertensive patients have been shown to have poorer prognosis for endodontically treated teeth as compared to controls.[14,30,33]

Coronary artery disease/atherosclerosis

A comparison of patients with cardiovascular disease (CVD) and cardiovascular risk factors (CVR) found that the number of RCT teeth, and teeth with AP was higher in CVD and CVR groups as compared to the control groups.[35] However, another study found no such difference in the endodontic outcome in patients having CVD and CAD, as well as presence of absence of periapical lesions.[24]

Autoimmune diseases

AP involves the same cells as autoimmune diseases[36,37] which is why there may be a direct association between endodontic disease and autoimmune diseases. Immune-suppressive agents prescribed to individuals with autoimmune disease can increase the susceptibility of an individual to increased risk of infection, which may negatively impact endodontic healing, yet some studies have shown that there is no effect of immune-suppressive agents on healing of periapical pathology.[14,38]

Rheumatoid arthritis

There are numerous studies which have reported individuals with rheumatoid arthritis (RA) have a greater risk of developing endodontic infection as well as persistence of endodontic pathology.[39–41] There is no evidence of rheumatoid-specific type of immune response in the periapical (PA) lesions of RA patients.[14]

Autoimmune hepatitis

There are no known studies regarding the outcome of endodontic treatment in patients with liver disease, but they do have an increased incidence of AP.[42] Patients with chronic liver disease also did not show compromised immune responses in periapical area.[43]

Irritable bowel disease

Irritable bowel disease (IBD) patients have more endodontically treated teeth with AP.[44] The prevalence and size of AP was found to be significantly higher in women taking biologic medications (BM), such as immunomodulators.[45] BMs may have a therapeutic effect in treating AP showing faster healing as compared to the control group.[46] The IBD group did not have a higher prevalence of AP.[47]

Systemic lupus erythematosus

Systemic lupus erythematosus (SLE) is an autoimmune disease in which the complement system triggers auto-antibodies to attract macrophages and neutrophils, which can eventually lead to vasculitis, fibrosis, and tissue necrosis. This results in an increased risk of systemic infection and developing AP.[48,49]

SLE patients are often on long-term corticosteroid therapy, which is associated with pulp obliteration.[48,50] Pulp obliteration may result in decreased pain sensation in the affected tooth, thereby masking the progression of dental diseases.[48,50] Pulp obliteration can further increase the level of difficulty in endodontic treatment, affecting prognosis.

Lyme disease

There are no studies that show a direct effect of Lyme disease (LD) on endodontic outcome. However, the musculoskeletal involvement in LD may lead to chronic orofacial pain, non-odontogenic toothache, and symptoms of temporomandibular disorder (TMD).[51]

Neuropathic symptoms of LD can present as tooth sensitivity or pulpitis-like pain, which can be misdiagnosed as endodontic pain.[52]

Undifferentiated orofacial pain or TMD can refer pain to the teeth which may mimic toothache and these signs and symptoms can influence the success of endodontic treatment.[53–55]

Osteoporosis

Osteoporosis and AP are characterized by a common feature of bone resorption.[56] There are minimal studies indicating the influence of osteoporosis on the healing of endodontically treated teeth. The altered bone density in osteoporotic patients was found to be associated with increased occurrence of AP.[4,57]

Renal disease

Inflammation and immune system activation are common underlying mechanisms for the development of renal disease.[58] During this process, systemic cytokine levels increase, which may play a role in the progression of both AP and chronic kidney disease (CKD).[58] CKD patients are almost 4 times more likely to have AP than individuals without CKD. The severity of AP has been positively associated with increases in serum creatinine, blood urea, and a decrease in estimated glomerular filtration rate. It has recently been hypothesized that AP may alter the progression of CKD.[58]

End-stage renal disease (ESRD) and uremia are associated with changes in the level of cytokines.[59] A study has also found that individuals diagnosed with ESRD are almost 3 times more likely to be diagnosed with AP.[60] However, a causal relationship has not been established.[60]

The treatment of AP through RCT appears to improve the survival of individuals with renal disease. A study of individuals receiving dialysis comparing those who received treatment of AP with RCT to those who did not receive RCT found a lower death rate.[61]

Blood dyscrasias

There are few studies evaluating blood disorders and endodontic outcomes. Inherited coagulation disorders, such as hemophilia A or B, or von Willebrand disease, can impair the nonspecific immune system impacting healing after endodontic treatment.[11]

Individuals with inherited coagulation disorders, such as hemophilia A, hemophilia B, or von Willebrand's disease, have shown twice the prevalence of radiographic

AP. It has been hypothesized that inherited coagulation disorders may be a risk factor for periapical disease.[62,63]

Sickle cell anemia (SCA) is associated with increased levels of inflammatory mediators and has also been investigated in the context of endodontic disease. Aseptic pulp necrosis appears to be the major endodontic complication noted in individuals with SCA.[64,65] Aseptic pulp necrosis is thought to occur in association with low oxygen saturation levels, with the occurrence of pulp necrosis 8.33 times higher in individuals with SCA as compared to controls.[65]

Nutritional deficiencies

Hypophosphatemic rickets is identified by low phosphate levels alongside normal or decreased serum vitamin D and calcium levels.[66] This condition often leads to developmental abnormalities in teeth, such as enlarged pulp chambers with increased pulp volume, a condition known as taurodontism. Additionally, it is marked by thin, underdeveloped enamel, dentinal defects, and abscesses occurring without the presence of cavities or trauma.[67] Case studies of individuals with hypophosphatemic rickets have demonstrated that even teeth displaying multiple radiolucencies and sinus tracts can be successfully treated with endodontics. As this population ages, there may be an increased need for endodontic treatment, particularly in posterior teeth.[68] Given the atypical morphology associated with this condition, it is advisable to refer such cases to specialists. RCT has proven effective in resolving the apical radiolucencies in 1-year and 2-year follow- up appointments.[69]

Other Systemic Factors Influencing the Outcome of Endodontic Treatment

Smoking

Smoking may be considered a modulating factor that negatively affects the healing of periapical tissues following endodontic therapy.[70,71] Emerging evidence shows that smoking tobacco has an adverse effect on the success of endodontically treated teeth by affecting vascular and immune systems.[5,71,72] There is a dose-dependent risk of persistent AP following RCT in smokers.[73]

Numerous studies have shown that the prevalence of AP is higher in smokers,[5,74,75] with increased number of root-filled teeth by 2-fold when compared to non-smokers.[4,76] A study revealed that the healing of periapical tissues following endodontic treatment was reduced by 30% in smokers when compared to non-smokers.[73]

Smokers have 3 times the risk of tooth extraction following endodontic treatment.[4,77] Extraction risk is further accelerated if a smoker's periodontal health is compromised.[78,79] However, the healing of periapical tissues following apical surgery is similar in both smokers and non-smokers having the same rate of success 1 year post-operatively.[80,81]

Bruxism

Bruxism has been associated with failure of restorations, which may also result in endodontic failure.[82] Bruxism can also lead to pulpal damage, as shown in a case study where patients developed apical periodontitis after a phase of intense bruxism.[83] Endodontically treated teeth have a reduced survival rate if they develop subsequent cracks.[84] Full cuspal coverage restorations on teeth with cracks are imperative after endodontic therapy to increase the survivability of endodontically treated teeth.[85]

Pregnancy

AP has been associated with adverse pregnancy outcomes in a limited number of studies.[86–88] During pregnancy, there are changes in the immune response. Adverse pregnancy events, such as stillbirth, early gestational age, neonatal death, low birth weight, pre-eclampsia, shorter head circumference, and preterm birth, have been associated with elevated maternal inflammatory mediators and AP.[86,87,89] Interestingly, AP was found to be predictive for pre-eclampsia.[88]

Aging

The effect of age on endodontic outcome has been evaluated across several studies. Although age could affect immune responsiveness, several systematic reviews have concluded that patient age is not a prognostic factor for the success of RCT[90–93] Additionally, research performed via the National Dental Practice Based Research Network has found that age not a predictor in the longevity of endodontically treated teeth.[92]

Bisphosphonates

Bisphosphonates are often used for osteoporosis and specific cancer treatments because they suppress the activity of osteoclasts.[94,95] Bisphosphonate-related osteonecrosis of the jaw (BRONJ) is a potential negative outcome after endodontic treatment which can be triggered by soft tissue damage during rubber dam and wedge placement, over-instrumentation, or apical extrusion.[94] Rinsing with chlorhexidine for a minute before starting, working under aseptic conditions, and using anesthetic without vasoconstrictors are recommended.[94,95]

Radiation therapy

High-dose radiotherapy is often used as treatment for oncologic patients in the head and neck region, but a long-term complication is osteoradionecrosis (ORN). A more modern technique, intensity-modulated radiotherapy (IMRT), has been shown to reduce oral side effects, including ORN.[96] IMRT limits the reparative capacity of osteoblasts, which slows down the bone adaptation, and may inhibit healing of AP.[96,97]

Chemotherapy

Common chemotherapy drugs, such as tamoxifen and aromatase inhibitors, can affect bone turnover and bone density.[98] This could affect the healing of AP in teeth in post-endodontic treatment. Chemotherapy drugs administered before the age of 10 have been associated with tooth abnormalities such as tooth size reduction, taurodontia, shorter roots, and root resorption.[99] The developmental stage of tooth formation is the most important factor in determining dental abnormalities.[100] The presence of dental anomalies can increase the difficulty of endodontic treatment and thereby impact on endodontic outcomes.

Blood thinners

It has been shown that traditional anticoagulants, such as warfarin, may cause delayed healing.[101] In recent years, more patients are being prescribed novel oral anticoagulants (NOAC) instead of traditional vitamin K antagonists, such as warfarin.[102] NOACs, such as dabigatran and apixaban, do not necessarily need to be discontinued for a dental procedure.[103] Further studies are needed to determine a protocol for which situations a NOAC needs to be discontinued[104] and what effect it would have on post-endodontic healing.

SUMMARY
Diabetes Mellitus

DM negatively affects endodontic outcomes.[10,12,14–16] Long-term diabetics and diabetics with poor glycemic control have decreased success of root canal therapy.[10,14,18,22,26,27]

Hypertension

Hypertension negatively affects endodontic treatment outcome by exaggerating the inflammatory response of periapical tissues and impairing the mineralization of bone in the process of healing.[32,56]

Coronary Artery Disease/Atherosclerosis

There are many studies that show a positive association between AP and CAD though very few studies evaluate the outcome of endodontic treatment in patients with CAD.[28]

Autoimmune Diseases

Some studies have shown a positive association between AP and autoimmune diseases, whereas other studies have shown no association.[14,38]

Rheumatoid Disease

Some studies have shown a positive association between rheumatoid disease and AP, whereas other studies have shown no correlation.[39,40]

Irritable Bowel Disease

There are limited studies regarding the outcome of endodontic treatment and irritable bowel disease, but there may be an increased incidence of AP in these individuals.[47]

Systemic Lupus Erythematosus

SLE patients are often on long-term corticosteroid therapy, which has been associated with pulpal obliteration,[48,50] leading to difficulty in endodontic diagnosis and treatment.[50]

Lyme Disease

LD has been associated with musculoskeletal involvement, which can cause referred pain to the teeth and mimic tooth pain.[51]

Osteoporosis

Studies have shown the prevalence of AP to be 3 times higher in osteoporotic patients than control groups.[4,57]

Renal Disease

Further studies are needed to evaluate the prognosis of endodontic treatment in patients with renal disease. Patients with chronic kidney disease and end-stage renal disease have been associated with having increased prevalence of AP.[58,60] Treating AP in individuals with renal disease may increase their survival.[61]

Blood Dyscrasias

Further studies are needed to evaluate the prognosis of endodontic treatment in patients with blood dyscrasias. Inherited coagulation disorders have shown to have a higher prevalence of AP.[62,63] Patients with sickle cell anemia have shown a higher prevalence of aseptic pulpal necrosis.[65]

Nutritional Deficiencies

Hypophosphatemic rickets affects the pulpal anatomy, making RCT more challenging. Further studies are needed to determine the prognosis of endodontic therapy in patients with hypophosphatemic rickets.[67]

Smoking

Tobacco smoking is considered a negative factor for the prognosis of endodontic treated teeth,[70,77,78] due to compromised immune response[74] and persistent destruction of bone.[4,77]

Bruxism

Patients with bruxism have more cracks in their teeth, which has been associated with poor survival rate in endodontically treated teeth.[84]

Pregnancy

Further studies are needed to evaluate the prognosis of endodontic treatment in pregnant patients.

Aging

Age is not a prognostic factor in the success of RCT.[90–93]

Radiation Therapy

Intensity-modulated radiotherapy may inhibit healing of RCT teeth with AP, but further investigation is needed.[96]

Chemotherapy

Further studies are needed to evaluate the prognosis of endodontic treatment in patients with chemotherapy.[100]

Blood Thinners

Anticoagulants can delay healing, but further studies are needed to specifically evaluate the prognosis of endodontic treatment in patients taking blood thinners.[101]

CLINICS CARE POINTS

- Diabetes mellitus is a negative prognostic factor of root canal therapy. Proper glycemic control is vital for a favorable endodontic treatment outcome.
- Healing of periapical tissues in root-filled teeth (RFL) is directly proportional to the dose of tobacco smoking.
- BRONJ/medication-related osteonecrosis of the jaw (MRONJ) can be triggered in patients taking bisphosphonates as a negative outcome after endodontic treatment, but by taking certain procedural precautions, this can be prevented.
- Patients with irritable bowel syndrome taking anti-tumor necrosis factor alpha biologic medications have been shown to have faster healing in treating apical periodontitis compared to control groups.
- Bruxism can cause cracks in teeth and full cuspal coverage on such teeth is imperative after endodontic therapy to increase the survivability of endodontically treated teeth.

DISCLOSURE

The authors have nothing to disclose.

REFERENCES

1. Tiburcio-Machado CS, Michelon C, Zanatta FB, et al. The global prevalence of apical periodontitis: a systematic review and meta-analysis. Int Endod J 2021; 54(5):712–35.
2. Sasaki H, Hirai K, Martins CM, et al. Interrelationship between periapical lesion and systemic metabolic disorders. Curr Pharmaceut Des 2016;22(15):2204–15.
3. Nair PN. On the causes of persistent apical periodontitis: a review. Int Endod J 2006;39(4):249–81.
4. Segura-Egea JJ, Cabanillas-Balsera D, Martin-Gonzalez J, et al. Impact of systemic health on treatment outcomes in endodontics. Int Endod J 2023;56(Suppl 2):219–35.
5. Pinto KP, Ferreira CM, Maia LC, et al. Does tobacco smoking predispose to apical periodontitis and endodontic treatment need? A systematic review and meta-analysis. Int Endod J 2020;53(8):1068–83.
6. Salles AG, Antunes LAA, Kuchler EC, et al. Association between apical periodontitis and interleukin gene polymorphisms: a systematic review and meta-analysis. J Endod 2018;44(3):355–62.
7. Lee LW, Lee YL, Hsiao SH, et al. Bacteria in the apical root canals of teeth with apical periodontitis. J Formos Med Assoc 2017;116(6):448–56.
8. Karamifar K, Tondari A, Saghiri MA. Endodontic periapical lesion: an overview on the etiology, diagnosis and current treatment modalities. Eur Endod J 2020;5(2):54–67.
9. Segura-Egea JJ, Cabanillas-Balsera D, Jimenez-Sanchez MC, et al. Endodontics and diabetes: association versus causation. Int Endod J 2019;52(6): 790–802.
10. Cintra LTA, Estrela C, Azuma MM, et al. Endodontic medicine: interrelationships among apical periodontitis, systemic disorders, and tissue responses of dental materials. Braz Oral Res 2018;32(suppl 1):e68.
11. Segura-Egea JJ, Martin-Gonzalez J, Castellanos-Cosano L. Endodontic medicine: connections between apical periodontitis and systemic diseases. Int Endod J 2015;48(10):933–51.
12. Segura-Egea JJ, Martin-Gonzalez J, Cabanillas-Balsera D, et al. Association between diabetes and the prevalence of radiolucent periapical lesions in root-filled teeth: systematic review and meta-analysis. Clin Oral Invest 2016;20(6): 1133–41.
13. Lima SM, Grisi DC, Kogawa EM, et al. Diabetes mellitus and inflammatory pulpal and periapical disease: a review. Int Endod J 2013;46(8):700–9.
14. Ye L, Cao L, Song W, et al. Interaction between apical periodontitis and systemic disease (Review). Int J Mol Med 2023;52(1).
15. Nagendrababu V, Segura-Egea JJ, Fouad AF, et al. Association between diabetes and the outcome of root canal treatment in adults: an umbrella review. Int Endod J 2020;53(4):455–66.
16. Ng YL, Mann V, Gulabivala K. A prospective study of the factors affecting outcomes of non-surgical root canal treatment: part 2: tooth survival. Int Endod J 2011;44(7):610–25.
17. Leite MF, Ganzerla E, Marques MM, et al. Diabetes induces metabolic alterations in dental pulp. J Endod 2008;34(10):1211–4.
18. Mesgarani A, Haghanifar S, Eshkevari N, et al. Frequency of odontogenic periradicular lesions in diabetic patients. Caspian J Intern Med. Winter 2014; 5(1):22–5.

19. Arya S, Duhan J, Tewari S, et al. Healing of apical periodontitis after nonsurgical treatment in patients with type 2 diabetes. J Endod 2017;43(10):1623–7.

20. Wang CH, Chueh LH, Chen SC, et al. Impact of diabetes mellitus, hypertension, and coronary artery disease on tooth extraction after nonsurgical endodontic treatment. J Endod 2011;37(1):1–5.

21. Britto LR, Katz J, Guelmann M, et al. Periradicular radiographic assessment in diabetic and control individuals. Oral Surg Oral Med Oral Pathol Oral Radiol Endod 2003;96(4):449–52.

22. Perez-Losada FL, Estrugo-Devesa A, Castellanos-Cosano L, et al. Apical periodontitis and diabetes mellitus type 2: a systematic review and meta-analysis. J Clin Med 2020;9(2).

23. Petean IBF, Kuchler EC, Soares IMV, et al. Genetic Polymorphisms in RANK and RANKL are Associated with Persistent Apical Periodontitis. J Endod 2019;45(5):526–31.

24. Laukkanen E, Vehkalahti MM, Kotiranta AK. Impact of systemic diseases and tooth-based factors on outcome of root canal treatment. Int Endod J 2019;52(10):1417–26.

25. Sanchez-Dominguez B, Lopez-Lopez J, Jane-Salas E, et al. Glycated hemoglobin levels and prevalence of apical periodontitis in type 2 diabetic patients. J Endod 2015;41(5):601–6.

26. Cintra LT, Samuel RO, Azuma MM, et al. Apical periodontitis and periodontal disease increase serum IL-17 levels in normoglycemic and diabetic rats. Clin Oral Invest 2014;18(9):2123–8.

27. Gupta A, Aggarwal V, Mehta N, et al. Diabetes mellitus and the healing of periapical lesions in root filled teeth: a systematic review and meta-analysis. Int Endod J 2020;53(11):1472–84.

28. Pinto KP, Serrao G, Alves Ferreira CM, et al. Association between apical periodontitis and chronic diseases: an umbrella review. Iran Endod J 2023;18(3):134–44.

29. Liu X, He G, Qiu Z, et al. Diabetes mellitus increases the risk of apical periodontitis in endodontically-treated teeth: a meta-analysis from 15 studies. J Endod 2023;49(12):1605–16.

30. Niazi SA, Bakhsh A. Association between endodontic infection, its treatment and systemic health: a narrative review. Medicina (Kaunas) 2022;58(7).

31. Fouad AF. Diabetes mellitus as a modulating factor of endodontic infections. J Dent Educ 2003;67(4):459–67.

32. Martins CM, Gomes-Filho JE, de Azevedo Queiroz IO, et al. Hypertension undermines mineralization-inducing capacity of and tissue response to mineral trioxide aggregate endodontic cement. J Endod 2016;42(4):604–9.

33. Martins CM, Sasaki H, Hirai K, et al. Relationship between hypertension and periapical lesion: an in vitro and in vivo study. Braz Oral Res 2016;30(1):e78.

34. Messing M, Souza LC, Cavalla F, et al. Investigating potential correlations between endodontic pathology and cardiovascular diseases using epidemiological and genetic approaches. J Endod 2019;45(2):104–10.

35. Dash G, Mishra L, Singh NR, et al. Prevalence and quality of endodontic treatment in patients with cardiovascular disease and associated risk factors. J Clin Med 2022;11(20).

36. Braz-Silva PH, Bergamini ML, Mardegan AP, et al. Inflammatory profile of chronic apical periodontitis: a literature review. Acta Odontol Scand 2019;77(3):173–80.

37. Chen E, Bakr MM, Firth N, et al. Inflammatory cell expression of Toll-like receptor-2 (TLR2) within refractory periapical granuloma. F1000Res 2018;7:1819.
38. Teixeira FB, Gomes BP, Ferraz CC, et al. Radiographic analysis of the development of periapical lesions in normal rats, sialoadenectomized rats and sialoadenectomized-immunosuppressed rats. Endod Dent Traumatol 2000; 16(4):154-7.
39. Karatas E, Kul A, Tepecik E. Association between rheumatoid arthritis and apical periodontitis: a cross-sectional study. Eur Endod J 2020;5(2):155-8.
40. Rotstein I, Katz J. Prevalence of periapical abscesses in patients with rheumatoid arthritis. a cross sectional study. Am J Dent 2021;34(4):211-4.
41. Oh WM, Hwang IN, Son HH, et al. Rapid periapical bone destruction during endodontic treatment of a patient with rheumatoid arthritis. J Endod 2008; 34(10):1261-3.
42. Lins L, Bittencourt PL, Evangelista MA, et al. Oral health profile of cirrhotic patients awaiting liver transplantation in the Brazilian Northeast. Transplant Proc 2011;43(4):1319-21.
43. Braga Diniz JM, Espaladori MC, Souza ESME, et al. Immunological profile of teeth with inflammatory periapical disease from chronic liver disease patients. Int Endod J 2019;52(2):149-57.
44. Segura-Sampedro JJ, Jimenez-Gimenez C, Jane-Salas E, et al. Periapical and endodontic status of patients with inflammatory bowel disease: Age- and sex-matched case-control study. Int Endod J 2022;55(7):748-57.
45. Piras V, Usai P, Mezzena S, et al. Prevalence of apical periodontitis in patients with inflammatory bowel diseases: a retrospective clinical study. J Endod 2017;43(3):389-94.
46. Cotti E, Mezzena S, Schirru E, et al. Healing of apical periodontitis in patients with inflammatory bowel diseases and under anti-tumor necrosis factor alpha therapy. J Endod 2018;44(12):1777-82.
47. Poyato-Borrego M, Segura-Egea JJ, Martin-Gonzalez J, et al. Prevalence of endodontic infection in patients with Crohn s disease and ulcerative colitis. Med Oral Patol Oral Cir Bucal 2021;26(2):e208-15.
48. Kudsi M, Nahas LD, Alsawah R, et al. The prevalence of oral mucosal lesions and related factors in systemic lupus erythematosus patients. Arthritis Res Ther 2021;23(1):229.
49. Hs S. Systemic lupus erythematosus in a 12-year-old boy: a rare entity in childhood. Int J Clin Pediatr Dent 2010;3(3):199-202.
50. Jiandong B, Yunxiao Z, Zuhua W, et al. Generalized pulp canal obliteration in a patient on long-term glucocorticoids: a case report and literature review. BMC Oral Health 2022;22(1):352.
51. Weise C, Schulz MC, Frank K, et al. Acute arthritis of the right temporomandibular joint due to Lyme disease: a case report and literature review. BMC Oral Health 2021;21(1):400.
52. Taheri JB, Anbari F, Sani SK, et al. A 10-year overview of chronic orofacial pain in patients at an oral medicine center in Iran. J Dent Anesth Pain Med 2022;22(4): 289-94.
53. Mello I, Peters J, Lee C. Neuropathy mimicking dental pain in a patient diagnosed with lyme disease. J Endod 2020;46(9):1337-9.
54. Renton T. Chronic pain and overview or differential diagnoses of non-odontogenic orofacial pain. Prim Dent J 2019;7(4):71-86.
55. De Laat A. Differential diagnosis of toothache to prevent erroneous and unnecessary dental treatment. J Oral Rehabil 2020;47(6):775-81.

56. Holland R, Gomes JEF, Cintra LTA, et al. Factors affecting the periapical healing process of endodontically treated teeth. J Appl Oral Sci Sep-Oct 2017;25(5): 465–76.
57. Lopez-Lopez J, Castellanos-Cosano L, Estrugo-Devesa A, et al. Radiolucent periapical lesions and bone mineral density in post-menopausal women. Gerodontology 2015;32(3):195–201.
58. Lamba J, Mittal S, Tewari S, et al. Association of apical periodontitis with different stages of chronic kidney disease measured by glomerular filtration rate and systemic markers: an observational study. J Endod 2023.
59. Kato S, Chmielewski M, Honda H, et al. Aspects of immune dysfunction in end-stage renal disease. Clin J Am Soc Nephrol 2008;3(5):1526–33.
60. Khalighinejad N, Aminoshariae A, Kulild JC, et al. Association of end-stage renal disease with radiographically and clinically diagnosed apical periodontitis: a hospital-based study. J Endod 2017;43(9):1438–41.
61. Chiu CC, Chang YC, Huang RY, et al. Investigation of the impact of endodontic therapy on survival among dialysis patients in taiwan: a Nationwide Population-Based Cohort Study. Int J Environ Res Publ Health 2021;18(1).
62. Castellanos-Cosano L, Machuca-Portillo G, Sanchez-Dominguez B, et al. High prevalence of radiolucent periapical lesions amongst patients with inherited coagulation disorders. Haemophilia 2013;19(3):e110–5.
63. Khalighinejad N, Aminoshariae MR, Aminoshariae A, et al. Association between systemic diseases and apical periodontitis. J Endod 2016;42(10):1427–34.
64. Souza SFC, Thomaz E, Costa CPS. Healthy dental pulp oxygen saturation rates in subjects with homozygous sickle cell anemia: a cross-sectional study nested in a cohort. J Endod 2017;43(12):1997–2000.
65. Costa CP, Thomaz EB, Souza Sde F. Association between sickle cell anemia and pulp necrosis. J Endod 2013;39(2):177–81.
66. Souza MA, Soares Junior LA, Santos MA, et al. Dental abnormalities and oral health in patients with Hypophosphatemic rickets. Clinics 2010;65(10):1023–6.
67. Sabandal MM, Robotta P, Burklein S, et al. Review of the dental implications of X-linked hypophosphataemic rickets (XLHR). Clin Oral Invest 2015;19(4): 759–68.
68. Andersen MG, Beck-Nielsen SS, Haubek D, et al. Periapical and endodontic status of permanent teeth in patients with hypophosphatemic rickets. J Oral Rehabil 2012;39(2):144–50.
69. Beltes C, Zachou E. Endodontic management in a patient with vitamin D-resistant Rickets. J Endod 2012;38(2):255–8.
70. Khalighinejad N, Aminoshariae A, Kulild JC, et al. The Influence of periodontal status on endodontically treated teeth: 9-year survival analysis. J Endod 2017; 43(11):1781–5.
71. Paljevic E, Brekalo Prso I, Hrstic JV, et al. Impact of smoking on the healing of apical periodontitis after nonsurgical endodontic treatment. Eur J Dermatol 2023.
72. Herbst CS, Schwendicke F, Krois J, et al. Association between patient-, tooth- and treatment-level factors and root canal treatment failure: A retrospective longitudinal and machine learning study. J Dent 2022;117:103937.
73. Majid OW. Dose-response association of smoking with delayed healing of apical periodontitis after endodontic treatment. Evid Base Dent 2023;24(4):174–5.
74. Aminoshariae A, Kulild J, Gutmann J. The association between smoking and periapical periodontitis: a systematic review. Clin Oral Invest 2020;24(2): 533–45.

75. Cheng LL. Smoking may increase the risk of periapical periodontitis. J Evid Base Dent Pract 2020;20(4):101500.
76. Sopinska K, Boltacz-Rzepkowska E. The influence of tobacco smoking on dental periapical condition in a sample of an adult population of the Lodz region, Poland. Int J Occup Med Environ Health 2020;33(1):45–57.
77. Cabanillas-Balsera D, Segura-Egea JJ, Bermudo-Fuenmayor M, et al. Smoking and radiolucent periapical lesions in root filled teeth: systematic review and meta-analysis. J Clin Med 2020;9(11).
78. Cabanillas-Balsera D, Segura-Egea JJ, Jimenez-Sanchez MC, et al. Cigarette smoking and root filled teeth extraction: systematic review and meta-analysis. J Clin Med 2020;9(10).
79. Mahmood AA, AbdulAzeez AR, Hussein HM. The effect of smoking habit on apical status of adequate endodontically treated teeth with and without periodontal involvement. Clin Cosmet Invest Dent 2019;11:419–28.
80. Sutter E, Valdec S, Bichsel D, et al. Success rate 1 year after apical surgery: a retrospective analysis. Oral Maxillofac Surg 2020;24(1):45–9.
81. Ogutlu F, Karaca I. Clinical and radiographic outcomes of apical surgery: a clinical study. J Maxillofac Oral Surg 2018;17(1):75–83.
82. Lobbezoo F, Jacobs R, A DEL, et al. [Chewing on bruxism: associations, consequences and management]. Ned Tijdschr Tandheelkd 2017;124(7–8):369–76. Kauwen op bruxisme. Associaties, gevolgen en behandeling.
83. Tang W, Wu Y, Smales RJ. Identifying and reducing risks for potential fractures in endodontically treated teeth. J Endod 2010;36(4):609–17.
84. de Toubes KMS, Soares CJ, Soares RV, et al. The correlation of crack lines and definitive restorations with the survival and success rates of cracked teeth: a long-term retrospective clinical study. J Endod 2022;48(2):190–9.
85. Olivieri JG, Elmsmari F, Miro Q, et al. Outcome and survival of endodontically treated cracked posterior permanent teeth: a systematic review and meta-analysis. J Endod 2020;46(4):455–63.
86. Harjunmaa U, Jarnstedt J, Alho L, et al. Association between maternal dental periapical infections and pregnancy outcomes: results from a cross-sectional study in Malawi. Trop Med Int Health 2015;20(11):1549–58.
87. Leal AS, de Oliveira AE, Brito LM, et al. Association between chronic apical periodontitis and low-birth-weight preterm births. J Endod 2015;41(3):353–7.
88. Khalighinejad N, Aminoshariae A, Kulild JC, et al. Apical periodontitis, a predictor variable for preeclampsia: a case-control study. J Endod 2017;43(10):1611–4.
89. Jakovljevic A, Sljivancanin Jakovljevic T, Duncan HF, et al. The association between apical periodontitis and adverse pregnancy outcomes: a systematic review. Int Endod J 2021;54(9):1527–37.
90. Gulabivala K, Ng YL. Factors that affect the outcomes of root canal treatment and retreatment-A reframing of the principles. Int Endod J 2023;56(Suppl 2):82–115.
91. Shakiba B, Hamedy R, Pak JG, et al. Influence of increased patient age on longitudinal outcomes of root canal treatment: a systematic review. Gerodontology 2017;34(1):101–9.
92. Thyvalikakath T, LaPradd M, Siddiqui Z, et al. Root canal treatment survival analysis in national dental PBRN Practices. J Dent Res 2022;101(11):1328–34.
93. Kytridou V, Gkikas I, Garcia MN, et al. A literature review of local and systemic considerations for endodontic treatments in older adults. Gerodontology 2023;40(4):410–21.

94. Moinzadeh AT, Shemesh H, Neirynck NA, et al. Bisphosphonates and their clinical implications in endodontic therapy. Int Endod J 2013;46(5):391–8.
95. AlRahabi MK, Ghabbani HM. Clinical impact of bisphosphonates in root canal therapy. Saudi Med J 2018;39(3):232–8.
96. Steiner SR, Saccardin F, Connert T, et al. Changes in periapical status of root canal-treated teeth after head and neck IMRT: a retrospective study. Swiss Dent J 2023;133(7).
97. Kielbassa AM, Attin T, Schaller HG, et al. Endodontic therapy in a postirradiated child: review of the literature and report of a case. Quintessence Int 1995;26(6): 405–11.
98. Handforth C, D'Oronzo S, Coleman R, et al. Cancer treatment and bone health. Calcif Tissue Int 2018;102(2):251–64.
99. Jodlowska A, Postek-Stefanska L. Systemic anticancer therapy details and dental adverse effects in children. Int J Environ Res Publ Health 2022;19(11).
100. Jodlowska A, Postek-Stefanska L. Duration and dose of chemotherapy and dental development. Dent Med Probl Jan-Mar 2022;59(1):45–58.
101. Butler AJ, Eismont FJ. Effects of anticoagulant medication on bone-healing. JBJS Rev 2021;9(5):e2000194.
102. Fortier K, Shroff D, Reebye UN. Review: An overview and analysis of novel oral anticoagulants and their dental implications. Gerodontology 2018;35(2):78–86.
103. Curto A, Albaladejo A. Implications of apixaban for dental treatments. J Clin Exp Dent 2016;8(5):e611–4.
104. Lopez-Galindo M, Bagan JV. Apixaban and oral implications. J Clin Exp Dent 2015;7(4):e528–34.

UNITED STATES POSTAL SERVICE ® — Statement of Ownership, Management, and Circulation (All Periodicals Publications Except Requester Publications)

1. Publication Title	2. Publication Number	3. Filing Date
DENTAL CLINICS OF NORTH AMERICA	566 – 480	9/18/2024

4. Issue Frequency	5. Number of Issues Published Annually	6. Annual Subscription Price
JAN, APR, JUL, OCT	4	$333.00

7. Complete Mailing Address of Known Office of Publication (Not printer) (Street, city, county, state, and ZIP+4®)

ELSEVIER INC.
230 Park Avenue, Suite 800
New York, NY 10169

Contact Person
Malathi Samayan
Telephone (Include area code)
91-44-4299-4507

8. Complete Mailing Address of Headquarters or General Business Office of Publisher (Not printer)

ELSEVIER INC.
230 Park Avenue, Suite 800
New York, NY 10169

9. Full Names and Complete Mailing Addresses of Publisher, Editor, and Managing Editor (Do not leave blank)

Publisher (Name and complete mailing address)

Dolores Meloni, ELSEVIER INC.
1600 JOHN F KENNEDY BLVD. SUITE 1600
PHILADELPHIA, PA 19103-2899

Editor (Name and complete mailing address)

JOHN VASSALLO, ELSEVIER INC.
1600 JOHN F KENNEDY BLVD. SUITE 1600
PHILADELPHIA, PA 19103-2899

Managing Editor (Name and complete mailing address)

PATRICK MANLEY, ELSEVIER INC.
1600 JOHN F KENNEDY BLVD. SUITE 1600
PHILADELPHIA, PA 19103-2899

10. Owner (Do not leave blank. If the publication is owned by a corporation, give the name and address of the corporation immediately followed by the names and addresses of all stockholders owning or holding 1 percent or more of the total amount of stock. If not owned by a corporation, give the names and addresses of the individual owners. If owned by a partnership or other unincorporated firm, give its name and address as well as those of each individual owner. If the publication is published by a nonprofit organization, give its name and address.)

Full Name	Complete Mailing Address
WHOLLY OWNED SUBSIDIARY OF REED/ELSEVIER, US HOLDINGS	1600 JOHN F KENNEDY BLVD, SUITE 1600 PHILADELPHIA PA 19103-2899

11. Known Bondholders, Mortgagees, and Other Security Holders Owning or Holding 1 Percent or More of Total Amount of Bonds, Mortgages, or Other Securities. If none, check box ▶ ☐ None

Full Name	Complete Mailing Address
N/A	

12. Tax Status (For completion by nonprofit organizations authorized to mail at nonprofit rates) (Check one)
The purpose, function, and nonprofit status of this organization and the exempt status for federal income tax purposes:
☒ Has Not Changed During Preceding 12 Months
☐ Has Changed During Preceding 12 Months (Publisher must submit explanation of change with this statement)

PS Form **3526**, July 2014 [Page 1 of 4 (see instructions page 4)] PSN: 7530-01-000-9931 PRIVACY NOTICE: See our privacy policy on www.usps.com.

---

13. Publication Title		14. Issue Date for Circulation Data below
DENTAL CLINICS OF NORTH AMERICA		JULY 2024

15. Extent and Nature of Circulation			Average No. Copies Each Issue During Preceding 12 Months	No. Copies of Single Issue Published Nearest to Filing Date
a. Total Number of Copies (Net press run)			139	120
b. Paid Circulation (By Mail and Outside the Mail)	(1)	Mailed Outside-County Paid Subscriptions Stated on PS Form 3541 (Include paid distribution above nominal rate, advertiser's proof copies, and exchange copies)	83	59
	(2)	Mailed In-County Paid Subscriptions Stated on PS Form 3541 (Include paid distribution above nominal rate, advertiser's proof copies, and exchange copies)	0	0
	(3)	Paid Distribution Outside the Mails Including Sales Through Dealers and Carriers, Street Vendors, Counter Sales, and Other Paid Distribution Outside USPS®	45	53
	(4)	Paid Distribution by Other Classes of Mail Through the USPS (e.g., First-Class Mail®)	8	6
c. Total Paid Distribution [Sum of 15b (1), (2), (3), and (4)]		▶	136	118
d. Free or Nominal Rate Distribution (By Mail and Outside the Mail)	(1)	Free or Nominal Rate Outside-County Copies included on PS Form 3541	2	1
	(2)	Free or Nominal Rate In-County Copies Included on PS Form 3541	0	0
	(3)	Free or Nominal Rate Copies Mailed at Other Classes Through the USPS (e.g., First-Class Mail)	0	0
	(4)	Free or Nominal Rate Distribution Outside the Mail (Carriers or other means)	1	1
e. Total Free or Nominal Rate Distribution (Sum of 15d (1), (2), (3) and (4))		▶	3	2
f. Total Distribution (Sum of 15c and 15e)		▶	139	120
g. Copies not Distributed (See Instructions to Publishers #4 (page #3))		▶	0	0
h. Total (Sum of 15f and g)		▶	139	120
i. Percent Paid (15c divided by 15f times 100)		▶	98.2%	98.33%

* If you are claiming electronic copies, go to line 16 on page 3. If you are not claiming electronic copies, skip to line 17 on page 3.

PS Form **3526**, July 2014 (Page 2 of 4)

16. Electronic Copy Circulation	Average No. Copies Each Issue During Preceding 12 Months	No. Copies of Single Issue Published Nearest to Filing Date
a. Paid Electronic Copies ▶		
b. Total Paid Print Copies (Line 15c) + Paid Electronic Copies (Line 16a) ▶		
c. Total Print Distribution (Line 15f) + Paid Electronic Copies (Line 16a) ▶		
d. Percent Paid (Both Print & Electronic Copies) (16b divided by 16c × 100) ▶		

☒ I certify that 50% of all my distributed copies (electronic and print) are paid above a nominal price.

17. Publication of Statement of Ownership

☒ If the publication is a general publication, publication of this statement is required. Will be printed in the OCTOBER 2024 issue of this publication. ☐ Publication not required.

18. Signature and Title of Editor, Publisher, Business Manager, or Owner	Date
Malathi Samayan	9/18/2024

Malathi Samayan - Distribution Controller

I certify that all information furnished on this form is true and complete. I understand that anyone who furnishes false or misleading information on this form or who omits material or information requested on the form may be subject to criminal sanctions (including fines and imprisonment) and/or civil sanctions (including civil penalties).

PS Form **3526**, July 2014 (Page 3 of 4) PRIVACY NOTICE: See our privacy policy on www.usps.com

Moving?

Make sure your subscription moves with you!

To notify us of your new address, find your **Clinics Account Number** (located on your mailing label above your name), and contact customer service at:

Email: journalscustomerservice-usa@elsevier.com

800-654-2452 (subscribers in the U.S. & Canada)
314-447-8871 (subscribers outside of the U.S. & Canada)

Fax number: 314-447-8029

Elsevier Health Sciences Division
Subscription Customer Service
3251 Riverport Lane
Maryland Heights, MO 63043

*To ensure uninterrupted delivery of your subscription, please notify us at least 4 weeks in advance of move.

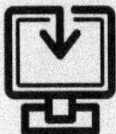

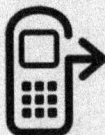

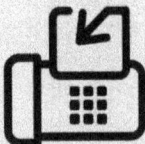

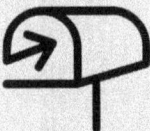

ELSEVIER

www.ingramcontent.com/pod-product-compliance
Lightning Source LLC
Chambersburg PA
CBHW082004190326
41458CB00010B/3064